THE YEAR IN GYNAECOLOGY 2001

THE YEAR IN GYNAECOLOGY

2001

JANET BARTER

and

NAOMI HAMPTON

CLINICAL PUBLISHING SERVICES

OXFORD

Clinical Publishing Services Ltd

Oxford Centre for Innovation
Mill Street, Oxford OX2 OJX, UK

Tel: +44 1865 811116
Fax: +44 1865 251550

Web: www.clinicalpublishing.co.uk

Distributed by:
Plymbridge Distributors
Estover Road
Plymouth PL6 7PY, UK

Tel: +44 1752 202300
Fax: +44 1752 202333
E mail: orders@plymbridge.com

First published 2001

A catalogue record for this book is available from the British Library

ISBN 0 9537339 2 0

The publisher makes no representation, express or implied, that the dosages in this book are correct. Readers must therefore always check the product information and clinical procedures with the most up-to-date published product information and data sheets provided by the manufacturers and the most recent codes of conduct and safety regulations. The authors and the publisher do not accept any liability for any errors in the text or for the misuse or misapplication of material in this work.

Commissioning Editor: Sheila Khullar
Typeset by Footnote Graphics, Warminster, Wiltshire
Printed in Spain by T G Hostench SA, Barcelona

Contents

Part III

Other gynaecology

Contributors

TR Adib, BSc, MRCOG, Gynaecological Oncology Research Fellow, Department of Obstetrics and Gynaecology, University College London Hospitals, Royal Free Hospital, Pond Street, Hampstead, London

Janet Barter, MRCOG, MFFP, Consultant and Honorary Senior Lecturer in Community Gynaecology, Department of Community Gynaecology, Royal Free Hospital, Pond Street, Hampstead, London

Deborah Bruce, HRT Research Unit, Guy's Hospital, St Thomas Street, London

Brianna Cloke, MA, MBBS, Senior House Officer, Department of Obstetrics and Gynaecology, Queen Charlotte's and Chelsea Hospital, Du Cane Road, London

David Crook, PhD, Senior Research Fellow, Department of Cardiovascular Biochemistry, St Bartholomew's and The Royal London School of Medicine and Dentistry, Charterhouse Square, London

Melanie Davies, MA, MRCP, MRCOG, Consultant and Subspecialist in Reproductive Medicine, Reproductive Medicine Unit, University College London Hospitals, Obstetric Hospital, Huntley Street, London

Colin Davis, MRCOG, Consultant in Obstetrics and Gynaecology, Subspecialist in Reproductive Medicine, St Bartholomew's and the Royal London Hospitals

Naomi Hampton, BSc, MRCOG, MFFP, Formerly Consultant in Reproductive Health Care and Community Gynaecology, Enfield Community Care NHS Trust, Ul Marecka 5, 04-717 Warsaw, Poland

Vik Khullar, BSc, MRCOG, MD, AKC, Senior Lecturer in Obstetrics and Gynaecology, Subspecialist in Urogynaecology, Department of Reproductive Science and Medicine, Imperial College School of Medicine, St Mary's Hospital, Norfolk Place, London

Usha Kumar, MRCOG, Specialist Registrar in Community Gynaecology, Community Health South London NHS Trust, Department of Reproductive Health, King's College Hospital, Denmark Hill, London

Jo Marsden, BSc, FRCS, Specialist Registrar in General Surgery, Department of Surgery, Royal Surrey County Hospital, Guildford, Surrey

Tim Mould, MA, DM, MRCOG, Consultant Gynaecological Oncologist, Department of Obstetrics and Gynaecology, University College London and Royal Free Hospitals, Royal Free Hospital, Pond Street, Hampstead, London

Chun Y Ng, MB, ChB, Specialist Registrar, Department of Obstetrics and Gynaecology, Queen Charlotte's and Chelsea Hospital, Du Cane Road, London

Caroline Overton, MD, MRCOG, Consultant in Obstetrics and Gynaecology and Sub-specialist in Reproductive Medicine and Surgery, Norfolk and Norwich University Hospital,

Nick Panay, BSc, MRCOG, MFFP, Consultant in Obstetrics and Gynaecology, Department of Obstetrics and Gynaecology, Queen Charlotte's and Chelsea Hospital, Du Cane Road, London

Pranav P Pandya, BSc, MRCOG, MD, Consultant in Foetal Medicine, Department of Foetal Medicine, University College London Hospital, Huntley Street, London

David J Perry, MD, PhD, FRCP, FRCPath, Senior Lecturer in Haemostasis and Honorary Consultant in Haematology, Department of Haemophilia and Haemostasis, Royal Free Hospital and University College London Medical School, Royal Free Hospital Campus, Pond Street, Hampstead, London

Janice Rymer, MD MRCOG FRNZCOG, Senior Lecturer/Consultant in Obstetrics and Gynaecology, UMDS, Guy's and St Thomas' Hospital Trust, HRT Research Unit, Guy's Hospital, St Thomas Street, London

Peter van den Hurk, MRCOG, Specialist Registrar in Obstetrics and Gynaecology, King George Hospital, Ilford

Barry White, Department of Haemophilia and Haemostasis, Royal Free Hospital and University College London Medical School, Royal Free Hospital Campus, Pond Street, Hampstead, London

Chris Wilkinson, MFFP, Consultant in Women's Sexual Health, Department of Reproductive Health, King's College Hospital, Denmark Hill, London

Foreword

The Year in Gynaecology 2001 provides a unique and comprehensive update for members of the Faculty of Family Planning & Reproductive Health Care of the Royal College of Obstetrics and Gynaecology, and others interested in our subject.

It is essential nowadays for people interested in this area of medicine to have an annual source of review of the key areas of new evidence and to be updated on a regular basis. I therefore look forward to the second volume of the excellent *The Year in Gynaecology*.

Other subjects are covered by their own yearbooks or annual reviews. However, our own subject has, in the past, missed out on this type of publication. Clearly, the book has to be read after studying more basic and postgraduate textbooks on family planning and reproductive health care, but it covers all essential aspects of these areas as a package, and deals with recent key papers in each field, having sections on reproductive health care, the menopause and other gynaecological relevant conditions.

Given that we all have an obligation to maintain personal development and revalidation, this approach allows an update in our own time, reading particular chapters that are of relevance to our own practice. Moreover, its style allows rapid assessment of recent papers and data, with each paper being discussed under 'background', 'interpretation' and 'comment'.

The book can be used to review a current subject, enabling one to obtain the recent references clearly and easily and read the original papers. It allows a rapid update or can be used as a reference book. Therefore, I believe that it is essential reading for those in family planning and reproductive health care, for those in primary care who have an interest in our subject, and similarly for those in hospital care working in gynaecology and related subjects. I also believe it is an excellent resource for those paramedical staff working in family planning and reproductive health care, particularly nurses, nurse specialists and nurse consultants. I am sure it will also be of interest to overseas readers working in the same area of medical care.

It is 'a must' for all those working in family planning and reproductive health care, and is essential reference material for libraries and postgraduate centres. I congratulate the editors and authors on producing an excellent *The Year in Gynaecology 2001* and look forward to the next issue.

Professor John Newton
Past President, Faculty of Family Planning &
Reproductive Health Care
Honorary Consultant in Gynaecology and
Community Gynaecology and Sexual Health
Birmingham, 2001

Preface

The purpose of this volume is to give a fairly concise overview of the developments in contraceptive care, the management of the menopause, and other aspects of gynaecology which affect the practice of those providing reproductive health care services in primary care and the community. The book is also useful as a summary text for mainstream obstetricians and gynaecologists, and trainees.

Chapter authors were given the brief of reviewing key papers published over the last few years. Some have selected not only papers published during the last year or so, but also older publications which have resulted in recent changes in practice, for example the licensing of a progestogen-only emergency contraceptive. This is particularly true of the chapters relating to contraceptive methods as there is a significant time-lag between the publication of efficacy data and the marketing of a product. In other areas with a wealth of publications, the authors have selected papers to bring the reader up to speed with what, in their opinion, are the most important developments. The chapters, whilst conforming to a model, manage to reflect the individual styles of the authors.

There is always discussion about what should and should not be included in a book of this type. To a large extent, the chapter list was planned to clarify areas of controversy and perhaps confusion, but this does result in some notable exclusions. Neither the treatment of benign gynaecological conditions such as fibroids and endometriosis nor the issues around therapeutic termination of pregnancy found their way on to the list. We very much wanted to include a chapter on abortion, as an intrinsic part of women's reproductive health, but since the subject has recently been extensively reviewed, it was difficult to add significantly to the body of literature currently available. We would therefore simply guide readers towards the excellent review in the dedicated supplement to the American Journal of Obstetrics and Gynaecology (Early medical abortion, coordinating editor Lauren Tews. Supplement to American Journal of Obstetrics and Gynaecology Aug 2000; Vol **183**(2): S1-S94). We would also recommend that readers refer to the January 2000 issue of the Journal of Family Planning and Reproductive Health Care for some key summary statements on family planning.

As editors we are very grateful to our chapter authors for tolerating our idiosyncrasies; we have learned a great deal from their work. We would also like to thank the Faculty of Family Planning and Reproductive Health Care for their support and for allowing us to reproduce the Emergency Contraceptive guidelines in Chapter 4.

Our thanks also go to our families for their love and support and for giving us enough time and space to see the book through to completion. We also wish to thank the staff at Clinical Publishing Services for keeping faith with the project.

Janet Barter and Naomi Hampton

Part I

Reproductive health care

1

Update on intrauterine devices

Introduction

The history of the intrauterine device (IUD) can be traced back to the insertion of pebbles into the uteri of camels to prevent conception during long trips across the desert. In 1909, the first human IUD was made from silkworm gut, followed in the 1920s by rings of silver or gold wire. The development of plastics technology allowed a device to be given memory of its shape after being stretched out into a linear form for insertion into the uterus. Zipper, impressed by the antifertility effect of copper in rabbits, introduced copper-bearing IUDs, which proved to be more effective. The first of the plastic, non-medicated/inert devices were the Margulies spiral and the Lippes loop. Other plastic devices followed (the Saf-T-coil, Dalkon Shield and Birnberg Bow). Closed devices became unpopular because of the potential for bowel obstruction should perforation occur. The Dalkon Shield was withdrawn from the market in 1975 as it was found to be associated with an increased risk of mid-trimester septic abortion and consequent deaths in the USA. The problem was thought to be due to the device's multifilament thread acting as a wick to ascending infection. Although the inert devices had low expulsion rates and low pregnancy rates, associated with a larger surface area of plastic, they were associated with high pain and bleeding rates. The addition of copper allowed a reduction in the girth of the plastic frame.

The IUD is the second most commonly used method of contraception in the world, after female sterilization. More than 106 million women world-wide use IUDs, about two-thirds of them in China. In western Europe, use in women aged 15–44 years is 7–19%, the highest rates of use are in southern Europe and Scandinavia. In the UK, use has declined somewhat over the past two decades to about 4% of women aged 15–49 years (see Fig. 1.1 for the IUDs, systems and implants currently in use in the UK). Usage in the USA was affected dramatically by adverse media publicity and litigation, particularly in relation to the Dalkon Shield; the effects of the 'bad press' have been long lasting.

It is not only in the design of IUDs that significant advances have been made over the last 30 years. The collection of reliable multicentre trial data has resulted in the calculation of accurate efficacy rates and the exploration of the historical association between IUD use and pelvic infection and ectopic pregnancy.

This chapter reviews recent IUD papers, starting with a study looking at antibiotic use at the time of IUD insertion. Individual copper-bearing IUDs (Gyne T

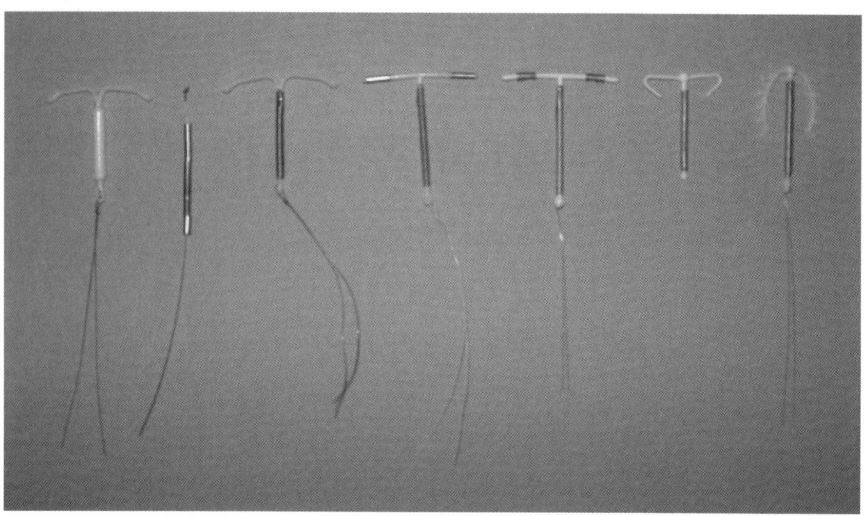

Fig. 1.1 Intrauterine devices, systems and implants currently in use in the UK. From left to right: Mirena®, GyneFix®, Nova T® 380, Gyne T 380™ (TCu 380S), T Safe® Cu 380A, Flexi-T 300, Multiload® Cu 375.

380™, Nova T 380®, Cu Safe 300 and GyneFix®) are then reviewed before the data looking at the contraceptive and gynaecological uses of the Levonorgestrel-releasing Intrauterine System (LNG-IUS) are examined.

IUDs and pelvic infection

Studies from the 1970s and early 1980s that demonstrated an increased risk of pelvic inflammatory disease (PID) in IUD users of up to 10-fold have now been shown to have methodological problems. It is now clear that PID is related to lifestyle and sexually transmitted infections (STIs). A landmark World Health Organization (WHO) paper |1| based on approximately 668 000 cycles of use showed that the risk of PID is increased by a factor of 6.3 in the 3 weeks after insertion (the insertion effect). Thereafter the risk is low for up to 8 years (the duration of the study) (see Table 1.1).

Up to one-third of European women using a reversible method of contraception use an IUD, whereas only 2% of American women use an intrauterine method. This low prevalence represents a considerable reduction from the high of approximately 10% in the 1980s. The decline of IUD use in the USA partly relates to issues of safety connected with IUD use and pelvic infection. As a result, less than a handful of clinical trials of IUDs have been performed in the USA during the last 25 years.

Table 1.1 Intrauterine devices and pelvic inflammatory disease (PID): subject characteristics and PID rates |1|

Characteristic	No. of insertions	Years of follow-up	PID cases	PID rate/1000 women-years
All women	22 908	51 399	81	1.58
Time after insertion				
≤ 20 days	22 908	1243	12	9.66
≥ 21 days	22 521	50 157	69	1.38
Age				
15–24 years	5006	9492	33	3.48
25–29 years	8287	18 292	23	1.26
30–34 years	6549	15 953	17	1.07
35+ years	3066	7663	8	1.04

Source: Farley *et al.* (1992).

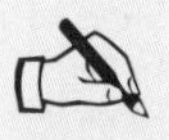

Randomised controlled trial of prophylactic antibiotics before insertion of intrauterine devices.

T Walsh, D Grimes, R Frezieres, *et al. Lancet* 1998; **351**: 1005–8.

BACKGROUND. The use of IUDs has been limited, in many countries, because of concern about the risk of infection of the upper genital tract. The administration of prophylactic antibiotics at suction termination of pregnancy strongly protects against postoperative infection and the possibility of producing a similar benefit in relation to IUD insertion prompted this study.

Previous studies had produced conflicting data. In a randomized trial in Kenya, participants received either doxycyline 200 mg or an identical placebo before IUD insertion. The women who received doxycyline had an apparently lower rate of PID than those who received the placebo, although the difference was not statistically significant. In contrast, a similar study in Nigeria, which stopped prematurely, found no benefit from using prophylactic doxycycline.

In North America, IUD use is generally restricted to women considered to be at low risk of STI. The authors considered that acute upper genital tract infection would be too rare an event to serve as the main outcome measure. They chose to use as an indicator of acute or subacute pelvic infection the rate of removal of the IUD within 90 days of insertion for reasons other than partial expulsion. The authors' principle aim was to determine whether antibiotic prophylaxis given before IUD insertion would affect the rate of early IUD removal. In addition, the seeking of medical attention after IUD insertion was assessed.

The authors undertook a pilot study to test the study protocol, randomization and masking procedures and the methods of data collection. A total of 447 IUD users were enrolled in the pilot study, they received either 200 mg doxycycline or identical placebos. Doxycycline use did not show any statistically significant effect and as a result the authors chose to use azithromycin for the full-scale investigation. They hoped that the long tissue half-life of azithromycin (2–4 days) would provide greater

protection than that seen with a single dose of doxycycline (half-life 24 hours). As the optimum dose of azithromycin needed for effective prophylaxis is unknown, the authors chose to use 500 mg—the loading dose recommended for multiple-dose therapy.

INTERPRETATION. Women requesting IUD insertion, who were considered to be at low risk of STI, were enrolled into the study from 11 clinic sites in southern California. Clinicians assessed the risk of STI according to the woman's self-reported medical history. All participants were screened for *Chlamydia trachomatis* and *Neisseria gonorrhoeae*. Seventy per cent of participants were screened at a pre-insertion visit and 30% were screened on the day of Gyne T 380™A insertion. No IUDs were inserted for emergency contraception.

Participants received either two capsules each containing 250 mg of azithromycin or two placebo capsules, identical in appearance and taste, 1 h before IUD insertion.

Standardized clinical criteria were used to define salpingitis—three points of pelvic tenderness (abdominal, uterine/cervical, adnexal) and at least one of the following: temperature above 38°C, white blood cell count above 10×10^9/litre, pus found in the peritoneal cavity on culdocentesis or laparoscopy, pelvic abscess or inflammatory complex on bimanual examination or ultrasonography or a positive gonorrhoea or chlamydia test result. These criteria were applied with masking maintained.

The primary outcome measure was IUD removal for any reason other than partial spontaneous expulsion within 90 days of insertion. The secondary outcome measure, use of medical services after IUD insertion, included unscheduled clinic visits as well as scheduled study visits at which the participant reported a gynaecological complaint for which she would have sought help.

The authors' a priori hypothesis was that the administration of antibiotic prophylaxis would reduce the rate of IUD removal during the first 90 days by 50% compared with placebo.

A total of 1985 women were randomly assigned to receive antibiotic or placebo. Of these, 94% (1867 women) had an IUD inserted; 933 received azithromycin and 934 received placebo. At least 90 days' follow-up information was obtained for approximately 98% of participants in both groups.

The rate of IUD removal within 90 days of insertion for any reason other than partial IUD expulsion was 3.8% (35/918) in the azithromycin group and 3.4% (31/915) in the placebo group [relative risk 1.1, 95% confidence interval (CI) 0.7–1.8]. The most common reasons for IUD removal were heavy menstrual bleeding and cramping or abdominal pain.

The rate of spontaneous IUD expulsion (complete and partial) was 3.5% in the antibiotic group and 3.4% in the placebo group; 92.7% of the women who received azithromycin and 93.2% of those who received placebo still had the IUD in situ at 90 days (relative risk 0.99, 95% CI 0.97–1.02).

Within 90 days of insertion, only one woman in each group had salpingitis which met the accepted diagnostic criteria. The woman who had received antibiotic prophylaxis had abdominal pain, bilateral adnexal tenderness and a temperature of 39.4°C. She was hospitalized and treated with intravenous antibiotics; she was discharged without complication. The woman who had received placebo experienced bilateral adnexal tenderness and leucocytosis; she received oral antibiotics as an out-patient and retained her IUD.

Six women in the antibiotic group (0.7%) and 12 in the placebo group (1.3%) were prescribed courses of antibiotics for uterine or adnexal tenderness, but there was no other evidence of infection and the accepted diagnostic criteria for salpingitis were not met.

Participants in the two groups sought help for gynaecological symptoms with the same frequency (38 visits per 100 participants). Clinically significant disorders were detected in 47% of visits made by the antibiotic group participants and 42% of visits by those in the placebo group.

Comment

This paper demonstrates that the administration of prophylactic azithromycin had no overall effect on IUD continuation rates at 90 days and, more significantly, that salpingitis or endometritis related to IUD use are very rare events.

In a population of 1833 women with careful follow-up, only two, one who had received antibiotic prophylaxis and one who had not, met the accepted diagnostic criteria for salpingitis. Fewer women in the antibiotic group (0.7%) than in the placebo group (1.3%) experienced pelvic tenderness for which they received antibiotics, but this difference was not statistically significant.

The excellence of the study design—triple-masked, randomized and placebo controlled—eliminated the potential for selection and confounding biases. The sample size was very large and the participants were a heterogeneous group representative of contemporary IUD users.

The authors' concluding paragraph aptly sums up the contribution made by this paper: 'In the absence of any demonstrable effect on IUD continuation rate, morbidity and use of medical services, routine antibiotic prophylaxis at IUD insertion seems unwarranted. In appropriate candidates for intrauterine contraception, infection of the upper genital tract is rare, with or without antibiotic prophylaxis'.

Gyne T 380™

The Copper T device was originally developed by the Population Council, it was subsequently improved by the addition of copper collars, either on the vertical arms (the Copper T 380 series) or on the vertical stem (the Copper T 220C). The Copper T 380A is identical in surface area and weight of copper to the Copper T 380S and the models have very similar clinical performances. The Copper T 380A has one of the lowest annual pregnancy rates of all IUDs and has become regarded as the 'gold standard' against which other devices must be judged.

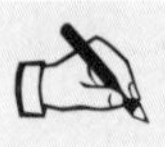

Long-term reversible contraception. Twelve years of experience with the TCu380A and TCu220C.

United Nations Development Programme/United Nations Population Fund/World Health Organization/World Bank, Special Programme of Research, Development and Research Training in Human Reproduction. *Contraception* 1997; **56**: 341–52.

BACKGROUND. Much of the literature relating to the safety and efficacy of the copper IUD comes from studies of less than 7 years' duration, with the majority relating to only the first 3 years of use. In many national family planning programmes there is a need for an effective, long-term (>7 years) non-hormonal method of fertility regulation which does not require repeated clinic visits.

This paper reports 12 years of experience with the TCu220C and TCu380A devices from two randomized, multicentre trials conducted in 24 centres among parous women. The devices were allocated at random, but because the devices were different in appearance and required different insertion techniques, the doctors inserting the devices could not be blind. The main endpoints were major complications associated with insertion; expulsions, perforation and pregnancy rates; and rates of removal for complaints of pain, bleeding, or other medical or personal reasons.

INTERPRETATION. A total of 3277 women using TCu220C and 1396 women using TCu380A were recruited between 1981 and 1986 and followed at 3, 6 and 12 months from insertion, then annually to 12 years. At the end of 12 years, 17 098 woman-years of experience had been accumulated for the TCu220C and 7159 woman-years for the TCu380A.

The cumulative 12-year intrauterine pregnancy rates were 7.0 per 100 women for the TCu220C [standard error (SE) = 0.6] and 1.9 for the TCu380A (SE = 0.5); $P < 0.001$. Pregnancy rates were highest in the first years after insertion for both devices and the TCu220C had a consistently higher annual pregnancy rate than the TCu380A at all intervals after insertion. In this study, in the first 5 years of use, the annual pregnancy rates for the TCu220C ranged from 1.6 at 2 years to 0.7 at 5 years. After this time, the annual rate was consistently less than 0.5 per 100 women. The annual pregnancy rates for the TCu380A were always 0.4 or less per 100 women and no pregnancies were reported with the TCu380A after 8 years of use. The cumulative ectopic pregnancy rates were 0.7 and 0.4 for TCu220C and TCu380A, respectively.

During the first year of use, the annual removal rate for medical reasons for the TCu380A was approximately 6%, between years 2 and 12 the annual rate remained constant at 4 per 100 women.

Although the majority of expulsions occurred in the first couple of years following insertion, some were still recorded between 8 and 12 years. The expulsion rate rose from 10.6% at 8 years of use to 12.5% at 12 years for the TCu220C.

Comment

The cumulative pregnancy rate for the TCu220C is low and comparable with other reversible methods of contraception at 12 years. However, as this device is currently only used in China, comments will be restricted to the data relating to the CuT380A.

The data show the TCu380A to be safe and effective for at least 12 years of use. The very high efficacy of the TCu380A confirms its place |2, 3| as the 'IUD of choice' for parous women and it should be considered as a reversible, non-surgical alternative to female sterilization for those requiring very long-term protection from pregnancy.

The cumulative ectopic pregnancy rate of 0.4 per 100 women at 12 years makes the TCu380A an appropriate option for women with a previous ectopic pregnancy.

Nova T® 380

The majority of copper-releasing IUDs of surface area 200 (Nova T®) to 250 mm^2 (Multiload® 250) have higher pregnancy rates |4| than higher load, more modern devices and are not suitable for long-term use. There is evidence to support the hypothesis that increasing the surface area of copper in IUDs improves contraceptive efficacy |3, 5|. The increase in concentration of ionized copper may explain this, as it has a direct effect on the fertilizing capacity of sperm.

The addition of a silver core to the copper wire in the Nova T® prevents fragmentation of the copper wire over long periods of use and increases the life span of devices. Adapting the concept of a larger copper surface area to improve contraceptive efficacy, the amount of copper has been increased from 200 mm^2 in Nova T® to 380 mm^2 in the new Nova T® 380.

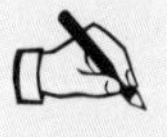

Two-year clinical experience with Nova T® 380, a novel copper–silver IUD.

I Batar, A Kuukankorpi, I Rauramo, M Siljander. *Adv Contracept* 1999; **15**: 37–48.

BACKGROUND. The Nova T® 380 is the logical development of the Nova T®, increasing the copper surface area from 200 to 380 mm^2 to aim to improve contraceptive efficacy. The Nova T® 380 is identical to the Nova T® except for the increased copper surface area, the diameter of the copper thread and the length of the loop. As a result of these changes, Nova T® 380 was expected to achieve higher contraceptive efficacy. This report presents the first results based on the initial 2 years of use.

INTERPRETATION. This study, started in 1992, was an open single-group phase III clinical trial at three centres in Hungary and Finland. Four hundred volunteer healthy, parous women aged 18–45 years with uteri of normal shape and size and relying solely on the IUD for contraception meeting the inclusion criteria were recruited. Exclusion criteria were a history of gonorrhoea, repeated episodes of PID or a single episode during the last 3 months, significant anaemia or severe dysmenorrhoea, postpartum endometritis or infected abortion during the last 3 months, pregnancy or previous ectopic pregnancy, use of chronic corticosteroid therapy or any contraindication to the use of a copper IUD. Eight per cent of the women were aged 40 years or more.

Unwanted pregnancy was the primary efficacy parameter with continuation being regarded as the secondary parameter.

By the cut-off date, 341 and 259 women had passed the 12- and 24-month visits, respectively. Exposure to the device was 8095 woman-months and the gross cumulative continuation rate at 24 months was 75.5 (CI 71.2–79.8) per 100 users.

Table 1.2 shows the number of cases of discontinuation, gross cumulative life-table rates, CI and Pearl indices by the type of discontinuation.

Two pregnancies occurred during the first year and a further three by the end of the second year, giving gross cumulative pregnancy rates of 0.5 (CI 0–1.3) and 1.6 (CI 0.2–3.0) per 100 users, respectively. The ages of the women at conception were 26, 26, 26, 31 and 43 years. In two of the pregnancies, the IUD had been either completely or partially expelled. No ectopic pregnancies were observed.

Four total and six partial expulsions were seen during the 24 months of follow-up. The gross cumulative expulsion rate per 100 women was 1.6 (CI 0.3–2.8) at the end of the first year and 2.8 (CI 1.1–4.6) at the end of the second year.

Thirty-one women terminated the study because of bleeding problems, 18 during the first year, giving gross cumulative discontinuation rates of 4.7 (CI 2.6–6.9) and 8.7 (CI 5.8–11.7) per 100 users after 1 and 2 years of use.

Comment

This preliminary report of the Nova T® 380 shows good protection from pregnancy, as evidenced by a gross cumulative pregnancy rate of 0.5 per 100 women at 1 year and 1.6 at the end of the second year. No ectopic pregnancies were reported. Cumulative pregnancy rates of 0.3–1.4 per 100 users at 1 year and 0.3–2.7 at 2 years have been reported for other IUDs with large copper surface areas |5–7|. Randomized comparative trials are needed to confirm whether the efficacy of the Nova T® 380 is similar to the Gyne T 380™ and the Multiload® 375.

Table 1.2 Number of cases of discontinuation, gross cumulative life-table rates, confidence intervals (CI) and Pearl indices by the type of discontinuation of the Nova T® 380

Reason for discontinuation	12 months				24 months			
	n	Gross rate	CI	Pearl rate	n	Gross rate	CI	Pearl rate
Overall discontinuation	43	11.0	7.9–14.1	11.7	93	24.5	20.2–28.8	13.8
Pregnancy	2	0.5	0–1.3	0.5	5	1.6	0.2–3.0	0.7
Expulsion	6	1.6	0.3–2.8	1.6	10	2.8	1.1–4.6	1.5
Bleeding problems	18	4.7	2.6–6.4	4.9	31	8.7	5.8–11.7	4.6
Pain	5	1.3	0.2–2.5	1.4	8	2.3	0.7–3.9	1.2

CI = confidence interval.

Source: Batar *et al.* (1999).

Gross cumulative expulsion rates of 1.6 and 2.8 per 100 women at 12 and 24 months are comparable with, or perhaps lower than, those reported for other IUDs with large copper surface areas.

Menstrual blood loss (MBL) was not measured in this study, but gross cumulative removal rates for bleeding of 4.7 and 8.7 per 100 users at 12 and 24 months suggest acceptable bleeding patterns and these results fall within the range reported for IUDs with less copper.

Gross cumulative continuation rates of 89.0 and 75.5 per 100 users at 12 and 24 months are comparable with those quoted for the Gyne T 380™.

As measured by pregnancy and continuation rates, the 2-year performance of the Nova T® 380 in this study is very promising. Contraceptive efficacy is comparable with other large copper surface area devices and continuation rates and bleeding problems are comparable with the Nova T®.

Data are now needed for use beyond 2 years and from comparative studies, particularly a study randomizing women to receive either Gyne T 380™ or Nova T® 380.

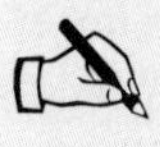

Clinical performance of the Nova T® 380 IUD in routine use by the UK Family Planning and Reproductive Health Research Network: 12 month report.

M Cox, S Blackwell. *Br J Fam Plann* 2000; **26**(3): 148–51.

B ACKGROUND . The Nova T® IUD, with a surface area of 200 mm² of copper, has been used extensively in the UK for more than 15 years. The development of a device, Nova T® 380, of the same size and with the same insertion technique, but with 380 mm² of copper, prompted this study to evaluate the pregnancy and complication rates of the new device in the clinical setting of general practice and family planning clinics within the UK; the findings to be compared with other published results. The principal investigators were 32 doctors working in general practice and at family planning clinics throughout the UK who collaborate in the UK Family Planning and Reproductive Health Research Network.

I NTERPRETATION . This study is an ongoing (5 years) open, single-group, multicentre phase III study in out-patients. A total of 572 Nova T® 380 IUDs were inserted 'according to the doctor's own clinical judgement' in healthy parous women aged 18–45 years with normal menstrual cycles requesting intrauterine contraception. Fourteen per cent of the women were aged 40 years or more. Thirty-three (6%) insertions were described as 'difficult' and 41 (7%) needed cervical dilatation.

Table 1.3 shows the Nova T® 380 to have a low pregnancy rate and a moderate expulsion rate at 12 months.

Four pregnancies occurred during the first 12 months, of which two were ectopic. Both intrauterine pregnancies were associated with partial expulsion.

Forty-six women had the device removed at or before 12 months of use following complaints about bleeding or bleeding and pain. Of these, 63% complained of heavier periods and 30% of continuous/persistent vaginal loss.

Table 1.3 Cumulative life-table gross rates per 100 users at 12 months for the Nova T® 380

	n	12 month gross rate	CI
Pregnancy	4	0.8	0.2–2.1
Expulsion	28	5.6	3.5–7.6
Bleeding problems	24	6.0	3.7–8.4
Pain	8	1.9	0.8–3.7
Bleeding and pain	22	5.3	3.1–7.4

CI = confidence interval.

Source: Cox *et al.* (2000).

Comment

The authors compare their results with data for the Nova T® at 12 months and conclude that neither their pregnancy rate of 0.8 with the Nova T® 380 nor Batar's rate of 0.5 is substantially better than reported rates of 0–1.8 at 12 months for the Nova T®. However, the effect of the increased surface area of copper must remain uncertain until comparative studies with the Nova T® are performed. With such low pregnancy rates, large, long-term studies are needed to detect difference.

The discontinuation rates for bleeding problems and pain and bleeding are higher than reported by Batar and the authors compare their figures for the Nova T® 380 unfavourably with their own work 10 years earlier with the Nova T®. They pose the question 'have British women become less tolerant of bleeding/pain problems over the last decade?' The role of the extra copper needs further elucidation as there is some evidence suggesting more bleeding problems occur with MLCu375 than MLCu250, but removal rates for TCu220C and TCu380A are similar.

The expulsion and removal rates for the Nova T® 380 in this study are similar to those seen with the Gyne T 380™. However, the gross cumulative pregnancy rate of 0.8 per 100 women compares unfavourably with the 0.3 per 100 users at 12 and 48 months widely quoted for the Gyne T 380™. Perhaps as Sivin postulates, it is the location of the copper on the transverse arms of the device, close to the fallopian tubes, which enhances contraceptive efficacy.

In this study, increasing the surface area of copper was not clearly associated with a reduction in pregnancy rate. However, it was not a comparative study with Nova T®. Although the insertion procedure for Nova T 380 is identical to that for Nova T®, it is questionable whether recent lack of experience with the latter device, as Gyne T 380™ is considered to be the 'gold standard', might have been a contributing factor, as both intrauterine pregnancies were associated with partial expulsion.

Studies like this, performed in general practice and family planning clinics rather than in research clinics, are important because they more accurately reflect the clinical outcomes women are likely to experience when requesting an IUD in everyday practice.

Cu Safe 300

The high efficacy, cost-effectiveness and long duration of action of modern copper IUDs are partly offset by the relatively high rates of expulsion and side-effects, mostly bleeding and/or pain, which result in early removal. Some IUD users who experience side-effects continue with the method, because of unhappiness with the other options, but fail to recommend the method to their friends. This is particularly significant in developing countries where reversible long-term methods are highly valued. In developing countries a complicated insertion technique also reduces distribution, as do problems with removal as a result of the threads breaking off or part of the device remaining in utero.

The Cu Safe 300 is a recent addition to the range of available IUDs and is marketed in the UK as Flexi-T 300®. It was specifically designed to decrease the unwanted side-effects of bleeding, pain and expulsion while providing a device which is easy to insert and remove and which provides good protection from pregnancy.

The Cu Safe 300 was designed with the specific purpose of reducing trauma to the endometrium. The design is based on long-term cavimetric investigations. The skeleton is made of polyethylene impregnated with X-ray opaque barium sulphate. The vertical stem is 1.5 mm in diameter and the horizontal arms are slightly thinner (1.15 mm diameter) and therefore more flexible. The arms are 23 mm wide and are bent inwards on both sides with the aims of reducing endometrial trauma and generating a fundal-seeking force. The 2.5-cm long vertical stem is wound with 32 cm of pure electrolytic copper wire which provides a copper surface area of approximately 300 mm^2. The monofilament polypropylene tail is moulded into the lower end of the vertical stem. The applicator has an outer diameter of 3.1 mm and contains no plunger. Insertion is performed using a simple push-in technique. The manufacturer recommends removal after 5 years.

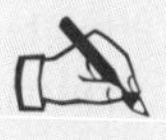

A randomized comparative study of the TCu380A and Cu Safe 300 IUDs.

HE Van Kets, H Van der Pas, W Delbarge, M Thiery. *Adv Contracept* 1995; **11**: 123–9.

BACKGROUND. The development of the Cu Safe 300 IUD, specifically designed to decrease the unwanted side-effects of bleeding, pain and expulsion prompted comparison with the 'gold standard' TCu380A.

INTERPRETATION. Recipients were nulliparous (n = 97) and parous (n = 503) healthy women between 18 and 45 years of age requesting an intrauterine contraceptive device, having a normal exposure to pregnancy and presenting no contraindications to IUD use. Allocation to receive a TCu380A or a Cu Safe 300 IUD was based on a randomization list prepared for each investigator.

An accidental pregnancy was defined as a conception with the IUD in situ or following unnoticed expulsion. Four pregnancies were observed during the first year in the Cu Safe cohort; one was ectopic. One pregnancy was observed during the second year of the study and two in the third year. In the TCu380A cohort, two women conceived in the first year, one after an unnoticed expulsion, and in the third year a ruptured tubal pregnancy was observed in this group.

Table 1.4 shows gross cumulative event rates per 100 users at 1, 2 and 3 years for interval insertion of the TCu380A and the Cu Safe 300.

After 12 months, the pregnancy rate was 0.8 in the TCu380A group and 1.5 in the Cu Safe 300 group; this difference was not statistically significant. After 3 years the rates were 1.5 and 2.5, respectively; this difference was also not statistically significant.

The expulsion rate at 1 year was 2.7 in the TCu380A group and 3.6 in the Cu Safe 300 group; not statistically significant. After 3 years the rates were 2.7 and 6.8, respectively ($P < 0.001$).

At 1 year the removal rates for bleeding and pain were 7.3 in the TCu380A group and 3.8 in the Cu Safe 300 group (not statistically significant). These rates rose to 15.6 and 10.4 after 3 years ($P < 0.05$).

There was no statistically significant difference in the continuation rates for the two devices at 3 years.

The authors also reported that all the investigators found the insertion and removal of the very flexible Cu Safe 300 to be easier than any IUD they had used previously, including the TCu380A.

Comment

This study demonstrates an improved tolerance for the Cu Safe 300 (cumulative removal rate for bleeding/pain 10.4 at 3 years versus 15.6 at 3 years for the TCu380A). However, this is at the expense of a significantly higher expulsion rate (6.8 for Cu Safe 300 compared with 2.7 for the TCu380A at 3 years). The pregnancy rate was slightly higher in the Cu Safe 300 users compared with the TCu380A users (cumulative rates at 3 years, 2.5 and 1.5, respectively).

The Cu Safe 300 would seem to present both advantages and disadvantages when compared with the 'gold standard' TCu380A. The device is less effective than the TCu380A, probably as a result of its tendency to be displaced downwards by uterine contractions against its very flexible plastic frame. Once the Cu Safe 300 has slipped into the cervical canal it is easily expelled due to the high flexibility of its frame.

It seems that the main advantage of the Cu Safe 300 is its easy insertion and removal. This may be especially significant in developing countries where para-medical staff are often required to perform IUD insertion in less than ideal circum-stances.

GyneFix®

While there have been significant improvements in the contraceptive efficacy of IUDs over the last 35 years, improvements in continuation rates have not been so

Table 1.4 Gross cumulative event rates per 100 users at 1, 2 and 3 years (95% confidence intervals in parentheses) for interval insertion of the TCu380A (n = 300) and the Cu Safe 300 (n = 300)

	1 year		2 years		3 years	
	T380A	**Cu Safe 300**	**T380A**	**Cu Safe 300**	**T380A**	**Cu Safe 300**
No. of insertions	223	234	161	195	107	110
Woman-months of use	3040	3107	5311	5643	6847	7330
Unplanned pregnancy	0.8 (0–3.0)	1.5 (0.4–3.7)	0.8 (0–3.0)	1.9 (0.6–4.4)	1.5 (0.3–4.4)	2.5 (0.9–5.4)
Expulsions	2.7 (1.1–5.5)	3.6 (1.7–6.7)	2.7 (1.1–5.6)	6.2 (3.2–9.2)	2.7 (1.1–5.5)	6.8 (3.6–10.0)
Removal for bleeding/pain	7.3 (4.1–10.5)	3.8 (1.8–7.6)	12.9 (8.6–17.2)	7.8 (4.4–11.2)	15.6 (10.7–20.4)	10.4 (6.3–14.5)
Continuation rate	81.5	85.3	69.6	75.5	64.2	68.1

Source: Van Kets *et al.* (1995).

dramatic. The main reasons for method discontinuation continue to be expulsion and client-requested removal for bleeding and/or pain.

GyneFix® is a new and innovative intrauterine contraceptive developed to address the problems of expulsion and removal for pain or bleeding. The concept of a frameless device was developed by the International Study Group on Intra-uterine Drug Delivery. The group looked at earlier work which had suggested incompatibility in size and shape between the IUD and the uterine cavity as a cause of problems with IUD performance. They also looked at the work in relation to efficacy and IUD location showing that optimal efficacy is achieved with fundal siting. GyneFix® is a device consisting of a thread with six copper sleeves attached. It is anchored by a knot embedded into the fundal myometrium. This unique anchoring mechanism allows retention of the copper within the uterine cavity without the need for a plastic frame. GyneFix® is both frameless and flexible.

GyneFix® consists of six copper sleeves, each 5 mm long, threaded on to a length of 00 monofilament polypropylene suture material. The first and last sleeves are crimped on to the suture thread. The total surface area of copper is 330 mm^2. At the far end of the thread is the knot, which is placed 9–10 mm into the fundal myometrium by the inserter mechanism.

At present there are three different versions of the GyneFix®: the interval version (described above), the postabortal version and the postpartum version. The postabortal implant GyneFix® PT is designed to be fitted immediately after ter-mination of pregnancy. The only difference from the interval implant is that the copper sleeves are held on thicker suture material (0 monofilament polypropylene) and hence the retaining knot is slightly larger. The postpartum version (GyneFix® PP) differs from the interval implant in that below the knot and threaded on to the suture material is a cone-shaped, biodegradable body with a 5-mm diameter at its base and a height of 4 mm. At insertion the cone and the knot are pushed into the fundal myometrium. The anchoring cone biodegrades over the next few weeks leaving the knot to anchor the implant once uterine involution is complete. Post-partum IUD insertions are common in many parts of the world. GyneFix® PP is currently not available in the UK.

The contraceptive efficacy of GyneFix® appears to compare favourably with the best of the current framed copper IUDs. The first randomized controlled trial was published in 1995 comparing the FlexiGard (same structure as GyneFix®, but using an earlier version of the insertion apparatus) with the TCu380A. The study con-ducted by WHO involved 4286 women with a total of 4777 woman-years of experi-ence. The cumulative pregnancy rates at 3 years were not statistically different between the two devices; both were shown to be highly effective at preventing preg-nancy. The 3-year cumulative pregnancy rate for the FlexiGard was 2.0 per 100 women and 1.7 per 100 women for the TCu380A. Beyond the first year of use, GyneFix® is certainly as effective as the TCu380A and may even be more effective. The high number of unnoticed expulsions, and their consequences, seen with the frameless device during the first year skew the cumulative pregnancy rates.

Performance of the TCu380A and Cu-Fix IUDs in an international randomised trial.

MJ Rosenberg, R Foldesy, DR Mishell, *et al. Contraception* 1996;
53: 197–203.

BACKGROUND. To assess the effectiveness, acceptability and safety of a new frameless, flexible IUD, the Cu-Fix, a randomized clinical trial comparing it with the TCu380A was performed in the USA and Europe.

INTERPRETATION. Data from 874 parous women aged 18–40 years recruited from 22 European and North American sites were analysed. Women were excluded from the study if they had clinical evidence or histories of ectopic pregnancy, PID or infection with *Niesseria gonorrhoeae* or *Chlamydia trachomatis*. Randomization to IUD type was performed using a computerized database on a block size of four. A diagnosis of PID was determined by the clinical judgement of the investigator.

Both devices provided effective protection against pregnancy. There were no pregnancies among the TCu380A users during the 2 years (5958 woman-months) of the study. Four pregnancies occurred in the Cu-Fix users, giving 1- and 2-year gross pregnancy rates of 1.0 and 1.5 per 100 women, respectively.

At 12 months the TCu380A expulsion rate was 2.0 per 100 women compared with 9.8 per 100 Cu-Fix users ($P < 0.001$, relative risk 5.4, 95% CI 2.4–12.2). No additional expulsions occurred in the TCu380A users after the first year, resulting in the same cumulative rate of 2.0 per 100 users, while the rate among the Cu-Fix users increased to 11.4 ($P < 0.001$, relative risk 5.9, 95% CI 2.7–13.2). Expulsion rates tended to decrease with increasing age and parity, but did not reach statistical significance.

Terminations for bleeding and/or pain were similar among the TCu380A and Cu-Fix users with rates of 6.9 per 100 TCu380A acceptors and 5.6 for the Cu-Fix users. Two-year rates were 11.4 per 100 women for the TCu380A and 8.3 for the Cu-Fix device.

First-year gross termination rates for PID were 1.0 per 100 women for the TCu380A and 1.1 for the Cu-Fix. When calculated as a rate per 1000 woman-years, the rates were similar at 6.0 per 1000 woman-years of use for the TCu380A and 8.3 per 1000 woman-years for the Cu-Fix. The four PID cases among the Cu-Fix users occurred at 7, 9, 12 and 16 months and the three among the TCu380A users occurred at 2, 12 and 13 months.

Comment

The gross termination rates for pregnancy in this study were in the lower range of reported values for high-load copper IUDs.

The Cu-Fix was associated with significantly more expulsions than the TCu380A and this study's rate was substantially higher than that reported by those responsible for the development of the Cu-Fix device. Whilst the Cu-Fix has the same structure as Gyne-Fix®, it has an earlier, inferior version of the insertion mechanism. The authors comment on the importance of the insertion technique and preliminary reports form a study with a redesigned inserter and substantially fewer expulsions.

An earlier randomized controlled trial |8| had also shown a statistically higher cumulative expulsion rate for the frameless device and an area which needs exploring is the learning curve for the new skill of inserting this type of device. Doctors unfamiliar with the insertion and implantation technique of GyneFix® are likely to have higher expulsion rates until they move along the learning curve for this new technique. Very experienced inserters are likely to make a significant contribution to the extremely low rates of expulsion reported in some of the early non-comparative work.

It was hoped that the absence of a frame would result in less bleeding and pain in GyneFix® users. Neither this study nor the earlier randomized trial |8| provide conclusive support for this and both have very similar discontinuation rates for pain or bleeding for GyneFix® and the CuT380A. However, both studies included only parous women and the problems of bleeding and pain associated with IUD use are most evident among nulliparous users. There are limited, but promising, data from a non-comparative cohort study which included more than 200 nulliparous women and had a removal rate of 1.2% at 3 years among the nulliparous women. There was no comparison group in this study and only limited information on the selection criteria and therefore any interpretation of the data should be cautious.

The overall PID rate from the study was higher than the WHO figure of 1.6 per 1000 woman-years. This is likely to be the result of the loose diagnostic criteria for PID used in this study. All but one case of PID occurred more than 6 months after IUD insertion, implying the new acquisition of a STI. Nevertheless the data support the statement that PID is an infrequent occurrence among appropriately selected candidates.

GyneFix® shares the general contraindications to use of copper IUDs. However, it could be argued that minor degrees of uterine cavity distortion are an indication to choose GyneFix® rather than a framed device, as could be previous expulsion or early intolerance/pain with a framed IUD. The small size and flexibility of Gyne-Fix® could provide nulliparous young women with some advantages over conventional framed devices and make the IUD an option for those appropriately screened and counselled about the STI acquisition risk.

It is the anchoring mechanism which makes GyneFix® unique and which marks a major development in intrauterine contraception and the potential for intra-uterine drug delivery.

The LNG-IUS and contraception

The LNG-IUS has many of the properties of an ideal contraceptive. It is highly efficient, has a long duration of action, requires minimal compliance, is independent of coitus, it is fully and immediately reversible, has non-contraceptive benefits and largely nuisance-only side-effects.

The LNG-IUS consists of a plastic T-shaped frame (32 mm in length and identical to that of the Nova T®) with a steroid reservoir around its vertical stem. This reservoir contains 52 mg of levonorgestrel/silastic mixture surrounded by a highly sophisticated rate-limiting polydimethylsiloxane membrane which regulates the release of levonorgestrel into the uterine cavity to 20 µg/24 h.

The LNG-IUS releases levonorgestrel into the uterine cavity where it is absorbed via the capillary network in the basal layer of the endometrium into the systemic circulation. Only 15 min after the insertion of the device levonorgestrel can be detected in plasma and maximum concentrations are reached after a few hours. Plasma levonorgestrel concentrations stabilize after the first few weeks at 0.3–0.6 nmol/litre and are lower than those seen in users of all other hormonal methods of contraception.

The LNG-IUS exerts its contraceptive effect by a strong progestational action on the endometrium, which is rendered thin and inactive, and on cervical mucus, which becomes thick and impenetrable to sperm; the effect on the endometrium is considered to be the main mode of action. Minor effects on ovulatory function have been reported, but ovulation is not normally inhibited. A form of 'foreign body reaction' with infiltration by leucocytes, plasma cells and macrophages is seen and there is a possible effect on sperm migration in the genital tract. The profound suppression of endometrial growth is seen after only a few months of use, but after removal of the LNG-IUS, the endometrium returns to normal and menstruation usually returns within the first month. Fertility also returns promptly, within 12 months 79–96% of women conceive.

The LNG-IUS is a very effective IUD. There is no statistically significant difference between it and the CuT380 at 7 years (see Table 1.5).

Table 1.5 Prolonged intrauterine contraception: a 7-year randomized study of the levonorgestrel 20 µg/day intrauterine device (IUD) and the copper T380Ag IUD |9|

	LNG-IUS	Standard error	CuT380Ag	Standard error
Pregnancies				
Total	1.1	± 0.5	1.4	± 0.4
Intrauterine	1.1		1.4	
Ectopic	0		†/*	
Expulsion	11.7	± 1.2	8.4	± 1.0
Medical removals				
Total	71.9		55.1	
Pain/bleeding	20.4**		30.0**	
Other	23.3		20.4	
Amenorrhoea	24.6***		1.1***	
Pelvic inflammatory disease	3.6		3.6	
Non-medical removals	44.9		48.0	
Woman-years of use	3371		3758	

*P < 0.05; **P < 0.01; ***P < 0.001.

†There were two cases of ectopic pregnancy, giving a rate of 0.05 per 100.

Source: Sivin *et al.* (1991).

Studies against other IUDs and Norplant®, lasting for up to 7 years collectively, report more than 12 000 woman-years of use and demonstrate very high effectiveness in preventing unwanted pregnancies (Pearl index 0–0.3, similar to female sterilization). Unlike all other methods of contraception, which become more effective as users age, the failure rate among women using the LNG-IUS is uniformly low.

The risk of ectopic pregnancy is strongly related to the total risk of pregnancy associated with IUD use. IUDs seem to prevent intrauterine pregnancy more effectively than extrauterine pregnancy and there is some evidence that this difference is more pronounced with the LNG-IUS. A European multicentre trial showed an incidence of ectopic pregnancy of only 0.02 per 100 women-years |10|. This represents an 80–90% reduction in risk compared with women not using contraception. Approximately 20% of conceptions with the LNG-IUS are ectopic |10| and the possibility of ectopic pregnancy should not be ignored in a woman with a LNG-IUS in situ. The high efficacy of the LNG-IUS makes it suitable for some women with a history of ectopic pregnancy.

Although the daily dose of levonorgestrel is low and there are no peaks in plasma concentrations, some women clearly feel the effect of the progestogen. Reported hormonal side-effects include headache, breast tenderness, nausea, hirsutism, acne and mood changes. Most of these symptoms are rare or mild, peak 3 months after insertion and reduce with time. Cumulative discontinuation rates for hormonal side-effects are low at 12.1 per 100 LNG-IUS users at 5 years |10|. A discussion about the potential for hormonal side-effects should always be included in pre-insertion counselling.

Menstrual irregularity, mostly frequent, irregular spotting, is common in the first few months after LNG-IUS insertion. From the fourth month onwards, however, a profound reduction in MBL is typical. With increasing duration of use an increasing number of women become amenorrhoeic. Around 25% of women are amenorrhoeic at 5 years. If counselled carefully about the reason for amenorrhoea it is usually very well tolerated; poorly counselled women may request removal because of concerns about amenorrhoea.

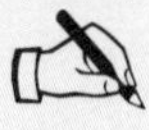

Clinical performance of the levonorgestrel intra-uterine system in routine use by the UK Family Planning and Reproductive Health Research Network: 12 month report.

M Cox, S Blacksell. *Br J Fam Plann* 2000; **26**(3): 143–7.

BACKGROUND. Prior to the introduction of the LNG-IUS in Finland in 1990 and its UK launch in 1995, a huge amount of clinical trial data have been published. This study was undertaken to determine the performance of the LNG-IUS in British women in routine clinical use, with particular regard to the nature and incidence of side-effects.

INTERPRETATION. This study is an ongoing, open, single-group, multicentre phase III study in out-patients. The 37 principal investigators work in general practice and at family planning clinics throughout the UK and co-operate in the UK Family Planning and Reproductive Health Research Network.

Selection for insertion was 'according to the doctor's own clinical judgement' in healthy parous women aged 18–45 years with normal menstrual cycles requesting intrauterine contraception. Before insertion all women were counselled about the likely menstrual changes. The subjects are being followed for 5 years from insertion. At the close of recruitment, 692 women meeting the inclusion criteria had been recruited.

Insertion of the LNG-IUS presented no difficulties in the majority of cases; the investigators reported 11% of insertions as difficult and there were 20 reported failed insertions. Only 14% of insertions required cervical dilatation; of these 93 cases only 30% were described as 'difficult' insertions by the investigator. LNG-IUS fitting was associated with no pain or mild pain in 78% of cases. The number of women offered or receiving analgesia or local anaesthesia is not known.

The cumulative gross rate for pregnancy was 0.6 (95% CI 0.1–1.7) at 12 months. Three pregnancies occurred; in one case the LNG-IUS was probably expelled prior to conception. Two conceptions ended in spontaneous abortion and one in a missed abortion.

Table 1.6 shows cumulative life-table closure rates per 100 users at 12 months (per protocol sample of 692).

Sixty women had their LNG-IUS removed at or before 12 months of use following a complaint of bleeding problems or bleeding and pain together. The mean length of use before removal for bleeding or pain and bleeding was 4.8 months. In 55% of removals the woman complained of continuous or persistent vaginal loss.

The rate of removal for other medical complaints was 7.4 at 12 months, most of these were due to a range of symptoms which may be related to systemic absorption of levonorgestrel. Included in this group were removals for oligo/amenorrhoea.

By 12 months six women had had their LNG-IUS removed following a diagnosis of PID. Diagnosis depended on the judgement of the clinician involved rather than predefined criteria and was recorded as being a 'doubtful' diagnosis in two cases. All cases were treated successfully.

Table 1.6 Cumulative life-table closure rates per 100 LNG-IUS users at 12 months (per protocol sample of 692)

	n	12 month gross rate	CI
Pregnancy	3	0.6	0.1–1.7
Expulsion	27	4.5	2.8–6.1
Bleeding problems	43	7.6	5.4–9.9
Pain	12	2.1	0.9–3.3
Bleeding and pain	17	2.9	1.5–4.2
Pelvic inflammatory disease	6	1.1	0.4–2.4
Other complaint associated with LNG-IUS	40	7.4	5.2–9.7
Continuation		70.6	

Source: Cox *et al.* (2000).

Two women required surgery for symptomatic ovarian cysts and in total 2% of women (15 subjects) developed ovarian cysts during the first 12 months of the study.

Comment

The results of this study are comparable with previously published data and demonstrate a very low pregnancy rate at 12 months. There were, however, more removals for bleeding and pain with bleeding in this study and the reason is not obvious. Perhaps the women were less tolerant of side-effects than in other studies or perhaps the large number of investigators precluded authoritative statements, based on own personal experience, about the transitory nature of many bleeding problems. Cultural factors may also have been important and one Muslim woman had her LNG-IUS removed at 2 months because long periods of bleeding interfered with prayer. While 10 women had their LNG-IUS removed for oligo/amenorrhoea during the first 12 months, many women commented favourably on the reduction in duration and quantity of menstrual bleeding. These results place very great emphasis on the need for very detailed counselling about likely menstrual changes and explanation about the origins of the oligo/amenorrhoea to help women persevere so that they can enjoy the longer-term benefits of the LNG-IUS.

The data reported in relation to PID diagnosis should be viewed with caution, as the diagnosis depended on clinical judgement and did not involve laparoscopy. There were also variations in pre-insertion screening practices with only some women being screened for *Chlamydia*. However, there did not appear to be an increased risk of PID soon after LNG-IUS insertion.

Most of the failed insertions were near the beginning of the study when many investigators were in the early phase of the learning curve for LNG-IUS insertion.

This study is important as it provides information about the LNG-IUS in routine clinical practice in the UK, rather than clinical trial populations in Scandinavia, on which general practitioners and family planning doctors can base accurate statements about the likely experience for the woman sitting across the consulting desk from them.

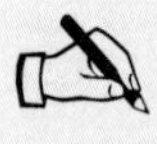

Length of use and symptoms associated with premature removal of the levonorgestrel intrauterine system: a nation-wide study of 17,360 users.

T Backman, S Huhtala, T Blom, R Luoto, I Rauramo, M Koskenvuo.
Br J Obstet Gynaecol 2000; **107**: 335–9.

BACKGROUND. Even though randomized clinical trials have provided ample evidence of the safety and efficacy of the LNG-IUS, an epidemiological study was undertaken to establish continuation rates and reasons for discontinuation among a large group of LNG-IUS users.

The objective of this study was to determine the overall continuation rates of the LNG-IUS in normal use and to evaluate the symptoms associated with the removal of

the system. Concomitantly with the launch of the LNG-IUS in Finland in 1990 a postmarketing survey was started. Women who had a LNG-IUS inserted between April 1990 and December 1993 were asked to participate in the survey. A total of 26 630 women agreed, representing 46% of all the LNG-IUS sold during this time period.

INTERPRETATION. Following two pilot studies to test the questionnaire and mailing system, a questionnaire with 75 questions was mailed to 23 885 women in April 1996. After three reminders a total of 17 914 questionnaires was returned, representing 75% of the mailed forms. After excluding women who had had their LNG-IUS removed because they were planning pregnancy, those over 48 years of age (as symptoms may be related to the menopause), and those where the identity of the person completing the form was in doubt (non-matching social security number and date of birth) or where consent to later collection of data was in doubt (no signature), 16 231 questionnaires were analysed. The analyses were interrupted at 5 years.

The LNG-IUS had been removed from 5175 women. The continuation rate was highest in the oldest cohort of women (39–48 years). The 1-, 2-, 3-, 4- and 5-year continuation rates for the LNG-IUS were 93, 87, 81, 75 and 65%, respectively.

A total of 108 women reported an unplanned pregnancy during the use of the LNG-IUS. Of these, 44 were ectopic. The Pearl index over 5 years of use was 0.18.

A multivariate analysis was performed using Cox's proportional hazard model to predict the premature removal of the LNG-IUS. Differences between groups were evaluated using risk ratios and 95% CI. A risk ratio smaller than one indicates a prolonged use of the LNG-IUS. Using this model, bleeding disorders (spotting and excessive bleeding) had the strongest association with premature LNG-IUS removal (relative risk 2.77, 95% CI 2.51–3.07). The following symptoms were also associated with a significantly higher risk of premature removal: pelvic infection (relative risk 1.40, 95% CI 1.25–1.57), pain (relative risk 1.32, 95% CI 1.23–1.42), depression (relative risk 1.33, 95% CI 1.24–1.43) and recurrent vaginal infections (relative risk 1.25, 95% CI 1.14–1.38).

The risk of premature removal of the LNG-IUS was significantly lower in women who had an occasional or total absence of menstruation (relative risk 0.46, 95% CI 0.43–0.50). Hormonal adverse effects such as loss of scalp hair, increased body hair and breast tenderness were associated with prolonged use of the LNG-IUS.

Comment

The very large population makes this study unique among contraceptive studies and its findings, based on routine clinical use, therefore significant. The Pearl index over 5 years of use was 0.18, which compares well with figures from earlier studies. The continuation rate in this study was as good or even better in routine clinical use than in earlier clinical trials. The authors state that, even if women planning pregnancy were included in the analysis, the continuation rates would continue to compare well with the clinical trial data.

In clinical trials the cumulative discontinuation rate due to amenorrhoea has been reported to be 1.5–4%, with very low removal rates in the more recent studies where women were adequately counselled about the benign nature of oligo/ amenorrhoea. In this study, the risk of premature removal was markedly lower among women who had occasional or total absence of menstruation. There was clearly a higher risk of having the LNG-IUS removed prematurely if excessive bleeding, spotting or PID were experienced. Bleeding disorders are the most common reason for discontinuing other intrauterine or long-acting progestogen-only methods. The frequency of 'hormonal' side-effects was very high in this study, although the removal rate was similar to results reported from earlier studies, supporting the fact that such symptoms are common irrespective of the contraceptive method in use and seldom lead to premature discontinuation as they do not seriously impact on quality of life.

This study of 17 360 LNG-IUS users confirms the LNG-IUS to have a high continuation rate for up to 5 years in routine use as well as the clinical trial situation. Oligo/amenorrhoea is associated with continuing use whereas bleeding disorders, pain and pelvic infection result in premature removal.

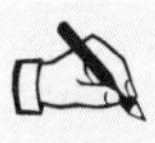

Health effects of long-term use of the intrauterine levonorgestrel releasing system. A follow-up study of 12 years of continuous use.

M Ronnerdag, V Odlind. *Acta Obstet Scand* 1999; **78**: 716–21.

BACKGROUND. Most of the studies published in relation to the LNG-IUS have looked at different aspects of the first 5 years of use. There are few studies concerning the long-term effects of LNG-IUS use. The aim of this study was to evaluate the effects of LNG-IUS use which had continued for more than two 5-year periods. The two principal objectives were to analyse various health parameters longitudinally to assess long-term effects and to assess the acceptability and bleeding pattern in women who became menopausal and began hormone replacement therapy (HRT) with the LNG-IUS still in situ.

INTERPRETATION. The report comprises LNG-IUS users from one Swedish centre who had participated in a large European multicentre study starting in 1983, in which women were randomized to receive either the Nova T® or the LNG-IUS. At the end of the 5-year study period, 109 of the 300 women originally allocated to the LNG-IUS were still using the device. No exchange LNG-IUS were available and all the 109 women were asked if they wished to extend use, under careful 3-monthly surveillance, for a further 18 months; 100 accepted to do so. When more LNG-IUS became available the second study period started, after a mean of 6.6 years (range 5.3–8.0) and 82 women accepted to have their first LNG-IUS exchanged for a second. None of the remaining 27 women terminated because of dissatisfaction with the LNG-IUS (15 had reached the menopause and 10 no longer needed contraception). The second segment of the study began in 1990 with 82 women who had had their second LNG-IUS inserted.

No pregnancies occurred during the follow-up. Five women (6%) discontinued LNG-IUS use during the second segment: one partial expulsion, one suspected PID, one was removed as the woman wished to conceive and two terminations for personal reasons. Four women were lost to follow-up as they moved away.

Of the 73 women still in the study at the end of the second segment, 69 had a third

LNG-IUS inserted. Two of the four women leaving the study wished for pregnancy, one woman became worried by her increasing haemoglobin (benign on full investigation) and one LNG-IUS had to be left in the uterus because large myomas made out-patient removal impossible; the woman declined surgery.

At the end of the first 5-year segment, 26% of the women were amenorrhoeic, 70% had scanty regular bleeds and 4% had infrequent scanty bleeds. Between 5 and 6.5 years only minimal changes in bleeding pattern were observed. When the second LNG-IUS was inserted many women became amenorrhoeic soon after insertion and the characteristic few months of spotting seen with first insertions did not recur. During the second segment of the study, 60% of the women became amenorrhoeic, but 8.5% of the women became menopausal.

There was a mean increase in haemoglobin concentration over the 12 years of 1.35 g/dl. There was a slight increase both in systolic and diastolic blood pressure; 4–10 mmHg systolic and 6–10 mmHg diastolic. There was an increase in body weight of 0.49 kg/year during the entire study period. Seventy-seven per cent of the women did not report any health problems during the entire follow-up period. One case of breast cancer and one osteosarcoma were reported. Seven women had laser conisations of the cervix and two women developed mild hypertension. Seven women (8.5%) between 46 and 50 years reached the menopause and were offered oestrogen replacement with oral or transdermal oestradiol and leaving the LNG-IUS in situ. They were amenorrhoeic when the menopause was diagnosed and remained so after the introduction of oestrogen replacement therapy.

There was a slight increase in the number of difficult fittings from the first to the third insertions, with the proportion of local anaesthesia use increasing from 6 to 13%. The third insertions were performed by a handful of very experienced inserters.

Comment

A study of extended use of the LNG-IUS showed high efficacy for up to 8 years with a single device. This study supports the LNG-IUS being effective for more than 5 years, providing at least 18 months' 'grace' beyond the recommended 5 years. The high continuation rate in this study is in part a reflection of the study design, as the women were already happy with the method and its effect on bleeding pattern. The authors comment that the women had always been encouraged to consider amenorrhoea as normal and to be expected with this method of contraception. The women never expressed any fears about untoward health consequences, with many choosing to continue with the LNG-IUS, because of oligo/amenorrhoea, even when the need for contraception had become less important. A comparative study is needed to determine whether there is a difference in quality of life in the later years with long-term LNG-IUS use.

Long-term use of the LNG-IUS allows a convenient transition from contraception to HRT in late reproductive life and the small number of women becoming menopausal in this study remained amenorrhoeic despite starting oestrogen replacement.

The increase in body weight is probably age related, as in the first 5 years of the study the women were compared with Nova T® users who showed the same weight gain. Whether the increase in blood pressure in this longitudinal study represents a significant change is unknown. The increase in difficulty re-inserting the LNG-IUS may be a consequence of the strong suppressive effect on the endometrium and the reduction in quantity of cervical mucus reducing the degree of cervical lubrication. Perhaps the use of intravaginal oestradiol prior to planned re-insertion might facilitate the fitting.

The long duration of this study suggests that the LNG-IUS remains a safe and effective method of contraception in the long term and which permits a bleed-free transition into hormone replacement.

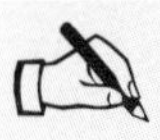

Levonorgestrel-releasing (20 μg/day) intrauterine systems (Mirena®) compared with other methods of reversible contraceptives.

RS French, FM Cowan, D Mansour, *et al. Br J Obstet Gynaecol* 2000; **107**: 1218–25.

BACKGROUND. The LNG-IUS is more expensive than copper-bearing IUDs (net cost £99 compared with approximately £9), but it offers considerable gynaecological benefits, particularly for women with heavy or painful menses. The LNG-IUS reduces MBL dramatically and is a rational alternative to surgery for many women with menorrhagia. The objectives of this systematic review were to assess the contraceptive efficacy, tolerability and acceptability of the LNG-IUS compared with other reversible methods of contraception, in women of reproductive age.

This systematic review included all randomized controlled trials where the study participants were of reproductive age, where the LNG-IUS was compared with another reversible method of contraception and predetermined outcomes were reported (pregnancy due to method or user failure and continuation of method use). Publications were sought through a variety of computerized databases and manual library searches, references were checked to identify further studies and requests for unpublished data made to individuals and organizations in the contraceptive field. All papers were blind for author and journal and the data were extracted independently by two reviewers. Single-decrement life-table probabilities (gross rates) with their standard errors and events per woman-month (akin to the Pearl index rate) were collected for each outcome at 1, 2, 3, 4 and 5 years. Quality was assessed independently in terms of general methodological factors which may bias study results, as well as some contraception-specific factors as recommended by Trussell. Menstrual changes were reported at 3-monthly intervals. Copper IUDs were divided into two categories based on the surface area of copper wire: >250 mm² (CuT380A and CuT380Ag) and ≤250 mm² (Nova T®, CuT200 and CuT220).

INTERPRETATION. The search strategy identified over 400 publications. Seven randomized controlled trials, reported in 23 publications, met the inclusion criteria. Six studies compared the LNG-IUS with copper IUDs—three with devices >250 mm² and three with devices ≤250 mm² (one study included devices with both copper loads). One study compared the LNG-IUS with Norplant® and another with the levonorgestrel intracervical device. The authors extracted appropriate data from five of the identified randomized controlled trials.

When compared with copper IUDs with >250 mm^2 copper there was no evidence to suggest that the LNG-IUS was relatively more or less effective in preventing pregnancy. No significant difference in contraceptive effect was found in the pooled life-table probability difference. However, the LNG-IUS was significantly more effective in preventing pregnancy than IUDs with ≤250 mm^2 copper at all follow-up points.

The relative risk for pregnancy after removal of the LNG-IUS was not significantly different when compared with non-hormonal IUDs. Data on hormonal side-effect outcomes could only be extracted from one paper comparing the LNG-IUS with the Nova T®. No significant differences were observed. At 5 years the relative risk (95% CI) for ovarian cysts was 1.5 (0.51–4.40), for headaches 1.71 (0.49–6.02), for breast tenderness
1.50 (0.31–7.17), for acne 5.56 (0.73–42.35), and for nausea 5.0 (0.24–103.86).

Amenorrhoea was shown to develop significantly more often in one study of LNG-IUS users compared with CuT380Ag users. At 3 months the relative risk (95% CI) was 2.25 (1.3–3.56) rising to 7.24 (4.14–12.55) at 3 years. No significant differences were noticed in prolonged bleeding. The authors were unable to extract data for any other of the specified menstrual outcomes.

LNG-IUS users were no more or less likely to experience device expulsion than users of copper IUD >250 mm^2 after 1 year, but were significantly less likely to have had an expulsion after 2 years than users of copper IUDs with ≤250 mm^2 copper.

Ectopic pregnancy risk could be examined using one study comparing the LNG-IUS with the CuT380Ag and two comparing the LNG-IUS with the Nova T®. No significant differences were found for the LNG-IUS versus CuT380Ag comparison. After 1 year there was no significant difference for the LNG-IUS versus Nova T® comparison, but after 3 years the rate ratio was 0.1 (0.02–0.62) and after 5 years 0.07 (0.01–0.41).

No significant differences were observed in the rates of PID; the authors were unable to use data suggesting lower PID rates among young LNG-IUS users in their analysis.

In general, LNG-IUS users were significantly more likely to discontinue use through hormonal side-effects than copper IUD users, but when compared with users of copper IUDs with >250 mm^2 copper a significant difference was not seen until 5 years. LNG-IUS users were significantly more likely to discontinue for menstrual disturbance than women using copper IUDs >250 mm^2. Further investigations revealed amenorrhoea to be the main cause for LNG-IUS discontinuations. In contrast, LNG-IUS users were significantly less likely to terminate use because of menstrual bleeding and pain.

When compared with users of copper IUDs with ≤250 mm^2 copper, LNG-IUS users showed no significant difference in discontinuation for menstrual change. However, discontinuations due to amenorrhoea were again significantly increased after 5 years.

The only trial meeting the inclusion criteria comparing the LNG-IUS with another reversible method of contraception was a comparison with Norplant®-2. No significant differences were observed for the following outcomes as reasons for discontinuation: pregnancy, continuation, expulsion, ovarian cysts, adverse events, menstrual disturbance and local device problems. However, LNG-IUS users were significantly more likely to experience oligo-amenorrhoea than Norplant®-2 users, but less likely to experience spotting and prolonged bleeding.

Comment

This meta-analysis concludes that at the present time there is no evidence to suggest that the LNG-IUS is any more or less effective than IUDs with >250 mm^2 of copper at preventing intrauterine and extrauterine pregnancies, but that it is significantly more effective than IUDs with ≤ 250 mm^2 of copper. The authors comment that there were little data available for these meta-analyses and that further comparative data on effectiveness will become available when the WHO LNG-IUS versus CuT380A multicentre trial reports. When comparing two highly effective methods of contraception, very large numbers of women need to be recruited into trials to ensure adequate power to detect significant differences.

Continuation rates for the LNG-IUS were significantly lower than those for copper IUDs with >250 mm^2 copper. The value of a contraceptive method, however effective, is greatly reduced if it is discontinued prematurely as an unintentional pregnancy may arise before another method is started. There are also financial considerations, particularly for the relatively more expensive methods.

The discontinuation rates for oligo/amenorrhoea highlight yet again the importance of counselling about menstrual change with the LNG-IUS. Women receiving adequate precontraceptive counselling may choose not to use a method if the side-effects are likely to concern them. More importantly, LNG-IUS users must be made aware of the aetiology of the oligo-amenorrhoea and that it has no adverse effects on health. There is some evidence to suggest that discontinuation rates for amenorrhoea are greatly influenced not only by cultural factors, but also by provider attitudes in different countries. More research is needed to assess the impact of counselling about menstrual change on user satisfaction and continuation rates.

The authors conclude that the LNG-IUS 'should be offered to women concerned about menstrual bleeding and pain associated with intrauterine device use, or who are experiencing heavy and painful menses'. I feel this is entirely appropriate and would add the category of client choice to their recommendation.

The LNG-IUS and menorrhagia

The strict definition of menorrhagia should be 'regular but heavy menstrual bleeding, usually >80 ml, from a secretory endometrium'. MBL exceeding 80 ml in most cycles for months or years may cause iron deficiency as the iron loss cannot be balanced by a normal dietary intake. However, objective measurements of MBL are not routinely performed in clinical practice and it is the woman's own perception of heavy blood loss which is usually the key determinant for the decision to treat. Idiopathic menorrhagia, when no underlying cause, such as fibroids or mild forms of Von Willebrand's disease, can be demonstrated, is the most common form. It is thought that heavy bleeding is the result of local defects in the haemostatic mechanisms within the endometrium.

More than 20 years ago the progesterone-releasing IUD Progestasert was shown to reduce MBL by 65% in menorrhagic women. The Progestasert was not widely used for this indication as it had to be replaced every 12 months when all the progesterone had been released. In an early study with the LNG-IUS, 20 women with proven menorrhagia had the LNG-IUS inserted, three women terminated the study (one expulsion and two cases of unacceptable intermenstrual bleeding), but in the remaining women the reductions in MBL were 86, 92 and 97% at 3, 6 and 12 months, respectively |**11**|.

The explanation for the therapeutic effect of the LNG-IUS in treating menorrhagia lies in the profound suppression of the endometrium produced. Levonorgestrel is much more potent than natural progesterone and has major effects on the stromal parts of the endometrium. In LNG-IUS users the endometrial concentration is about 1000 times higher than the circulating concentration which is very low. Despite normal plasma oestradiol levels in the presence of the LNG-IUS, the proliferation/stimulation effect of oestrogen on the endometrium is inhibited and the normal cyclic changes induced by ovarian steroids during ovulatory cycles are absent.

The endometrium exposed to intrauterine levonorgestrel shows atrophy of the endometrial epithelium, both luminal and glandular, and a strong decidual reaction in the stroma. The stroma is swollen and fibroblast-like stromal cells are differentiated into decidual cells. The decidual cells are morphologically similar to those in premenstrual and early pregnancy endometrium. The LNG-IUS also affects the vascular system in the endometrium; the changes include thickening of the arterial walls, suppression of the spiral arteries and capillary thrombosis. During the first few months of use an inflammatory reaction has also been reported within the endometrium with increased numbers of neutrophils, lymphocytes and plasma cells.

The morphological changes can be detected only 1 month after LNG-IUS insertion, are uniform within three cycles and are similar in the first and seventh years of use. The changes return to normal in most cases within a month of removal. The anti-oestrogenic effect is assumed to be due to an effect on endometrial oestrogen and progesterone receptors, but very little is known about the interaction between levonorgestrel and its endometrial receptors and its effect on gene transcription. In addition to steroid receptors, levonorgestrel may affect other local factors that mediate hormone-dependent events in the endometrium, either directly or indirectly.

Perhaps the best characterized growth factor system in the endometrium is the insulin-like growth factor (IGF) system. It includes IGF-I and IGF-II, their receptors and soluble IGF-binding proteins (IGFBPs). The LNG-IUS causes alterations in the endometrial IGF system. When the LNG-IUS is in utero IGF-I-mediated oestrogenic effects are inhibited. In the endometrium of LNG-IUS users, both for contraception and HRT, there is a suppression of IGF-I and abundant production of IGFBP-I by decidualized stromal cells; this may be one of the molecular mechanisms responsible for the suppression of endometrial epithelial growth during this treatment.

In the future it is likely that a great many levonorgestrel-induced changes in endometrial gene expression and the production of factors important for cell growth and differentiation or regulation of menstrual flow will be discovered to explain the antiproliferative and blood loss reducing effects of the LNG-IUS. Intensive research is being undertaken.

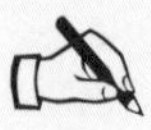

Randomised comparative trial of the levonorgestrel intrauterine system and norethisterone for treatment of idiopathic menorrhagia.

GA Irvine, MB Campbell-Brown, MA Lumsden, *et al. Br J Obstet Gynaecol* 1998; **105**: 592–8.

BACKGROUND. Sixty per cent of women with menorrhagia referred to gynaecologists undergo hysterectomy within 5 years. Whilst hysterectomy provides an effective cure for menorrhagia it involves major surgery and is only suitable for women who have completed their family. Endometrial ablation has much lower postoperative morbidity than hysterectomy, but again is unsuitable for women wishing to preserve their fertility; the long-term effects of endometrial ablation are not yet known. Most women with excessive loss have no demonstrable organic pathology and are said to have dysfunctional uterine bleeding. Pharmacological management can be effective in reducing MBL: prostaglandin synthetase inhibitors (25% reduction), inhibitors of fibrinolysis (50% reduction), combined oral contraceptive pill (40% reduction), danazol (80% reduction) and gonadotrophin-releasing hormone analogues (75% reduction). There may be contraindications to the use of some of these regimens in women in their fifth decade and the long-term use of some is prohibited by their side-effects. The most commonly prescribed drug in the UK for the treatment of menorrhagia is norethisterone, but recent studies have shown it to be ineffective in its currently recommended dosage.

Local progestogen, levonorgestrel delivered by the LNG-IUS, has been shown to be effective in the treatment of dysfunctional uterine bleeding in comparative studies with flurbiprofen and tranexamic acid, but there have been no comparative studies of the effectiveness of local and systemic progestogens in the management of dysfunctional uterine bleeding. This randomized trial was designed to compare the effectiveness of the LNG-IUS with norethisterone in the management of idiopathic menorrhagia. The norethisterone regimen chosen (5 mg three times daily from day 5 to day 26 of the cycle) represents an increase in dose and duration from that usually recommended, but had been demonstrated to be effective in a small study in Australia.

INTERPRETATION. To be eligible for the trial, women had to be parous, aged 18–45 years, in good general health, with a regular menstrual cycle, a normal pelvic examination (with a sound measurement of the uterus of <10 cm), negative cervical cytology and a measured MBL (using the alkaline haematin method) >80 ml.

MBL was recorded over one pretreatment cycle and the women were issued with menstrual diaries in which to record bleeding patterns and menstrual pain.

The women were randomized, using computer-generated numbers, to receive either norethisterone 15 mg daily from day 5 to day 26 of the cycle or to have a LNG-IUS inserted between days 1 and 7 of a cycle. A symptom questionnaire was completed at entry and the women were asked to collect their menstrual loss after their first and third treatment cycles. At the third cycle visit, or premature termination, the women's satisfaction with their treatment was assessed and they were given the option of continuing with the treatment. Haemoglobin and serum ferritin levels were measured at study entry and at 3 months/premature termination.

Forty-four women enrolled in the trial and the randomization process successfully created two groups of women with similar prognostic factors. Of the 44 women who entered the trial, eight withdrew before the end of the 3-month follow-up period. Three because of unacceptable drug-related side-effects (two in the norethisterone group, one in the LNG-IUS group), two because of perceived treatment failure (both in the norethisterone group), one because of prolonged amenorrhoea (norethisterone group) and one woman in the norethisterone group defaulted her final study visit. One woman expelled her LNG-IUS during the third treatment cycle. Two women in the norethisterone group did not make a final collection of their menstrual loss. Twenty women in the LNG-IUS group and 16 women in the norethisterone group completed the trial. No serious adverse events related to either treatment were reported.

MBL was significantly reduced following treatment compared with baseline for both the LNG-IUS group ($P < 0.001$) and the norethisterone group ($P < 0.001$). The median reduction in MBL from baseline to cycle three was not statistically significant between the treatment groups. The median MBL was reduced to normal (<80 ml) in both groups by the first cycle of treatment.

By 3 months the LNG-IUS had reduced MBL by 94% (median reduction 104 ml). The norethisterone regimen had produced an 87% reduction in MBL (median reduction 95 ml). Six of the 19 women (32%) in the LNG-IUS group were amenorrhoeic after three cycles. None of the women remaining in the norethisterone group was amenorrhoeic at 3 months. Following treatment there was no significant change in mean haemoglobin and ferritin levels in either group.

At baseline, 11 of the 22 women in the LNG-IUS group and eight of the 22 in the norethisterone group experienced intermenstrual bleeding. After three cycles of treatment, 10 of the 19 LNG-IUS users experienced intermenstrual bleeding compared with only two of the 12 women taking norethisterone. Five of the 11 women with the LNG-IUS had similar bleeding at baseline and cycle three compared with none of the eight women taking norethisterone.

Symptoms such as headache, acne, abdominal or back pain, nausea, oedema, weight gain, decreased libido, sweating, hair loss or greasy hair and increase in body hair were unchanged between baseline and cycle three. There was no difference between the groups. A small, but significant, weight gain was seen in both groups, 1.1 kg in the norethisterone group and 0.6 kg in the LNG-IUS group; this was not perceived by the women. There was a significant reduction in the incidence of mood swings in each group from baseline to cycle three, but there was no difference between the groups. There was also a significant reduction in the incidence of breast tenderness in each group from baseline to the end of treatment, but the LNG-IUS users were more likely to experience breast tenderness during treatment than the women taking norethisterone. In both groups the women stated that menstruation interfered with daily life less after three cycles of treatment than at baseline.

In the LNG-IUS group, 64% of the women liked the treatment 'well' or 'very well' and 17 of 22 (77%) elected to continue with the system at the end of the 3-month study. In the norethisterone group, 44% reported that they liked the treatment 'well' or 'very well' and four of 18 (22%) elected to continue with the treatment.

Comment

This randomized trial shows both the LNG-IUS and oral norethisterone at a dose of 15 mg daily for 21 days per cycle to be highly effective in reducing MBL by 3 months. Intermenstrual bleeding occurred more frequently among the LNG-IUS users, but this could be expected to settle during the next few months.

Studies using norethisterone for 6–10 days in the late luteal phase have shown at best a 20% reduction in MBL. This study has shown that, given in high enough doses from early in the cycle, norethisterone is effective at reducing MBL; only one woman still had loss >80 ml after 3 months of treatment. This dose regimen also produced a significant reduction in intermenstrual bleeding.

In recruiting for this study, 41 of 89 women referred with excessive loss, who collected MBL, were found to have loss <80 ml supporting previous observations that half the women who complain of heavy periods have menstrual loss within the normal range. This has important implications in respect of over-treatment, as many women perceived as having 'failed medical treatment' may have blood loss within the normal range. These women may seek a permanent surgical cure with its associated risks.

In this study, both the LNG-IUS and the norethisterone regimen used compare favourably with other currently available medical treatments. The LNG-IUS was well tolerated and more than three-quarters of the women wished to continue with it in the long term. It is also a highly effective contraceptive and once inserted frees the user from the need for daily compliance with a drug-taking regimen. It would seem to offer an effective and acceptable long-term alternative to surgery for women with menorrhagia.

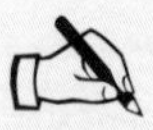

Open randomised study of use of levonorgestrel releasing intrauterine system as alternative to hysterectomy.

P Lahteenmaki, M Haukkamaa, J Puolakka, *et al*. *Br Med J* 1998; **316**: 1122–6.

BACKGROUND. **Many women scheduled for hysterectomy as the final treatment for excessive menstrual loss might still prefer a conservative alternative. Women who had already decided to undergo hysterectomy were invited to participate in a randomized study comparing the LNG-IUS with their current medical treatment. The primary aim of the study was to assess, after 6 months, whether the LNG-IUS could provide an alternative to hysterectomy in the management of excessive uterine bleeding with or without dysmenorrhoea.**

The authors recruited women with spontaneous cycles scheduled to undergo hysterectomy from hospital waiting lists. Women were excluded from the study if they

had one fibroid greater than 3 cm in diameter or ultrasonic evidence of more than three fibroids, a history or current clinical evidence or suspicion of malignancy or active liver disease, adnexal tumours or cysts or PID within the preceding 12 months. If the women were prepared to accept a further attempt at medical management they were enrolled into the study.

INTERPRETATION. The study was an open phase III randomized multicentre study (three Finnish hospitals) with two parallel groups: a LNG-IUS group and a control group who continued with their existing medical management for excessive uterine bleeding with/without dysmenorrhoea.

The women were randomly allocated to the LNG-IUS and control groups using a randomization table, the randomization being balanced in blocks of four. The primary efficacy measure was the woman's decision at 6 months, at discontinuation or when hysterectomy became available, whether she wished to continue with her current treatment or undergo hysterectomy. If she chose to continue with her current treatment she was asked again 12 months later. Two years after enrolment was completed, hospital records were checked to see how many women had undergone hysterectomy.

A visual analogue scale was used at screening, 6 and 12 months/discontinuation to assess the degree of disturbance caused by menstrual bleeding and/or pain on general well-being, work performance, physical activity, sexual activity, general leisure time activity. Menstrual diary cards were also used to record bleeding and spotting.

When designing the study, the authors expected that 40% of the women in the LNG-IUS group and 10% of the women in the control group would cancel the hysterectomy, a power calculation allowing for discontinuation suggested 60 women per group to provide a power of 95. The study started in two clinics and a third was included because the rate of recruitment was slower than expected. During the study, the waiting time for hysterectomy shortened from over 12 months to under 6 months in two hospitals and as the ethics committees had requested that the women should be offered hysterectomy once it became available, recruitment to a 6-month study became complicated. By this time, 28 women had been recruited into each group, giving a power of 70%.

A total of 56 women were randomized, 28 into each group. Three women withdrew before enrolment, two from the control group and one from the LNG-IUS group.

Eighteen of the 28 women in the LNG-IUS group and four of the 28 women in the control group cancelled their hysterectomy at 6 months ($P < 0.001$). In the control group, two women wished to continue with their existing prostaglandin synthetase inhibitors and two decided to switch to the LNG-IUS.

At 12 months, 12 women (57%) in the LNG-IUS group had discontinued treatment and undergone hysterectomy. Of these, seven women discontinued LNG-IUS use because of prolonged bleeding/spotting and/or pain; four were found to have adenomyosis and/or fibroids on histological assessment of the hysterectomy specimen, one to have chronic endometritis and in two no pathology was found. Another woman with pain was found to have adhesions. Two women with symptoms potentially attributable to levonorgestrel absorption had normal histology and fibroids, respectively. Two women who wanted hysterectomy for personal reasons were found to have adenomyosis. By the end of 1995, 48% of the women continued to use the LNG-IUS with an average follow-up time of 3 years (range 23–49 months).

The visual analogue scores were unchanged in the control group at 6 months, whereas they were significantly improved in each category in the study group at 6 and 12 months.

Comment

This study suggests that the LNG-IUS gives good short-term results in the management of excessive menstrual loss among women already scheduled for hysterectomy. Two-thirds of the LNG-IUS group cancelled their hysterectomy at 6 months compared with 14% in the control group. Half the LNG-IUS users chose to continue with this treatment option.

There was no improvement in the menstrual disturbance score in the control group whereas it improved significantly in the LNG-IUS users in all areas evaluated, despite the characteristic increase in spotting days seen on insertion of the LNG-IUS.

In this study, a placebo effect cannot be excluded. The nature of the device makes a blind comparative study with other medical treatments impossible and the LNG-IUS was already receiving favourable publicity in Finland at the time of the study.

This study suggests that women considering hysterectomy for menorrhagia with/without dysmenorrhoea should be offered the LNG-IUS before a final decision about hysterectomy is reached. A reduction in the annual number of hysterectomies, even by less than half, would be a considerable achievement and if the LNG-IUS was an earlier management option then even greater reductions could be achieved. The benefits of the LNG-IUS in preserving potential fertility should not be ignored.

This study was well designed with an easily identified study population, but by limiting recruitment to women awaiting hysterectomy we are not able to conclude that women would find the LNG-IUS an attractive alternative to all surgical approaches. The threshold for surgical intervention may be lower for minimally invasive techniques. The early data provided here demonstrate that the LNG-IUS clearly has great potential in the management of menorrhagia, but further studies are needed to evaluate the long-term clinical effectiveness and cost-effectiveness of using the LNG-IUS.

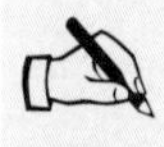

A randomised study comparing levonorgestrel intrauterine system (LNG-IUS) and transcervical resection of the endometrium (TCRE) in the treatment of menorrhagia: preliminary results.

N Kittelsen, O Istre. *Gynaecol Endosc* 1998; **7**: 61–5.

BACKGROUND. The length of hospital stay, subsequent sick leave and complication rates associated with hysterectomy motivated research into alternative, less invasive procedures such as transcervical techniques to remove the endometrium with the aim

of decreasing menstrual bleeding. The LNG-IUS seems to be an important alternative to oral therapy and to hysterectomy in the management of menorrhagia. This study was designed to compare the effectiveness of transcervical resection of the endometrium (TCRE) and the LNG-IUS in the treatment of menorrhagia.

The study was performed at a gynaecological clinic in Oslo, Norway, specializing in operative hysteroscopy. All TCREs were performed by one surgeon experienced in the technique. All the women had been referred after failed attempts at medical management and were initially prepared to undergo hysterectomy. A diagnosis of excessive uterine bleeding was based on history and a pictorial blood loss assessment score. All women were premenopausal, had not used hormonal treatment during the preceding 3 months and had no history of thromboembolism or liver disease. Women uncertain about their future wish for pregnancy were also excluded.

Thirty women were randomized into each treatment group; they were comparable in age, weight and height. One woman in the TCRE group refused treatment, otherwise the operative procedures and data collection were uneventful. Prior to study entry, all women had a pelvic examination and a cervical smear, endometrial biopsy (Pipelle) and transvaginal ultrasound (to excluded visible fibroids and to record the endometrial thickness) were performed.

The TCRE was performed using a Storz resectoscope and an 8-mm resection loop. The LNG-IUS was inserted within the first 7 days of the menstrual cycle.

The study participants were seen at 3, 6 and 12 months. Ferritin levels were recorded, pictorial blood loss assessment charts were reviewed and transvaginal ultrasound was performed to measure endometrial thickness.

INTERPRETATION. In the LNG-IUS group, six women discontinued treatment, three women for persistent bleeding/spotting after 9 months, two for pelvic pain (one at 17 days and one after 5 months) and one device was expelled after 3.5 months. The other 24 women in this randomization arm completed the study. At 12 months the pictorial blood loss assessment score had decreased from 418 [standard deviation (SD) 349] at baseline to 42 (SD 99.7).

In the TCRE group, one of the 29 women withdrew after randomization for personal reasons. Premature interventions such as dilatation and curettage, cervical blocking or repeat resection were taken as failure of TCRE even though the women continued in the study. Four women underwent repeat resection during the 2-year follow-up period. Two of these women had haematometra and completed the study without further complication following repeat resection at 16 and 20 months, respectively. Two women had continuous bleeding problems and had repeat resections at 8 and 15 months, respectively; in one, a 3-cm fibroid was found and resected. Two women became menopausal and were withdrawn from the study. No women underwent hysterectomy during the follow-up. At 12 months the bleeding tendency was significantly less in the TCRE group, 70% of the women were amenorrhoeic compared with 36% of the women in the LNG-IUS group.

Comment

The same dramatic reduction in MBL with the LNG-IUS was seen in this study as previously reported in the management of menorrhagic women. However, significantly less bleeding was seen in the TCRE group than the LNG-IUS group.

The authors suggest that 60–70% of women currently scheduled for operative procedures might be treated successfully by the LNG-IUS. They point out that the LNG-IUS has the major advantage of reversibility in contrast to the methods involving destruction or resection. The provision of adequate contraception is also relevant, as despite the pre-operative coagulation of the tubal ostia, women cannot be guaranteed infertility after TCRE.

The authors conclude that the LNG-IUS is an appropriate first-line agent in the management of menorrhagia in younger women. Whilst endometrial resection is even more effective at reducing bleeding, it requires day surgery, is irreversible and is associated with a need for repeated resection.

The unique mode of action of the LNG-IUS is likely to expand its therapeutic use as the mechanism of common gynaecological conditions such as fibroids, endometriosis and adenomyosis are better understood.

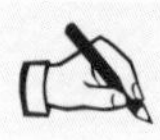

A levonorgestrel-releasing intrauterine system for the treatment of dysmenorrhoea associated with endometritis: a pilot study.

P Vercellini, G Aimi, S Panazza, *et al. Fertil Steril* 1999; **72**(3): 505–8.

BACKGROUND. Dysmenorrhoea is by far the most frequent symptom reported by women with endometriosis and whilst surgical ablation of lesions is usually effective, postoperative relapse is quite common. Symptomatic relief can be produced by drugs such as danazol and gonadotrophin-releasing hormone agonists inducing anovulation and hypo-oestrogenism, but pain often recurs at resumption of ovulation when the drugs are withdrawn after a few months because of side-effects and/or cost considerations. The identification of safe long-term treatment options is a key point in current clinical research on symptomatic endometriosis.

As a result of their limited side-effects, the use of progestogens is being investigated. However, tolerance is variable and the possibility of aiming therapeutic action at specific organs and reducing the general metabolic impact would be interesting.

A pilot study was designed to evaluate the tolerability and efficacy of the LNG-IUS in the long-term treatment of recurrent dysmenorrhoea associated with endometriosis. This prospective, non-comparative study was conducted in a tertiary care and referral academic centre for patients with endometriosis to assess variations in dysmenorrhoea intensity and patient satisfaction after 1 year of therapy using the LNG-IUS.

Parous women under 40 years who had undergone conservative surgery for endometriosis during the previous 12 months who did not want further surgery and who were assessed to have recurrent moderate to severe dysmenorrhoea were considered for enrolment.

Symptom intensity was assessed using a visual analogue scale and a three-point verbal rating scale which grades dysmenorrhoea according to loss of work efficiency and need for bed rest. Women were also requested to compile pictorial blood loss assessment charts for two consecutive cycles.

Subjects were eligible if they had at least moderate pain on both scales and a normal uterus and adnexa on clinical examination and transvaginal ultrasonography. Women were excluded if they had received treatment other than non-steroidal anti-inflammatory drugs during the preceding 3 months, if they had contraindications to progestin use, a history of PID, an unwillingness to tolerate menstrual changes or a wish to conceive.

After insertion of the LNG-IUS, the women were seen every 2 months, at which time the pictorial blood loss assessment chart scores were reviewed and variations in menstrual pain intensity were recorded. At the final 12-month visit the women were requested to rate their overall degree of satisfaction with their treatment (very satisfied, satisfied, uncertain, dissatisfied).

INTERPRETATION. Twenty parous women with a mean ± SD age of 34 ± 4 years were recruited. LNG-IUS insertion was uneventful. Two women withdrew from the study, one requested LNG-IUS removal because of weight gain and bloating and one expelled her device 3 months after insertion; one woman was lost to follow-up after she became amenorrhoeic and was satisfied with treatment, but before the 12-month evaluation. These women were classed as treatment failures, but were excluded from the pain and blood loss analyses because diary data were incomplete.

Of the remaining 17 women, 24% were amenorrhoeic, 47% had light bleeds or spotting and 29% had normal flow at 12 months. There was a significant reduction in pictorial blood loss chart scores and visual analogue and verbal rating scores between baseline and 12 months. Only 29 and 24% of women, respectively, were considered to have moderate and severe menstrual pain according to the visual analogue and verbal rating scales.

At 12 months, four women (20%) were very satisfied with the treatment, 11 (55%) were satisfied, two (10%) were uncertain and three (15%) were dissatisfied.

Comment

In this pilot study, the use of the LNG-IUS greatly reduced menstrual pain associated with endometriosis and offered a high degree of patient satisfaction. The authors considered that this was mainly the result of the oligo/amenorrhoea induced in most women by the local action of progestogen, with a corresponding 76% mean reduction in pictorial blood loss assessment chart scores.

The non-comparative study design and the small sample size undoubtedly limit the strength of the findings, but this was a small pilot study designed to determine what effect the LNG-IUS might have on endometriosis-associated dysmenorrhoea. Further trials are needed to determine whether the good results achieved at 12 months are maintained in the longer term and to determine whether effectiveness is maintained outside this selected population (parous women, not wanting to conceive and who had dysmenorrhoea as their only or main symptom). Effectiveness also needs to be assessed, in comparison with other treatment options, in the management of dyspareunia and non-menstrual pelvic pain.

The LNG-IUS and HRT

The use of unopposed oestrogen in women with intact uteri is strongly and consistently associated with the risk of endometrial hyperplasia and malignancy. The use of progestogen effectively opposes the stimulatory effect of oestrogen, but concern has been expressed that the addition of progestogen reduces the beneficial effect of oestrogen on the cardiovascular system, especially in relation to lipoproteins. The addition of progestogen to HRT preparations may also contribute to the side-effect profile. Compliance with HRT is poor and the duration of use seldom long enough to achieve and maintain long-term benefit. Women post-hysterectomy are far more likely to use HRT, which may be explained by the absence of bleeding and progestogen-related side-effects. At the present time the endometrium is regarded as being the only target organ requiring the use of progestogen in HRT and therefore the smallest dose of progestogen necessary to oppose oestrogenic endometrial stimulation should be used. In continuous combined oral therapy, endometrial stimulation is successfully avoided and less progestogen is required to achieve this than in sequential preparations, but bleeding patterns are rarely acceptable in perimenopausal women.

Experience using the LNG-IUS in fertile women has demonstrated a profound local suppressive effect on the endometrium and reduced bleeding. The development of the LNG-IUS to oppose oestrogen replacement therapy was therefore a logical step. In 1992 Andersson published the first data relating to the use of the LNG-IUS in 18 perimenopausal women receiving oral oestrogen therapy. At 12 months 83% of women were amenorrhoeic and endometrial samples showed a pronounced progestogenic effect with stromal decidualization. Similar histology and patterns of bleeding were seen when the LNG-IUS was used in combination with non-oral routes of oestrogen administration.

Spotting and bleeding are seen during the first few months of use as with oral continuous combined regimens and when the LNG-IUS is used for contraception. True bleeding is very rare after the first 6 months of use and the LNG-IUS induces amenorrhoea effectively in both peri- and postmenopausal women.

The Levonorgestrel intrauterine system in menopausal hormone replacement therapy: five year experience.
E Suvato-Luukkonen, A Kauppila. *Fertil Steril* 1999; **72**(3): 161–3.

BACKGROUND. The LNG-IUS, originally developed as a contraceptive, has also been used successfully to deliver the progestogen element of HRT in combination with oestrogen administered orally, transdermally via a patch, as a subdermal implant or percutaneously as a gel. Most reports relate to short follow-up periods. The authors present their 5-year experience using an oestradiol gel and the LNG-IUS.

Twenty menopausal volunteers aged 45–61 years (median 52 years) were accepted into the study. All had an intact uterus, no contraindications to HRT, a serum follicle-stimulating hormone level >20 IU/litre and their last menstrual period at least 6 months prior to study entry. All the women used 2.5 g of an oestradiol gel percutaneously that delivered 1.5 mg oestradiol per day, together with the LNG-IUS.

INTERPRETATION. During the first year, two women discontinued treatment, one because of abdominal pain 2 weeks after insertion and the other because of irregular bleeding. During the second to fifth years, a further six women withdrew from the study, three had irregular spotting, two believed that they no longer needed HRT and one woman left the study because she underwent hysterectomy for uterine prolapse. At 5 years, 12 women were still continuing with the treatment regimen.

During the first 3–6 months spotting was common, but by 12 months 80% of the women were amenorrhoeic. Amenorrhoea rates were largely unchanged through the next 4 years with the exception of two women who had a few days of spotting during the second year and one woman who had 55 days of bleeding and spotting during the second year; she discontinued the study. No side-effects were reported.

The median endometrial thickness measured using vaginal ultrasonography was 2.3, 3.0, 3.2 and 3.0 mm after 2, 3, 4 and 5 years of the study, respectively. Annual endometrial samples using the Pistolet technique showed epithelial atrophy and stromal decidualization in all the women. Plasma cells or giant cells were seen in some samples, but no clinical endometritis was seen and no LNG-IUS were removed prematurely.

Comment

Long-term compliance among users of sequential HRT is relatively low as a result of monthly bleeds and many women would welcome amenorrhoea-inducing regimens. The long-term endometrial effects of continuous combined oral preparations are promising and the LNG-IUS offers an alternative delivery route for progestogen which may, due to lower circulating levels, have fewer systemic side-effects.

In this study of 5 years' duration, the results in terms of clinical compliance, bleeding pattern and endometrial response were promising. The uniform endometrial suppression with epithelial atrophy and stromal decidualization reflects the much higher tissue concentrations of progestogen achieved with local administration than systemic therapy and explains the high rate of amenorrhoea.

The exact menopausal status of these women at study entry is unclear, some may have been perimenopausal; it is perhaps this group for whom the intrauterine administration of progestogen from a LNG-IUS is most appropriate as it also abolishes irregular anovulatory bleeding and provides highly effective contraception.

Conclusion

In 1993 David Bromham wrote 'The intrauterine contraceptive device (IUD) is a highly effective and safe form of reversible contraception. It does not cause pelvic inflammatory disease, ectopic pregnancy or infertility; it could be used by most nulligravidae. In its latest form (LNG-IUS) it can be used to treat excessive menstrual loss and it acts by preventing fertilisation not implantation'. In the years since his untimely death, publications have not only confirmed his statement, but added to the range of conditions which can be managed by the intrauterine administration of therapeutic agents.

References

1. Farley TNM, Rosenberg MJ, Rose PJ, *et al.* Intrauterine devices and pelvic inflammatory disease: an international perspective. *Lancet* 1992; **339**: 785–8.

2. Sivin I, Stern J, Coutinho E, *et al.* Prolonged intra-uterine contraception: a seven year randomized study of the levonorgestrel 20 mcg/day (LNg 20) and the copper T380Ag IUDs. *Contraception* 1991; **44**: 473–80.

3. World Health Organization Special Programme of Research, Development and Research Training in Human Reproduction. Task Force on the Safety and Efficacy of Fertility Regulating Methods. The TCu380A, TCu220C, Multiload 250 and Nova T IUD at 3, 5 and 7 years of use—results from three randomized multi-centre trials. *Contraception* 1990; **42**: 141–58.

4. Rowe PJ. Clinical performance of copper IUDs. In: Wayne Bardin C, Mishell DR (eds): *Proceedings of the 4th International Conference on IUDs.* Butterworth Heinemann, London, 1994, pp. 13–31.

5. Wilson JC. A New Zealand randomized comparative study of three IUDs (Nova T, MLCu375, MLAgCu250): 1, 2 and 3 year results. *Adv Contracept* 1992; **82**: 153–9.

6. Sastravinata S, Farr G, Prihadi SM, *et al.* A comparative trial of the TCu 380A, Lippes Loop D and Multiload Cu375 IUDs in Indonesia. *Contraception* 1991; **44**: 141–54.

7. Sivin I, Diaz S, Pavez M, *et al.* Two year comparative trial of the Gyne T 380 Slimline and Gyne T 380 intrauterine copper devices. *Contraception* 1991; **44**: 481–7.

8. IUD Research Group. The TCu380A IUD and the frameless IUD 'the Flexigard': interim three-year data from an international multicenter trial. UNDP, UNFPA and WHO Special Programme of Research, Development and Research Training in Human Reproduction, World Bank. *Contraception* 1995; **52**(2): 77–83.

9. Sivin I, Stern J, Coutinho E, *et al.* Prolonged intrauterine contraception—a 7 year study of Levonorgestrel IUCD 20 µg/day and the Copper T 380Ag. *Contraception* 1991; **44**: 473–80.

10. Andersson K, Odlind V, Rybo G. Levonorgestrel-releasing and copper-releasing (Nova T) IUDs during five years of use: a randomised comparative trial. *Contraception* 1994; **49**: 56–72.

11. Andersson K, Rybo G. Levonorgestrel-releasing intrauterine device in the treatment of menorrhagia. *Br J Obstet Gynaecol* 1990; **97**: 690–4.

2

Oral contraceptives and thrombosis

Introduction

The combined oral contraceptive (COC) pill is effective, convenient and reversible. For most women it is also remarkably safe. However, since the early 1960s use of the COC has been associated with an increased risk of myocardial infarction (MI), stroke and venous thromboembolism (VTE). The suggestion that the risk of thrombosis was related to the oestrogen content led to the development of second and third generation COCs which contained lower doses of ethinyl oestradiol [1]. Second generation COCs contain 20–35 μg of ethinyl oestradiol with levonorgestrel or norethisterone. Third generation COCs contain 20–35 μg of ethinyl oestradiol with either gestodene, desogestrel or norgestimate. The progestogens in the third generation preparations are associated with an improved lipid profile and were expected to reduce the risk of arterial thrombosis [2].

In 1995 and 1996, four studies (with cohort and/or case–control design) demonstrated an approximately two-fold increased risk of VTE in patients receiving third generation COCs in comparison with second generation preparations [3–6]. These studies have been the subject of sustained criticism and re-analysis and the debate as to whether third generation COCs are associated with an excess risk of VTE remains unresolved [7]. There were two key criticisms of these studies. First, the excess risk of VTE associated with third generation pills may have reflected the type of patient who received the preparation rather than the medication itself. For instance, patients at increased risk of VTE may have been prescribed third generation pills because of the perception, at that time, that they would be associated with a lower risk of thrombosis. Second, no plausible biological explanation had been provided to explain the excess risk associated with the third generation preparations.

There has been no convincing evidence that the more favourable lipid profile associated with third generation COCs decreases the risk of MI or ischaemic stroke. An initial case–control study found no difference in the rate of MI between the two types of COC preparation [8]. A subsequent case–control study demonstrated lower incidence of MI in association with the third generation pills, but this study has been criticized because of the failure of the investigators to adjust for the measurement of blood pressure prior to starting the COC [7]. Similarly, while the use of

COCs has been associated with an increased risk of stroke, it is unclear whether there is a differential effect between the second and third generation COCs |9|.

The absence of oestrogen and the minimal activation of the coagulation cascade in patients receiving progestogen-only contraceptives suggest that this preparation may be associated with a reduction in thrombosis risk. However, this hypothesis has not been assessed in clinical studies. Similarly, there are no available data on the risk of thrombosis associated with progestogen-only emergency contraception.

Over the past 3 years a number of key publications have addressed the following issues regarding thrombosis and the use of COCs:

1. The risk of VTE associated with second and third generation COCs, combined oestrogen and progestogen postcoital pills and progestogen-only contraceptives.
2. The identification of the haemostatic mechanism(s) responsible for the observed difference in thrombotic risk associated with second and third generation COCs.
3. The risk of MI and ischaemic stroke associated with second and third generation COCs.
4. The risk of VTE associated with the use of COCs in patients with inherited pro-thrombotic defects.

The risk of VTE associated with COCs, combined oestrogen and progestogen postcoital pills and progestogen-only contraceptives

Comparison of the risk of VTE associated with second and third generation COCs

Two recent analyses of the General Practice Research Database (GPRD) have assessed the risk of VTE associated with second and third generation COCs and produced conflicting results. The GPRD contains information from general practitioners within the UK who have been trained to record medical information using a standard protocol.

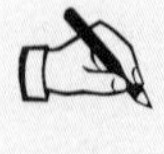

Effect of 1995 pill scare on rates of venous thromboembolism among women taking combined oral contraceptives: analysis of General Practice Research Database.

RD Farmer, TJ Williams, EL Simpson, AL Nightingale. *Br Med J* 2000; **321**: 477–9.

BACKGROUND. The objective of this study was to compare the incidence of VTE among women taking COCs before and after the October 1995 'pill scare'.

INTERPRETATION. There was no significant change in the incidence of VTE between the two time periods (January 1993 to October 1995 and November 1995 to December 1998) after adjusting for age (incidence ratio 1.04, 95% CI 0.78–1.39). This is despite a fall in the prescription of third generation pills from 53 to 14% of total use after the 'pill scare'. The findings are thus not compatible with the assertion that third generation oral contraceptives are associated with a two-fold increase in risk of VTE compared with older progestogens.

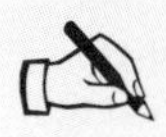

Risk of venous thromboembolism among users of third generation oral contraceptives compared with users of oral contraceptives with levonorgestrel before and after 1995: cohort and case–control analysis.

H Jick, A James, JA Kaye, C Vasilakis-Scaramozza, SS Jick. *Br Med J* 2000; **321**: 1190–5.

BACKGROUND. The objective of this study was to compare the risk of idiopathic VTE among women taking third generation oral contraceptives (with gestodene or desogestrel) with that among women taking oral contraceptives with levonorgestrel. Cohort and case–control analyses were derived from the GPRD.

INTERPRETATION. The adjusted estimates of relative risk for VTE associated with third generation oral contraceptives compared with oral contraceptives with levonorgestrel were 1.9 (95% CI 1.3–2.8) in the cohort analysis and 2.3 (95% CI 1.3–3.9) in the case–control study. The estimates for the two types of oral contraceptive were similar before and after the warning issued by the Committee on Safety of Medicines in October 1995. These findings are consistent with previously reported studies which found that, compared with oral contraceptives containing levonorgestrel, third generation oral contraceptives are associated with around twice the risk of VTE.

Comment

Part of the explanation for the discrepant findings from two studies using the same database must lie in the methods and the design. The study by Farmer *et al.* assessed changes in the use of second and third generation COCs before and after the 'pill scare' in 1995, and also assessed the incidence of venous thrombosis between these two periods. This study only adjusted for age and some concerns have been expressed as to whether this was adequately performed. On the other hand, Jick *et al.* replicated this approach for the purpose of comparison but also presented cohort and nested case–control analysis. They uncovered important confounding factors, which may have limited the reliability of the Farmer *et al.* study. The reduction in use of third generation oral contraceptives mainly involved young women (who were at lowest risk of venous thrombosis) and doctors tended to avoid prescribing third generation preparations to obese women and smokers. Clearly only one study can have the right answer and the superior design of the Jick *et al.* study suggests that there is an increased risk associated with third generation COCs.

The risk of VTE in users of postcoital contraceptive pills (PCP)

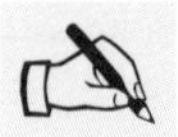

The risk of venous thromboembolism in users of post-coital contraceptive pills.

C Vasilakis, SS Jick, H Jick. *Contraception* 1999; **59**(2): 79–83.

BACKGROUND. **PCP (as per the Yuzpe regimen) has recently been approved for use as emergency contraception in the USA. The objective of this study was to assess the risk of idiopathic VTE in relation to exposure to PCP, and to quantify better the risk of idiopathic VTE associated with COC use and pregnancy. A population-based cohort study with a nested case–control analysis was conducted using women from the UK GPRD.**

INTERPRETATION. There were no women with an outcome of idiopathic VTE with current exposure to PCP (100 615 prescriptions). The incidence rates for various exposures were 3.0/100 000 person-years for the unexposed, 5.3/100 000 person-years for second generation COCs, 10.7/100 000 person-years for third generation COCs, and 15.5/100 000 person-years in pregnant (or postpartum) women. The relative risk estimates were 1.7 (95% CI 0.3–10.5) for second generation COCs, 4.4 (95% CI 1.0–18.7) for third generation COCs, and 6.3 (95% CI 1.2–33.5) for pregnancy. Short-term use of PCP is not associated with a substantially increased risk of developing VTE.

Comment

This study also supports the previous published data by the authors, using the same database and an overlapping time period, which demonstrated an excess risk of VTE in association with the use of third generation COCs |3|.

The risk of VTE associated with PCP was assessed by a population-based cohort study with nested case–control analysis. The cohort study documented the episodes of VTE per year of patient exposure to PCP from data obtained from the GPRD. Each prescription for the PCP was assigned an exposure time of 45 days. Exposure to pregnancy/postpartum (assigned an exposure time of 1 year) and COCs (assigned an exposure time of 30 days per pill pack) was also recorded. Cases of VTE were then matched with controls (six when possible) which had been corrected for difference in age, geography, calendar time, smoking and body mass index.

Despite the large number of subjects included in this study, the absolute baseline risk of VTE in this population is so small that a review of 100 000 prescriptions for PCP is insufficient to provide a definitive assessment of thrombotic risk. Nevertheless the data are reassuring and suggest that the risk of VTE is not substantially higher than for COCs despite the higher dose of oestrogen used in PCP.

Cardiovascular risk factors and use of oral and injectable progestogen-only contraceptives and combined injectable contraceptives

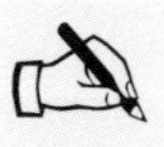

Cardiovascular risk factors and use of oral and injectable progestogen-only contraceptives and combined injectable contraceptives.

World Health Organization Collaborative Study of Cardiovascular Disease and Steroid Hormone Contraception. *Contraception* 1998; **57**(5): 315–24.

BACKGROUND. This report describes the first study to evaluate the risks of cardiovascular disease (CVD) associated with the use of oral and injectable progestogen-only and combined injectable contraceptives.

INTERPRETATION. Although limited by the small number of cases and control subjects using the types of contraceptives under investigation, these data suggest that there is little or no increased risk of stroke, VTE or MI associated with the use of oral or injectable progestogen-only or combined injectable contraceptives. However, further investigation into a possible adverse effect on stroke risk of progestogen-only contraceptives used by women with a history of high blood pressure is indicated.

Comment

This was a hospital-based case–control study conducted by the WHO and involving 21 centres throughout Africa, Asia, Europe and Latin America. Each centre recruited cases and control subjects from variable numbers of collaborating hospitals. Eligible cases were women aged 22–44 years (15–49 years in three centres) who had been admitted to collaborating hospitals and, in the opinion of the responsible physician, had one of three CVD (VTE, ischaemic stroke or MI). A monitoring system was set up in each centre to notify all eligible cases. For each case, one to three sex- and age-matched controls were recruited. All cases and control subjects were interviewed in hospital in a standard manner with the same questionnaire. Cases and controls were excluded if they had a past history of a transient ischaemic attack, stroke, MI or VTE, or if they had a history in the previous 6 weeks of pregnancy, surgery or a major illness causing bed rest for greater than 1 week. Cases and controls had similar mean ages and body mass index, but cases were more likely to have a history of cardiovascular risk factors including hypertension, diabetes, rheumatic heart disease, and smoking.

Among 3697 cases of cardiovascular events (59% stroke, 31% VTE and 10% MI), 53, 37 and 13 women were current users of oral progestogen-only, injectable progestogen-only and injectable combined contraceptives, respectively. The adjusted odds ratios for all cardiovascular events were 1.4 (95% CI 0.79–1.63), 1.02 (95% CI 0.68–1.54) and 0.95 (95% CI 0.49–1.86) for users of oral progestogen-only, injectable progestogen-only and injectable combined contraceptives, respectively. There was no significant increase in the odds ratio for stroke or MI. However, a small non-significant increased risk of VTE was apparent for oral and injectable progestogen-only contraceptives, with adjusted odds ratios of 1.74 (95% CI 0.76–3.9) and 2.19 (95% CI 0.66–7.2), respectively. Among women with a history of hypertension, the odds ratio for stroke rose from 7.2 (95% CI 6.1–8.5) among non-users to 12.4 (95% CI 4.1–37.6) among users of oral progestogen-only contraceptives.

Grouping all cardiovascular complications together for the purpose of analysis may have been necessary because of the small sample size, but the interpretation of these data is severely limited by the major differences in the pathophysiological mechanisms responsible for VTE, MI and stroke. A definitive assessment of each of these complications separately is impossible because of the very wide confidence intervals. However, they identify an increased risk of stroke (primarily haemorrhagic) in hypertensive patients receiving oral progestogens, which is potentially important given that this form of contraception is frequently advocated for high-risk individuals.

The limited size of the study means that it provides only minimal reassurance about the risk of thrombosis associated with progestogen-only contraception. Further studies are required to provide a more definitive risk assessment.

Identification of the haemostatic mechanism(s) responsible for the observed difference in thrombotic risk associated with second and third generation oral contraceptives

The following papers were published from data generated from a single cross-over study involving women who received two consecutive cycles of a second generation oral contraceptive containing levonorgestrel and a third generation oral contraceptive containing desogestrel separated by two pill-free cycles.

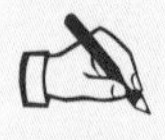

Low-dose oral contraceptives and acquired resistance to activated protein C: a randomised cross-over study.
J Rosing, S Middeldorp, J Curvers, *et al. Lancet* 1999; **354**: 2036–40.

BACKGROUND. These authors had previously reported a study which suggested that, compared with the use of second generation oral contraceptives, the use of third generation oral contraceptives was associated with increased resistance to the anticoagulant action of activated protein C (APC). They did, however, criticize their own study in that its cross-sectional design may have allowed unknown bias or uncontrolled effects of the menstrual cycle. This study was a cycle-controlled randomized cross-over trial with the aim of overcoming these sources of bias.

INTERPRETATION. Oral contraceptive treatment diminished the efficacy with which APC down-regulated in vitro thrombin formation. This phenomenon, which the authors designated 'acquired APC resistance', was more pronounced in women using desogestrel-containing oral contraceptives than in women using levonorgestrel-containing preparations. The authors comment that the issue of whether or not this acquired APC resistance induced by oral contraceptives explains the increased risk of VTE in oral contraceptive users remains to be established.

Comment

The cross-over design of this study virtually excludes the possibility that this difference is caused by uncontrolled cycle effects or variability between individuals. Therefore, the plasma from women using desogestrel-containing oral contraceptives is substantially more resistant to the anticoagulant action of APC than the plasma from women using levonorgestrel-containing contraceptives. APC resistance was quantified on the basis of endogenous thrombin potential. Resistance to APC is an independent risk factor for venous thrombosis even in non-carriers of factor V Leiden |10|. However, whether the increased resistance to APC is sufficient to explain the observed excess of VTE associated with third generation oral contraceptives remains to be proven.

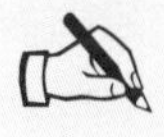

Effects on coagulation of levonorgestrel and desogestrel containing low dose oral contraceptive: a cross over study.

S Middledorp, J Meijers, A van den Ende, *et al. Thromb Haemost* 2000; **84**: 4–8.

BACKGROUND. This randomized cycle-controlled cross-over study of 28 healthy volunteers was designed to assess potential differences between the effects of a COC containing 150 μg of levonorgestrel and 150 μg of desogestrel in combination with 30 μg of ethinylestradiol on several coagulation factors and markers of thrombin formation.

INTERPRETATION. The authors conclude that there are differences between the effects of levonorgestrel- and desogestrel-containing COCs on some coagulation factors, but cannot say whether or not this explains the reported difference in thromboembolic risk. They comment that more work is needed to examine the various haemostatic systems, in case there are changes in several which could combine to affect the haemostatic balance towards a prothrombotic state, and may lead to overt clinical VTE.

Comment

The plasma concentrations of factors II, VII, X and fibrinogen significantly increased during use of levonorgestrel- and desogestrel-containing COCs. The plasma concentrations of factor VIII increased and factor V decreased, but these changes only reached statistical significance during the use of desogestrel-containing COCs. During exposure to desogestrel-containing COCs, as compared with levonor-gestrel-containing COCs, factor VII and factor II were significantly increased (factor VII, 32 and 12%, respectively; $P < 0.001$; factor II, 16 and 12%, respectively; $P = 0.048$), whereas factor V was significantly decreased (-11 to -3%; $P = 0.01$). Only one of the markers of ongoing thrombin generation (prothombin fragment 1+2) showed a significant increase during COC use and there was no difference between the different COCs.

This study confirms earlier observations of potentially important alterations in plasma concentrations of coagulation factors induced by the use of COCs and indicates that the increase in factors VII and II and the decrease in factor V were more pronounced when desogestrel-containing COCs were used. The difference for factor VII was considerable, but the blood level of this factor has not been associated with risk of VTE. There was also a significant difference for factor V, but neither high nor low levels of this factor have been associated with VTE. While elevated factor II levels have been associated with VTE |11|, the magnitude of the difference between the two generations of COCs is rather small. The potential clinical significance of the changes reported in this study is further undermined by the failure to demonstrate a difference in markers of thrombin generation between the second and third generation oral contraceptives.

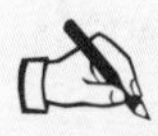

A randomized cross-over study on the effects of levonorgestrel and desogestrel containing oral contraceptives on anticoagulant pathways.

G Tans, J Curvers, S Middledorp, *et al. Thromb Haemost* 2000; **84**: 15–21.

BACKGROUND. It is recognized that the use of COCs causes disturbances of procoagulant, anticoagulant and fibrinolytic pathways of blood coagulation which may contribute to the increased risk of venous thrombosis associated with COC therapy. This cycle-controlled randomized cross-over study looked at the effects of second and third generation COCs on a number of anticoagulant parameters.

INTERPRETATION. The study findings indicate that the activity of the anticoagulant pathways in plasma from users of the desogestrel-containing COC is more extensively impaired than in the plasma from users of the levonorgestrel-containing COC.

Comment

The anticoagulant parameters determined were: antithrombin, α_2-macroglobulin, α_1-antitrypsin, protein C inhibitor, protein C, total and free protein S and APC sensitivity ratios as measured by two functional APC resistance tests which quantify the effect of APC on either the activated partial thromboplastin time or on the endogenous thrombin potential. COC use was associated with increased resistance to APC, using both assay systems, which is consistent with the previously discussed data. A decrease in free and total protein S was associated with desogestrel but not levonorgestrel. Compared with levonorgestrel, desogestrel-containing COCs caused a significant decrease in total ($P < 0.005$) as well as free protein S ($P < 0.0001$) and more pronounced APC resistance in both the activated partial thromboplastin time ($P = 0.02$) and endogenous thrombin potential ($P < 0.0001$) APC resistance tests.

The mechanism responsible for the occurrence of acquired APC resistance during COC use and the difference between the two generations of COC have not been established. The reduction in protein S may contribute to APC resistance in patients receiving third generation COCs. However, other mechanisms are clearly responsible for the increased APC sensitivity ratios associated with COC use, as levonorgestrel results in APC resistance without any change in protein S levels. The reduction in protein S in patients receiving third generation COCs may still contribute to the increased risk of VTE as protein S deficiency has been associated with an increased risk of VTE |**12**|.

Summary

These data clearly demonstrate that third generation COCs elicit a different haemostatic response to second generation preparations. The reduction in protein S and the increased resistance to APC are plausible biological mechanisms to explain the clinical observation that third generation COCs are associated with an increased risk of venous thrombosis.

The risk of MI and ischaemic stroke associated with second and third generation oral contraceptives

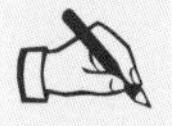

Oral contraceptives and myocardial infarction: results of the MICA case–control study.
N Dunn, M Thorogood, B Faragher, *et al. Br Med J* 1999; **318**: 1579–84.

BACKGROUND. This was a retrospective community-based case–control study with data being obtained from interviews and general practice records in England, Wales and Scotland. The aim was to determine the association between MI and the use of different types of oral contraception in young women.

INTERPRETATION. No significant association was seen between the use of oral contraceptives and MI and no significant difference was found between second and third generation products. The modest and non-significant point estimates for this association have wide confidence intervals.

Comment

This was a community-based retrospective case–control study undertaken in the populations of England, Scotland and Wales. Cases were identified from hospital in-patient episode statistics, the deaths register of the Office for National Statistics for England and Wales, the Information and Statistics Division of the Department of Health and the Registrar General's Office in Scotland. Diagnostic information for each potential case was extracted from hospital notes, and these data were submitted to a panel of three cardiologists, blind to exposure status, for confirmation of diagnosis. Age- and sex-matched control women were selected from the same general practice as the index case. There was good agreement between interview data and general practitioner records. The power of the study to detect a two-fold increased risk of MI associated with second and third generation COCs was 96 and 81%, respectively, at the 5% significance level. The second generation COCs used in the study contained norethisterone or levonorgestrel, while the third generation COCs contained gestodene or desogestrel.

The adjusted odds ratio for MI was 1.4 (95% CI 0.78–2.52) for combined COC users, 1.1 (95% CI 0.52–2.3) for second generation users and 1.96 (95% CI 0.87–4.39) for third generation users. The adjusted odds ratio for third generation users versus second generation users was 1.78 (95% CI 0.66–4.83). The modest increases in the odds ratio had wide confidence intervals and were not statistically significant.

The potential limitations of this study included low interview rates and the potential for the misclassification of COC exposure and selection bias. Seventy-three per cent of the survivors of MI were interviewed, but proxy interviews were only obtained in 20% of cases of fatal MI. Misclassification of exposure may have occurred because interviewees were asked to recall contraceptive habits. The adverse publicity about third generation contraceptives may have biased responses to the questions. However, this is unlikely to have had a major impact because there was good agreement between data obtained from the medical records and result of interviews.

This well-designed study is an important and reassuring contribution to the literature. The power of the study suggests that second and third generation COCs are either not associated with an increased risk of MI or if such a risk exists then it is associated with an odds ratio of less than two. There was no evidence of any advantage of third generation over second generation contraceptives in the rate of MI.

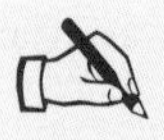

Effect on stroke of different progestagens in low oestrogen dose oral contraceptives. WHO Collaborative Study of Cardiovascular Disease and Steroid Hormone Contraception.

NR Poulter, CL Chang, TM Farley, MG Marmot, O Meirik. *Lancet* 1999; **354**: 301–3.

BACKGROUND AND INTERPRETATION. This multicentre WHO collaborative case–control study had limited power to differentiate stroke risks by progestagen

component in low-dose COCs. Given this caveat, odds ratios for ischaemic, haemorrhagic, and all strokes combined associated with use of oral contraceptives containing desogestrel or gestodene ('third generation') were found to be similar to those containing levonorgestrel in this study.

Comment

The differential risk of stroke association with use of second and third generation oral contraceptives was assessed with data obtained from a multicentre WHO collaborative study assessing the risk of CVD in patients receiving steroid hormone contraceptives.

The use of COCs was associated with an increased risk of ischaemic and haemorrhagic stroke [odds ratio 2.85 (95% CI 2.09–3.58) and 1.73 (95% CI 1.31–2.29), respectively]. There was no difference in the adjusted odds ratio for all strokes or haemorrhagic strokes between third and second generation COCs. The odds ratio for ischaemic stroke was greater among users of levonorgestrel-containing COCs than third generation preparations [odds ratio 2.70 (95% CI 1.77–4.14) and 1.75 (95% CI 0.59–5.16), respectively]. However, this difference was reduced among women who reported that their blood pressure had been measured before starting this episode of oral contraceptive use. The adjusted odds ratios were 1.63 (95% CI 0.43–6.61) and 1.95 (95% CI 1.06–3.58) for second and third generation preparations, respectively.

Although large, this study had limited powder to evaluate and compare risk estimates for stroke associated with oral contraceptives containing different progestogens which is reflected in the wide confidence intervals especially in patients using third generation preparations. Major differences in either direction between products could not be excluded and therefore the results presented in this report must be interpreted with great caution.

Summary

There was no difference in the risk of ischaemic stroke or MI between second and third generation COCs in patients without additional risk factors for CVD, although the stroke study had limited power. Further studies are required to compare the two preparations especially in at-risk individuals. The reportedly lipid-friendly third generation products were expected to be associated with fewer adverse arterial events. However, the epidemiological evidence supporting a reduction in arterial ischaemic events associated with these products is lacking.

The risk of VTE associated with the use of oral contraceptives in patients with inherited prothrombotic defects

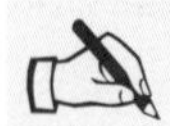

Interaction between the G20210A mutation of the prothrombin gene and oral contraceptive use in deep vein thrombosis.

I Martinelli, E Taioli, P Bucciarelli, S Akhavan, PM Mannucci. *Arterioscl Thromb Vasc Biol* 1999; **19**: 700–3.

BACKGROUND. It is recognized that single point mutations in the gene coding for prothrombin (factor II:A20210) or factor V Leiden (factor V:A1691) are associated with an increased risk of VTE. The use of oral contraceptives is also a strong independent risk factor for the disease, and the interaction between factor V:A1691 and oral contraceptives greatly increases the risk. In order to investigate whether there is a similar interaction between oral contraceptives and the mutant prothrombin gene, this study investigated 148 women with a first, objectively confirmed episode of deep venous thrombosis of the lower limbs and 277 healthy women as controls.

INTERPRETATION. The authors conclude that carriers of the prothrombin mutation who use oral contraceptives have a markedly increased risk of deep venous thrombosis, much higher than the risk conferred by either factor alone.

Comment

This was a case–control study of women referred for thrombophilia testing because of a first, objectively confirmed episode of deep venous thrombosis of the lower limbs. The control population consisted of healthy women who were friends or partners of any of the patients referred to the centre for investigation. They were not genetically related to the patients being investigated. After exclusion of 19 patients who were pregnant or postpartum at the time of the thrombosis, 64% of the patients and 25% of the controls had been using a COC until 2 weeks or less before the thrombotic episode. Of the COCs used, third generation preparations were the most common, being used in 73% of COC-using cases and 80% of COC-using controls.

After adjustment for the presence of other thrombophilic conditions, the odds ratio for prothrombin mutation was 5.7 (95% CI 2.2–14.6) and for factor V Leiden was 9.7 (95% CI 3.9–23.8). The risk conferred by the oral contraceptive was 5.6 (95% CI 3.3–9.6). The risk for women who used oral contraceptives and who were carriers of a mutation was 16.3 (95% CI 3.40–79.1) for the prothrombin mutation and 20 (95% CI 4.2–94.3) for the factor V Leiden mutation in comparison with non-users with normal genotype.

It has been previously reported that women with factor V Leiden who use oral contraceptives have an increased risk of venous thrombosis (30-fold) in comparison with non-users with normal genotype |**13**|. This paper found a similar effect between factor V Leiden and COCs and also demonstrated a synergistic interaction between the mutant prothrombin allele and the risk of thrombosis associated with oral contraceptives (16-fold increased risk).

The major limitation of this study was the small number of patients and controls using COCs, which is reflected in the wide confidence intervals of the odds ratios. The size of the study also prevented comparison of the interaction between second and third generation COCs and prothrombin mutation. Furthermore, while pulmonary embolus is the most significant presentation of VTE, only patients with deep venous thrombosis were included in this study. Nevertheless this paper represents an important contribution to the literature and represents the first and at present the only data assessing the interaction between COCs and the prothrombin mutation.

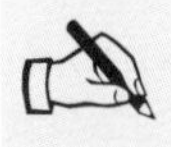

Selective screening for the factor V Leiden mutation: is it advisable prior to the prescription of oral contraceptives?

CM Schambeck, S Schwender, I Haubitz, U Geisen, R Grossmann, F Keller.
Thromb Haemost 1997; **78**: 1480–3.

BACKGROUND. As there is a cumulative thrombotic risk of factor V Leiden and oral contraceptives, the question is often raised as to whether screening for the mutation should be performed before prescription of COCs. Assuming that a family history of thrombosis increases the risk of likelihood of a patient bearing factor V Leiden, selective screening would be expected to be more useful than universal screening. The aim of this study was to test whether screening for factor V Leiden on the basis of a family history of thrombosis would be effective.

INTERPRETATION. Family history of thrombosis was found to be an unreliable criterion to detect factor V Leiden carriers.

Comment

This was a case–control study involving 101 cases (aged 15–45 years) who developed a first episode of deep venous thrombosis or pulmonary embolus while using oral contraceptives and who were referred to a thrombosis centre. One hundred and one age- and sex-matched controls from the same geographical area as the cases, who did not have a history of VTE, were recruited by four gynaecologists. The controls completed a standard questionnaire regarding the use of COCs, family history of venous thrombosis and acquired risk factors. Family history in a first-degree relative was considered positive if any parent or sibling had a previous VTE.

There was no significant relationship between family history of venous thrombosis in a first-degree relative and occurrence of factor V Leiden. The positive predictive value of family history in a first-degree relative was only 12% for controls and 14% for patients with a history of venous thrombosis. This study demonstrates that screening for factor V Leiden in patients with a family history of VTE in a first-degree relative is unjustified.

Venous thrombosis, oral contraceptives and high FVIII levels.

KW Bloemenkamp, FM Helmerhorst, FR Rosendaal, JP Vandenbroucke.
Thromb Haemost 1999; **82**: 1024–7.

BACKGROUND. Elevated plasma levels of factor VIII have been described as a strong risk factor for venous thrombosis. This study analysed the data from the Leiden Thrombophilia Study, a population-based case–control study on the cause of venous thrombosis, to verify whether the risk due to oral contraceptive use was higher in women with higher factor VIII levels. The study also investigated the joint risk of high factor VIII levels and oral contraceptive use.

INTERPRETATION. There was an increase in risk associated with contraceptive use in women with higher factor VIII levels and both factors have additive effects.

Comment

The cases for this study included 155 women aged 15–49 years at the time of a first episode of objectively confirmed deep venous thrombosis. One hundred and sixty-nine age- and sex-matched controls were selected. Elevated factor VIII was defined as a value of greater than 150 U/dl. Of the 155 cases, 109 (70%) had used oral contraceptives during the month preceding the deep venous thrombosis in contrast to 65/169 (38%) control subjects, yielding an odds ratio for venous thrombosis of 3.8 (95% CI 2.4–6.0). Elevated factor VIII was associated with an odds ratio of 4.5 (95% CI 2.1–10.2). The combination of COC use and elevated factor VIII was associated with an odds ratio of 8.8 (95% CI 4.1–18.8).

The interaction between elevated factor VIII and COCs appears to be additive. However, like so much literature in this area, the wide confidence intervals limit definitive interpretation of the true nature of the relationship. Furthermore, while this study represents the analysis of the interaction between elevated factor VIII and COC use, no information is provided on the different types of COC used or on the risk associated with pulmonary embolus.

Overall summary

Inherited thrombophilia defects are associated with an increased risk of COC-induced VTE. There are no data on the risk of thrombosis associated with the use of emergency contraception or progestogen-only preparations in patients with thrombophilia. The demonstration of an excess risk of VTE associated with COC use in patients with thrombophilia supports the current practice of avoiding COCs in these patients. However, because of the low absolute risk of VTE, even in those patients with thrombophilia, it may be appropriate to use oral contraception, especially progestogen-only preparations, in individual cases.

The demonstration that progestogen-only contraceptives were not associated with an increased risk of thrombosis is reassuring, although further data are required. Similarly, the combined postcoital pill (Yuzpe regimen) was not associated with VTE in a single study which excluded patients at increased risk of thrombosis.

The excess risk of VTE associated with third generation COCs has never been satisfactorily explained on the basis of bias or confounding. The recent demonstration that third generation preparations are associated with a reduction in protein S and a more significant increase in APC resistance provides a plausible biological mechanism to explain how these preparations could be associated with increased risk of VTE. Furthermore, third generation COCs have not been associated with a reduction in the rate of MI or ischaemic stroke. Because desogestrel- and gestodene-containing COCs appear to be associated with an increased risk of VTE without any apparent reduction in arterial thrombosis, they should probably be considered second line to levonorgestrel- and norethisterone-containing pills at the present time.

References

1. Inman WH, Vessey MP, Westerholm B, Engelund A. Thromboembolic disease and the steroidal content of oral contraceptives. A report to the Committee on Safety of Drugs. *Br Med J* 1970; **2**: 203–9.

2. Godsland IF, Crook D, Simpson R, *et al.* The effects of different formulations of oral contraceptive agents on lipid and carbohydrate metabolism. *N Engl J Med* 1990; **323**: 1375–81.

3. Jick H, Jick SS, Gurewich V, Myers MW, Vasilakis C. Risk of idiopathic cardiovascular death and nonfatal venous thromboembolism in women using oral contraceptives with differing progestagen components [see comments]. *Lancet* 1995; **346**: 1589–93.

4. Spitzer WO, Lewis MA, Heinemann LA, Thorogood M, MacRae KD. Third generation oral contraceptives and risk of venous thromboembolic disorders: an international case–control study. Transnational Research Group on Oral Contraceptives and the Health of Young Women [see comments]. *Br Med J* 1996; **312**: 83–8.

5. Anonymous. Effect of different progestagens in low oestrogen oral contraceptives on venous thromboembolic disease. World Health Organization Collaborative Study of

Cardiovascular Disease and Steroid Hormone Contraception [see comments]. *Lancet* 1995; **346**: 1582–8.

6. Bloemenkamp KW, Rosendaal FR, Helmerhorst FM, Buller HR, Vandenbroucke JP. Enhancement by factor V Leiden mutation of risk of deep-vein thrombosis associated with oral contraceptives containing a third-generation progestagen [see comments]. *Lancet* 1995; **346**: 1593–6.

7. Lewis MA, Heinemann LA, Spitzer WO, MacRae KD, Bruppacher R. The use of oral contraceptives and the occurrence of acute myocardial infarction in young women. Results from the Transnational Study on Oral Contraceptives and the Health of Young Women. *Contraception* 1997; **56**: 129–40.

8. Anonymous. Acute myocardial infarction and combined oral contraceptives: results of an international multicentre case–control study. WHO Collaborative Study of Cardiovascular Disease and Steroid Hormone Contraception [see comments]. *Lancet* 1997; **349**: 1202–9.

9. Anonymous. Haemorrhagic stroke, overall stroke risk, and combined oral contraceptives: results of an international, multicentre, case–control study. WHO Collaborative Study of Cardiovascular Disease and Steroid Hormone Contraception [see comments]. *Lancet* 1996; **348**: 505–10.

10. de Visser MC, Rosendaal FR, Bertina RM. A reduced sensitivity for activated protein C in the absence of factor V Leiden increases the risk of venous thrombosis. *Blood* 1999; **93**: 1271–6.

11. Simioni P, Tormene D, Manfrin D, *et al.* Prothrombin antigen levels in symptomatic and asymptomatic carriers of the 20210A prothrombin variant. *Br J Haematol* 1998; **103**: 1045–50.

12. Comp PC, Esmon CT. Recurrent venous thromboembolism in patients with a partial deficiency of protein S. *N Engl J Med* 1984; **311**: 1525–8.

13. Vandenbroucke JP, van der Meer FJ, Helmerhorst FM, Rosendaal FR. Factor V Leiden: should we screen oral contraceptive users and pregnant women? [see comments]. *Br Med J* 1996; **313**: 1127–30.

3

Progestogen-only methods of contraception

Introduction

A progestogen-only method is ideal for women who have contraindications to the use of oestrogen-containing products—women with previous venous thrombo-embolism (VTE), women with conditions aggravated by oestrogen (e.g. systemic lupus erythematosus) or those with risk factors for venous thrombosis (e.g. severe obesity). Progestogen-only methods are also suitable for women with risk factors for arterial disease—smokers over 35 years of age, women with hypertension or diabetes mellitus and women with migraines with aura or severe migraine.

Progestogen-only pills (POPs)

POPs have been used in the UK for many years, but continue to have limited acceptability by both clients and doctors. POPs account for only 8% of the current UK oral contraceptive market and only 1–2% of couples rely on POPs. In addition to the general indications for use of progestogen-only methods, POPs can also be used postpartum, as they have no effect on milk volume or content.

The failure rate of the POP (0.7–1.8/100 woman-years) is higher than that of the combined oral contraceptive pill (0.17–0.41/100 woman-years) which is one of the disadvantages of its use in women for whom pregnancy represents a serious threat to health. The need for consistent timing of tablet ingestion, and hence compliance, contributes to the failure rate of both combined and POPs and the higher method failure rate with the POP may relate to ovulation not being consistently inhibited. A new POP which consistently inhibits ovulation would be a valuable addition to the currently available progestogen-only methods of contraception.

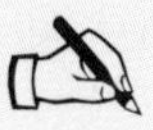

Ovarian activity and vaginal bleeding patterns with a desogestrel-only preparation at three different doses.

C Rice, S Killick, D Hickling, H Coelingh Bennink. *Hum Reprod* 1996; **11**(4): 737–40.

BACKGROUND. Ovulation inhibition is incomplete with established POP regimens, but with more complete inhibition of ovulation contraceptive efficacy could be further enhanced. A major limiting factor in the use of POPs is the disruption seen to the normal bleeding pattern. This randomized, double-blind, group-comparative study was designed to study the effects at three different dose levels of desogestrel on ovarian function and vaginal bleeding. Desogestrel is well known in combination with ethinyloestradiol, but had not previously been studied as a POP.

Forty-four apparently healthy women with ovulatory cycles of between 24 and 35 days were recruited from an out-patient clinic in a British university hospital. The women were randomly allocated, by means of a computer randomization code, to receive 30, 50 or 75 μg of desogestrel daily without interruption for six cycles of 28 days (168 days). The volunteers were instructed to use barrier methods of contraception, condoms or diaphragm without spermicide (to avoid interference with cervical mucus scoring) during screening and for the full period of the study.

After physical examination, transabdominal ultrasonography was performed between days 10 and 16 of a spontaneous screening cycle. Follicles with a mean diameter ≥15 mm were scanned daily until rupture. If ovulation was observed and all other screening data were considered normal, the volunteer was given her desogestrel therapy in coded bottles, in order to maintain the double-blind design of the study. Treatment was started on the first full day of menstruation. Ultrasound examination and serum oestradiol were performed twice weekly during two assessment periods, the first 56 days and the last 28 days of the study period. Cervical mucus was assessed by Insler scoring when indicated by the presence of a follicle ≥15 mm. The volunteers kept a daily record of their vaginal bleeding. Therapy was stopped after 6 months. Ultrasound scanning and endocrine monitoring were continued until normal menstruation was established. The bleeding patterns were analysed using two reference periods of 84 days.

INTERPRETATION. Forty-three of the 44 women randomized received treatment. Another woman who was accepted into the 75 μg group despite ovulation not being proven in the screening cycle, left the study after 17 days for reasons not related to the treatment. Eleven of 14 women completed six cycles of 75 μg of desogestrel and 13 of 15 women taking 50 μg and 11 of 14 women taking 30 μg completed the study period.

A dose response was observed for maximum progesterone concentrations. No progesterone concentrations >10 nmol/litre were seen in the 75 μg desogestrel group and none >30 nmol/litre in the 50 μg group. However, in the 30 μg group, maximum progesterone levels in the postovulatory range >30 nmol/litre were seen in four cases (three subjects in the first assessment period and one in the second).

An apparent dose response was also seen for the mean oestradiol concentrations for each assessment period by dosage group with the levels being inversely related to the desogestrel dose.

Follicular development >10 mm was seen in the majority of women in all three dosage groups. However, in more than one-third of the women in the lowest dose group follicles reached a diameter >30 mm, while in the highest dose group this did not occur during the first assessment period and occurred in just two women during the second assessment period. The presence of persistent follicles was more common in all dosage groups during the first assessment period than the second.

Cervical mucus was only assessed in the presence of a follicle ≥15 mm. A maximum Insler score < 9 was obtained in approximately 80% of women during each treatment period, equally divided between the treatment groups. A maximum Insler score ≥9 was seen in 20%, also equally distributed.

In view of the small sample size of the study, no statistical analysis was performed on the bleeding pattern data. A trend towards less bleeding/spotting for the 75 µg group was observed. Two women in the 50 µg group and one in the 30 µg group discontinued the study because of unacceptable vaginal bleeding, whereas none of the subjects in the high-dose group withdrew for this reason. A trend was also seen between the first and the second 84-day reference periods. A large reduction in bleeding/spotting was seen in the 75 µg group and to a lesser extent in the 50 µg group.

Among this well motivated group of women the acceptability of the desogestrel preparations was good, as measured through the recording of adverse events. Four women experienced adverse events which may or may not be related to the treatment; one case of depression in the 75 µg group (subject withdrew during the first 28 days of treatment), two cases of alopecia [one in the 50 µg group and one in the 30 µg group (withdrew from the study)] not associated with increased testosterone or reduced sex hormone binding globulin levels. Three women found the altered bleeding pattern unacceptable and withdrew from the study (two in the 50 µg group and one in the 30 µg group). Five of the eight women not completing the study withdrew because of adverse events.

Spontaneous menstruation returned promptly after cessation of use in almost all cases and three volunteers conceived in the post-treatment cycle before the onset of menses.

Comment

The assessment schedule of twice-weekly ultrasound scans did not allow for accurate diagnosis of ovulation, but an overall view of ovarian activity could be reached. The 75 µg desogestrel preparation showed better suppression of ovarian function. Although some follicular activity was seen on ultrasound, serum progesterone concentrations did not exceed levels of 10 nmol/litre, indicating absence of luteinization. Follicles >30 mm diameter were only seen in a relatively low percentage of women and the incidence of persistent follicles was lowest in this group. In contrast, the 30 µg group showed most ovarian activity, both by ultrasound and progesterone measurements; persistent follicles were diagnosed more commonly. The 50 µg group showed intermediate results.

The mean oestradiol concentrations showed an inverse response to the desogestrel doses, again indicating greater ovarian suppression with increasing doses. The cervical mucus showed a low maximum Insler score in 80% of all analyses indicating the contraceptive effect of desogestrel on the cervix.

The 75 μg desogestrel preparation gave a more regular bleeding pattern, which was found acceptable by the women participating in this study. It also showed a marked improvement over time with a reduction in bleeding and spotting, but the small sample size of the study prohibits firm conclusions to be drawn. All three doses were well tolerated with minimal side-effects.

The authors concluded that the 75 μg desogestrel preparation showed considerable benefits over other POPs and was the most promising dose for further clinical development as a contraceptive, the first stage being to perform randomized double-blind studies with other POPs.

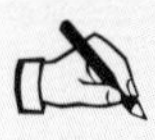

A comparison of the inhibition of ovulation achieved by desogestrel 75 μg and levonorgestrel 30 μg daily.

CF Rice, SR Killick, T Dieben, H Coelingh Bennink. *Hum Reprod* 1999; **14**(4): 982–5.

BACKGROUND. Desogestrel administered at a daily dose of 60–75 μg has been shown to inhibit ovulation completely, suggesting that it should be a more effective POP than levonorgestrel 30 μg/day which prevents ovulation in only 40% of cycles and which relies upon mucus hostility, endometrial changes and alterations in Fallopian tube motility for its contraceptive effect. This study was designed to compare desogestrel 75 μg/day with a currently available preparation of levonorgestrel 30 μg/day in their ability to inhibit ovulation in healthy female volunteers.

Seventy-one female volunteers with regular cycles and established ovulation by ultrasonography and serum progesterone concentrations were recruited from an out-patient clinic at a university hospital in the UK and randomly allocated to receive either desogestrel 75 μg/day or levonorgestrel 30 μg/day for 13 treatment periods of 28 days.

The subjects were between 18 and 40 years and were in good physical health with normal ovulatory cycles (mean length 24–35 days). Body weight was between 80 and 120% of ideal body weight. None of the subjects had used injectable hormonal contraceptives for the preceding 6 months or oral hormonal contraceptives for the two menstrual cycles prior to the study.

Ovulation was confirmed prior to the start of the study by transvaginal ultrasound on alternate days from day 10 until the dominant follicle reached 15 mm in diameter, from which time the scans were performed daily until follicular rupture. Blood was taken at each visit for 17β oestradiol, luteinizing hormone (LH) and follicle stimulating hormone (FSH) determination. At 4, 7 and 10 days postovulation, blood was assayed for progesterone concentration as well as oestradiol. The women who had demonstrated ovulatory cycles were asked to start medication on the first day of their next menstrual cycle. The tablets were taken daily with no break between packets.

The women were reviewed after 3 months and evaluated throughout the seventh and 12th treatment cycles. During these treatment periods they attended twice weekly and underwent ultrasound examination to assess follicular development. When a follicle greater than 15 mm was measured, the scans were performed daily until

follicular rupture or until the measurements had been static for three consecutive days. The scans were then continued twice weekly. A blood sample was taken for analysis of serum progesterone, oestradiol, FSH and LH concentrations at every visit.

INTERPRETATION. After the initial visit, 71 women were randomized, seven were found to be unsuitable due to anovulation or cyst formation during the screening cycle or a prolonged menstrual cycle. The 64 eligible women started the medication on the first day of their next menses, 33 women in the desogestrel group and 31 in the levonorgestrel group. Of these, 29 women in the desogestrel group and 28 women in the levonorgestrel group completed the 12 treatment cycles. Of the seven women who withdrew, most did so because of adverse events. In the desogestrel group, one woman withdrew because of depression, fatigue and headache, two for bleeding disturbances and one developed an intercurrent illness. In the levonorgestrel group, one woman withdrew because of premenstrual tension, one because of bleeding disturbances and one moved abroad during the trial.

All 64 women demonstrated ovulation on ultrasonography during the screening cycle. Ultrasound observations from the two assessment periods were used to rank the degree of ovarian suppression achieved by each preparation at both 7 and 12 months. Decreasing rank order was taken to be from no follicular activity to persistent follicles (15–30 mm) to cyst formation ($\geq$30 mm) to follicular rupture.

In treatment period seven, no follicular activity was seen in five women in both treatment groups, although in treatment cycle 12 this had increased to nine subjects in the levonorgestrel group. Follicular rupture was seen in 19 cycles in the levonorgestrel group compared with only three in the desogestrel group. The number of persistent follicles was greater in the desogestrel group.

A comparison of ovarian suppression was also made using serum progesterone levels during the seventh and 12th treatment cycles. Decreasing rank order was taken to be from progesterone values <10 nmol/litre to a value 10–30 nmol/litre to levels >30 nmol/litre. The difference between the desogestrel and levonorgestrel groups for a maximum progesterone level >30 nmol/litre was statistically significant ($P \leq 0.001$) for both assessment periods.

When the ultrasound findings were combined with the progesterone results, a more accurate indication of ovulation was obtained. Ovulation was defined as follicular rupture followed by a rise in the serum progesterone level to $\geq$30 nmol/litre. In the cycles studied, levonorgestrel was found to have a greater percentage of ovulatory cycles. Table 3.1 combines the results from both treatment periods for each treatment group.

Table 3.1 Follicular rupture and maximum serum progesterone concentrations (nmol/litre) per treatment group in the cycles studied

		Desogestrel		Levonorgestrel	
		n	**%**	**n**	**%**
Follicular rupture	Progesterone $\geq$ 30	1	(1.7)	16	(28)
Follicular rupture	Progesterone 10–30	1	(1.7)	2	(3.5)
Follicular rupture	Progesterone $\leq$ 10	1	(1.7)	1	(1.7)

Source: Rice *et al.* (1999).

In the women who demonstrated persistent follicles or cysts, none of the desogestrel group had raised progesterone values, whereas in the levonorgestrel group, 39% with persistent follicles and 42% with cysts had raised progesterone values, i.e. luteinized unruptured follicles. None of the persistent follicles or cysts caused any clinical symptoms and resolved spontaneously.

The maximum LH levels were significantly lower in the desogestrel group compared with the levonorgestrel group, although there was no significant difference between the FSH values in either treatment cycle. The maximum oestradiol values during both treatment periods were significantly lower in the desogestrel group than the levonorgestrel group as were the mean oestradiol levels.

Comment

This study followed follicular development for two 4-week periods at 7 and 12 months and combined these results with those for serum oestradiol, progesterone and LH/FSH measurements to provide a comprehensive insight into ovarian function during the use of two POPs. Defining ovulation as follicular rupture on scan followed by a rise in serum progesterone value, the desogestrel 75 μg/day preparation demonstrated a significantly greater effect on the inhibition of ovulation. Only one woman ovulated in the desogestrel group during the 59 cycles studied, whereas 16 of 57 (28%) levonorgestrel cycles were shown to be ovulatory. These results strongly suggest that a 75 μg/day desogestrel POP should be a more reliable contraceptive.

The decrease seen for LH in both study periods was significantly greater in the desogestrel group indicating that the suppression of the hypothalamic–pituitary axis is more profound with desogestrel than levonorgestrel. Whilst a similar number of women in both the desogestrel and levonorgestrel groups formed persistent follicles, none of those seen in women taking desogestrel showed any evidence of luteal activity compared with a 40% incidence of luteinized unruptured follicles in the levonorgestrel group.

The maximum and mean oestradiol levels were significantly lower in the desogestrel group compared with the levonorgestrel group, but hypo-oestrogenism was not observed in the study population and the oestradiol levels were above those which might lead to concern about osteoporosis risk.

The authors concluded that their results confirm earlier studies about the mechanism of contraceptive action of levonorgestrel POPs being the creation of an abnormal luteal phase and inadequate cervical mucus rather than consistent inhibition of ovulation. Desogestrel 75 μg/day produced a significant inhibition of ovulation in comparison with levonorgestrel and should therefore be expected to have a lower failure rate than the currently marketed POPs.

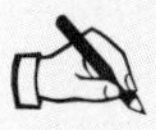

A double-blind study comparing the contraceptive efficacy, acceptability and safety of two progestogen-only pills containing desogestrel 75 μg/day or levonorgestrel 30 μg/day.

Collaborative Study Group on the Desogestrel-containing Progestogen-only Pill. *Eur J Contracept Reprod Health Care* 1998; **3**: 169–78.

BACKGROUND. Currently marketed POPs contain levonorgestrel, norethisterone, lynestrenol or ethynodiol diacetate and have a multifaceted mode of action. Inhibition of ovulation is achieved in about half of all cycles and contributes only partly to the effectiveness of the method. Compared with the combined oral contraceptive pill, traditional POPs have a slightly lower contraceptive efficacy, a higher incidence of irregular bleeding and a higher rate of ectopic pregnancy. A newly developed POP improving one or more of these drawbacks could be a valuable addition to the existing range.

Desogestrel is a selective progestogen with less androgenicity than the progestogens traditionally used in POPs. A dose high enough to inhibit ovulation is not likely to trigger androgen-related side-effects.

The objective of this study was to evaluate contraceptive efficacy, bleeding pattern, acceptability and safety of a pill containing 75 μg/day desogestrel compared with 30 μg/day levonorgestrel in healthy female subjects.

The design was a double-blind, randomized, group-comparative, multicentre trial for 13 consecutive treatment periods of 28 days. The subjects were recruited in 44 centres in Germany, the UK, the Netherlands, Norway, Finland and Sweden.

The study was designed to enrol up to 1200 healthy female volunteers (900 on desogestrel 75 μg/day and 300 on levonorgestrel 30 μg/day) who were willing to use a POP for 12 months. The sample size was chosen to achieve a follow-up of at least 500 women for 12 months in the desogestrel group. The volunteers were randomized in a double-blind manner and classified into three strata: 'breast-feeding women', 'switchers' (users of oral contraceptives within the last 2 months, not breast feeding) or 'starters' (not a switcher, not breast feeding).

The study subjects were women between 18 and 45 years in good health, who were sexually active and of child-bearing potential, with normal cycles with a mean length of between 24 and 35 days (with an individual variation of ±3 days). Body weight was between 80 and 130% of ideal and the women had to be willing to fill in the diary card with daily information about pill taking and bleeding pattern. Contraindications to the study were history of ectopic pregnancy and history or presence of pelvic inflammatory disease or functional ovarian cysts.

After general and pelvic examination, the subjects were randomly allocated to receive either 75 μg/day desogestrel or identical looking tablets containing 30 μg/day levonorgestrel. The tablets were to be taken daily during 13 consecutive treatment periods of 28 days. The subjects were instructed to take a tablet at about the same time every day. At the end of three, seven and 13 treatment periods, body weight, blood pressure and pregnancy status were assessed and the subject was questioned about adverse experiences and the use of concomitant medication. Completed diary cards were collected. The evaluation of bleeding patterns was based

on the daily diaries and the analysis was based on 90 consecutive day reference periods.

Contraceptive efficacy was based on the occurrence of pregnancy during the period of drug administration. Pregnancy rate was expressed by calculating the Pearl index. The Pearl index was also calculated excluding the exposure during breast feeding as the duration of breast feeding was known for almost all lactating women.

INTERPRETATION. The study population analysed consisted of 979 women who received 75 µg/day desogestrel and 327 women who received 30 µg/day levonorgestrel. Approximately one-third of the treated subjects in each group were breast feeding at the start of the study. Both treatment groups were comparable with respect to age, body mass index, number of pregnancies and menstrual characteristics. In total, the exposure to desogestrel 75 µg/day was 728 woman-years and to levonorgestrel 30 µg/day was 258 woman-years. There were no statistically significant differences between the groups for study discontinuations.

Seven pregnancies were reported during the study period, three in the desogestrel group and four in the levonorgestrel group. This gives a crude Pearl index of 0.41 (95% CI 0.085–1.204) for the desogestrel group and of 1.55 (95% CI 0.422–3.963) for the levonorgestrel group. When documented gross non-compliance with tablet ingestion is taken into account, one in-treatment pregnancy during the use of desogestrel 75 µg/day and three during the use of levonorgestrel 30 µg/day remain, resulting in Pearl indices of 0.14 (95% CI 0.003–0.766) and 1.17 (95% CI 0.240–3.406), respectively. Because contraceptive efficacy could have been enhanced by the high numbers of women breast feeding, Pearl indices were also calculated excluding exposure to breast feeding. Based on one pregnancy during desogestrel use (600 woman-years) and three during levonorgestrel use (213 woman-years) the Pearl indices were 0.17 (95% CI 0.004–0.928) and 1.41 (95% CI 0.290–4.116), respectively. The differences in Pearl indices between desogestrel and levonorgestrel presented were not statistically significant.

Bleeding pattern analysis was based on 90-day reference periods. The relative risk of women experiencing infrequent bleeding, frequent bleeding and prolonged bleeding near the start of the study was 1.5–2 times higher for the desogestrel users compared with the levonorgestrel users. The analysis of the incidence of amenorrhoea showed a significant treatment–stratum interaction with non-breast-feeding women using desogestrel having a relative risk of 3.44 compared with levonorgestrel users; for breast-feeding women there was no difference between the treatment groups. The proportion of women experiencing amenorrhoea or infrequent bleeding among desogestrel users increased with time, with about half the women in the desogestrel group experiencing either amenorrhoea or infrequent bleeding compared with about 10% of the levonorgestrel users during the last 90 days of the study. The proportion of women in the desogestrel group experiencing frequent bleeding decreased steeply with time and became lower than in the levonorgestrel group towards the end of the study period. The incidence of prolonged bleeding also decreased with time in both groups, but remained higher in the desogestrel group than in the levonorgestrel group. Among the desogestrel users, the trend towards less frequent bleeding could not solely be attributed to study discontinuation by women with bleeding. Breast-feeding women with both preparations had a higher incidence of amenorrhoea and lower incidence of frequent bleeding than 'switchers' or 'starters'.

The percentage of women discontinuing the study due to 'irregular bleeding' was slightly higher for desogestrel 75 μg/day (22.5%) than for levonorgestrel 30 μg/day (18%), but this was not statistically significant. The percentages of women with adverse and serious adverse experiences were comparable for desogestrel (41.8 and 1.4%, respectively) and levonorgestrel (41.3 and 1.8%, respectively). Four serious adverse events, all ovarian cysts, were considered to be possibly related to the use of desogestrel; two serious adverse events, one ovarian cyst and one ectopic pregnancy, were considered to be possibly related to the use of levonorgestrel. No major differences were seen for any of the adverse experiences reported. Specifically there was no difference between the occurrence of acne and dysmenorrhoea between users of desogestrel and levonorgestrel. The discontinuation rates due to adverse experiences were similar for the two groups: 10.5% for desogestrel users and 9.2% for levonorgestrel users.

Comment

In this double-blind, randomized, group-comparative multicentre study it appears that the contraceptive efficacy of desogestrel 75 μg/day is better than that of levo-norgestrel 30 μg/day. The Pearl index for desogestrel 75 μg/day excluding gross non-compliance and including breast feeding, was 0.14, which is within the range quoted for low-dose combined oral contraceptives, whilst in this directly comparative study, the Pearl index for levonorgestrel 30 μg/day was well above this range. This can be explained by the more pronounced suppression of the hypothalamic–pituitary–ovarian axis and consistent inhibition of ovulation seen with desogestrel 75 μg/day. No ectopic pregnancies were reported among desogestrel users, but because of the low overall pregnancy rate and consequent very low incidence of ectopic pregnancies, more extensive data are needed before definitive conclusions can be drawn.

The higher progestogen dose in desogestrel 75 μg/day did not lead to a remarkable change in the pattern or incidence of adverse events compared with levonorgestrel 30 μg/day and specifically not with a typical androgen-related experience like acne.

In spite of the relatively high proportions of desogestrel 75 μg/day users experiencing amenorrhoea, infrequent bleeding, frequent or prolonged bleeding compared with users of levonorgestrel 30 μg/day, the percentage of women discontinuing treatment because of irregular bleeding seems to be comparable. In this study there was a shift in time towards less bleeding among the desogestrel users which was not seen with the levonorgestrel users. This information can be used to counsel women about improvements in bleeding pattern with time, which may increase the acceptance of the bleeding pattern. Traditional 'targets' for POPs are breast-feeding women and women approaching the menopause, groups who do not usually expect to have regular cycles and who may be inclined to accept a more variable bleeding pattern in exchange for improved contraceptive efficacy.

The results of this comparative study show desogestrel 75 μg/day to have a higher contraceptive efficacy than traditional POPs, supporting the consistent inhibition of ovulation. The incidence and pattern of adverse events were similar for 75 μg/day desogestrel and 30 μg/day levonorgestrel, as was the discontinuation rate for adverse events. The bleeding pattern for desogestrel 75 μg/day was more variable than that seen with levonorgestrel 30 μg/day, but tended to settle with time. In choosing a POP, the advantage of increased contraceptive efficacy for desogestrel 75 μg/day will need to be balanced against its more variable bleeding pattern.

In June 2000, data were presented at the European Society of Contraception in Ljubljana, that the use of a 75 μg/day desogestrel pill by lactating women in Iceland had no adverse effect on milk quantity and quality. In a study comparing 42 desogestrel POP users with 41 copper intrauterine device users, breast milk quantity was assessed by weighing infants before and after each 24-hour feeding period at baseline and at the end of the first and fourth 28-day study cycles. Breast milk quality was evaluated by analysing levels of triglyceride, protein and lactose. Infant growth was monitored over 2.5 years. The quantities of breast milk produced were not statistically significantly different at either assessment and there were no differences in milk quality between the groups or between baseline and the assessments. The growth of the infants was similar in both groups when evaluated after 1.5 and 2.5 years. No clinically relevant differences were observed between the infants in the two treatment groups.

In 1999, 75 μg/day desogestrel was marketed in Germany as Cerazette™ (Organon). Within 12 months it had already taken 90% of the market for POPs. It is hoped that Cerazette™ will become available in the UK during 2001 or early 2002.

Injectables

Depot medroxyprogesterone acetate (DMPA) has been widely used throughout the world for more than 30 years as a highly effective long-term reversible method of contraception. It acts by inhibiting ovulation and by rendering the endometrium atrophic. Since the early 1990s, when a case–control study suggested an association between DMPA use and lowered bone density, questions have remained about the long-term use of DMPA.

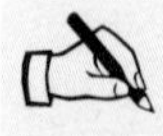

Bone density in long term users of depot medroxyprogesterone acetate.

B Gbolade, S Ellis, B Murby, S Randall, R Kirkman. *Br J Obstet Gynaecol* 1998; **105**: 790–4.

B ACKGROUND . Amenorrhoea is seen in 45% of women after 10–12 months of DMPA use and this proportion is maintained with prolonged use. In 1991, Cundy *et al.* |1| found that bone density among long-term users of DMPA was intermediate between those of normal premenopausal and postmenopausal controls, although no correlation

was found between bone density and duration of DMPA use. Cundy's study caused concern among family planning doctors as DMPA is often used in women who lead irregular lifestyles and who may not be in the best of health. This study was designed to address this concern. The authors performed a cross-sectional study of DMPA users amenorrhoeic for more than 12 months or those who had used the method for more than 5 years to identify women thought to be most at risk of decreased bone density.

All women attending two large family planning centres in Manchester and Portsmouth, UK, for repeat DMPA injections fulfilling the above criteria had blood taken for serum oestradiol determination and were offered an appointment for the bone density of their femoral neck and lumbar spine to be measured. At the densitometry visit, height and weight were measured, ethnic group noted and details of smoking habits and concomitant medication were obtained. The duration of DMPA use, medical details and menstrual history were obtained from case records. Bone density of the left femoral neck and lumbar spine was measured using dual-energy X-ray absorptiometry (DEXA) scanners. The two scanners were cross-calibrated and found to give identical measurements.

INTERPRETATION. Eighty-two of the 96 women offered bone density appointments in Manchester and 103 of the 107 women offered appointments in Portsmouth attended for bone densitometry. Ethnic group was predominantly Caucasian, but the study group included three Afro-Caribbean and five Asian women. The study group contained 95 smokers and 88 non-smokers (the smoking habits of two women were not documented). The duration of DMPA use ranged from 1 to 16 years with a median of 5 years. There was no statistically significant difference between the measurements made at the two centres in any decade and therefore all the results are for the combined group.

For each woman the bone mineral densities (BMD) measured at the lumbar spine and left femoral neck were compared with age-matched normal values. The difference between each measured value and the mean of the normal population was then calculated as a Z score; 95% of the normal population have Z scores between -2 and $+2$ and an individual with the same BMD as the normal mean has a Z score of 0. The use of Z scores removes the age dependence of the normal range from the data and allows women of different ages to be combined into a single, large study group, with the women grouped by decade (see Table 3.2).

There was a small (3.32%) but statistically significant difference ($P < 0.001$) in lumbar spine BMD between the study group and age-matched controls. There was no statistically significant difference between femoral neck values. Correlation analysis was performed to assess whether prolonged DMPA use caused progressive loss of BMD in the lumbar spine. There was a very weak negative correlation, but without statistical significance. There was also no clear relationship between serum oestradiol levels and duration of DMPA use.

As a serum oestradiol level of 150 pmol/litre has been found to maintain bone density adequately in hormone replacement therapy, the data were subdivided into less than and more than 150 pmol/litre for comparison of Z scores for the lumbar spine. A total of 149 women had serum oestradiol levels <150 pmol/litre and 32 women had levels >150 pmol/litre. The data showed no statistically significant difference between the Z scores for the two groups in the lumbar spine or the femoral neck. The small decrease in lumbar spine BMD resulting from DMPA use occurred equally in both groups of women and appeared independent of the serum oestradiol level. Correlation analysis

Table 3.2 Deviation of measured bone mineral density (BMD) in the depot medroxyprogesterone acetate (DMPA) study group from age-matched controls. Values are given as mean (95% confidence intervals)

	Age range (years)				Total
	20–29	30–39	40–49	50–59	20–59 years
No. of women	63	73	41	4	181
Lumbar spine					
BMD (g/cm^2)	1.138 (0.850 to 1.426)	1.173 (0.907 to 1.439)	1.144 (0.827 to 1.462)	1.318 (1.047 to 1.589)	–
Z score	–0.516 (–0.812 to –0.219)	–0.226 (–0.480 to 0.029)	–0.417 (–0.825 to –0.009)	1.488 (0.300 to 2.676)	
P (compared with normal)	<0.01	0.08	0.05	–	<0.001
Femoral neck					
BMD (g/cm^2)	0.959 (0.708 to 1.210)	0.958 (0.749 to 1.166)	0.962 (0.683 to 1.241)	1.034 (0.804 to 1.264)	–
Z score	–0.257 (–0.512 to 0.001)	–0.109 (–0.307 to 0.089)	0.096 (–0.266 to 0.458)	1.065 (0.088 to 2.042)	–0.088 (–0.237 to 0.060)
P (compared with normal)	0.12	0.31	0.61	–	0.25

Source: Gbolade *et al.* (1998).

confirmed that there was no significant relationship between BMD and serum oestradiol level.

Comment

These data were not collected as part of a formal research study; bone density was measured because of clinical concern about osteoporosis and DMPA use. By selecting very long-term users of DMPA and amenorrhoeic women, the authors hoped to identify the women most likely to exhibit an adverse effect. Using these criteria, most women had low levels of oestradiol, but the results indicate that there is no clinically important adverse effect on bone density of the lumbar spine or femoral neck from long-term use of DMPA.

The findings of this study contradict Cundy *et al.* |**1**|, but this study was larger and involved consecutive women, thus reducing the probability of selection bias. Cundy *et al.*'s finding of no correlation between bone density and duration of DMPA use is confirmed. The findings of this study are supported by a small Swedish study which found no significant change during the first 6 months of DMPA use |**2**| and two Thai studies which compared bone density among intrauterine device, Norplant® and DMPA users.

Within any population there is a broad distribution of bone densities. Therefore, densitometry will identify some women who are osteopenic whether or not they are using DMPA. This study indicates that inducing amenorrhoea by using DMPA does not put women at any significant risk of further bone loss and there is strong evidence to support bone density being maintained in a steady state when DMPA is used for longer than 12 months. The authors comment that they can see no indication for bone-conserving measures among DMPA users, such as adding back oestrogen.

Because cardiovascular events have a low incidence in women of child-bearing age and relatively few women use injectable and progestogen-only contraception (12–13 million users out of a total of 100 million hormonal contraception users), previous studies have not been large enough to evaluate the risks of cardiovascular disease associated with the use of these products.

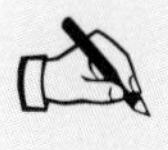

Cardiovascular disease and use of oral and injectable progestogen-only contraceptives and combined injectable contraceptives. Results of an international, multicentre, case–control study.

World Health Organization Collaborative Study of Cardiovascular Disease and Steroid Hormone Contraception. *Contraception* 1998; **57**: 315–24.

BACKGROUND. The World Health Organization (WHO) Collaborative Study of Cardiovascular Disease and Steroid Hormone Contraception was designed to evaluate

whether currently used steroid hormone contraceptives continued to be associated with increased risk of cardiovascular disease despite changes in the dose and composition of preparations and the cardiovascular risk profile of users. The results of the VTE, stroke and acute myocardial infarction (AMI) components of the study in relation to combined oral contraceptive use have been reported previously.

The study was a multicentre, hospital-based case–control study performed in 21 centres in 17 countries in Africa, Asia, Europe and Latin America. Eligible cases were women aged 20–44 years who had been admitted with, in the opinion of the responsible physician, a venous thrombotic episode, a stroke or an AMI. Women were excluded if they had suffered a transient ischaemic attack, had died within 24 h of admission, had a history of VTE, stroke, AMI, or natural or surgical menopause; or had a history during the previous 6 weeks of pregnancy, a major illness that resulted in bed rest for more than 1 week or surgery. VTE cases were classified as definite, probable, possible or other, stroke cases as one of seven subgroups of stroke and AMI cases as definite, possible or other. Cases classified as other were excluded from all analyses. For each case, up to three female control subjects matched by a 5-year age band were recruited. All cases and controls were interviewed in hospital in a standard manner using the same questionnaire.

INTERPRETATION. A total of 3697 cases were included in the analyses. Of these, 2196 women (59%) had suffered a stroke, 1137 (31%) had experienced VTE and 364 (10%) had had an AMI. Among stroke cases, 29, 25 and nine women were current users of oral and injectable progestogen-only and combined injectable contraceptives, respectively. For VTE, the numbers were 21, 11 and three, respectively, and for AMI were three, one and one. A total of 9997 control subjects were matched to 3697 cases, with an average of 2.8, 2.6 and 2.6 control subjects per case with stroke, VTE and AMI, respectively.

Overall the cases and control subjects had similar mean ages and body mass indices, but cases were, not surprisingly, more likely to have a history of other cardiovascular risk factors, e.g. hypertension and diabetes, and were more likely to be smokers.

Crude and adjusted odds ratios associated with the current use of oral progestogens or progestogen-only or combined injectables compared with non-users were not significantly increased or decreased for stroke, VTE, AMI or a combination of all three disorders. No differences were observed between odds ratios associated with current use of any type of steroid hormone contraceptives in Europe and the developing countries.

Table 3.3 shows odds ratios stratified by reported history of hypertension for all cardiovascular diseases combined, stroke, VTE and AMI. Among users of any type of steroid hormone contraception, a self-reported history of high blood pressure, excluding hypertension in pregnancy, was associated with a significant increase in odds ratio for stroke and AMI, but not VTE. Odds ratios for stroke among women with a history of high blood pressure, compared with non-users of steroid hormone contraceptives with no history of hypertension, rose from 7.21 (6.10–8.52) among non-users to 12.4 (4.09–37.6) among users of all oral progestogens. No such trend was apparent for VTE or AMI. In addition, among women exposed to progestogen-only injectables there were five stroke patients giving a combined risk estimate of 15.7 (5.45–45.0) for all progestogen-only contraceptive methods. This was 2.2 (0.75–6.22) times the risk for non-users with a history of hypertension. The excess risk of stroke appeared to be due

Table 3.3 Adjusted odds ratios [95% confidence intervals (CI)] for all cardiovascular diseases combined: stroke, venous thromboembolism (VTE) or acute myocardial infarction (AMI) in relation to current use of progestogen-only and injectable steroid hormone contraceptives

	No history of hypertension				History of hypertension			
	Cases	Controls	Odds ratio	(95% CI)	Cases	Controls	Odds ratio	(95% CI)
Cardiovascular diseases combined (stroke, VTE and AMI)								
Non-users	1939	7721	1.00	(Reference)	718	540	5.87	(5.12–6.73)
Oral progestogens (all)	36	130	1.11	(0.74–1.65)	17	11	7.58	(3.19–18.0)
Continuous POP only	35	118	1.20	(0.79–1.81)	16	11	6.78	(2.82–16.3)
Progestogen-only injectable	30	120	1.01	(0.67–1.55)	5	2	7.16	(1.32–38.7)
All stroke								
Non-users	1193	4811	1.00	(Reference)	571	368	7.21	(6.10–8.52)
Oral progestogens (all)	15	63	0.85	(0.46–1.58)	14	7	12.4	(4.09–37.6)
Continuous POP only	14	53	0.95	(0.49–1.82)	13	7	10.9	(3.55–33.8)
Progestogen-only injectable	18	81	0.80	(0.46–1.39)	5	0	–	–
VTE								
Non-users	439	1667	1.00	(Reference)	41	91	1.52	(0.98–2.36)
Oral progestogens (all)	9	22	1.88	(0.80–4.45)	1	2	1.18	(0.06–23.7)
Continuous POP only	9	21	1.99	(0.83–4.74)	1	2	1.18	(0.06–23.7)
Progestogen-only injectable	6	15	2.92	(0.84–10.2)	0	1	–	–
AMI								
Non-users	175	742	1.00	(Reference)	84	53	8.05	(4.89–13.3)
Oral progestogens (all)	2	6	1.40	(0.21–9.34)	1	1	2.04	(0.10–41.3)
Continuous POP only	2	5	1.72	(0.24–12.5)	1	1	1.90	(0.09–38.4)
Progestogen-only injectable	1	7	0.67	(0.07–6.11)	0	0	–	–

POP = progestogen-only pills.
Source: WHO (1998).

primarily to an increase in haemorrhagic stroke. Smoking among non-users of steroid hormone contraceptives was associated with a small but significant increase in odds ratios for stroke and AMI, but not for VTE. The use of oral progestogens was associated with a small increase in odds ratios among smokers for all three diseases. However, injectables had small and inconsistent effects on the odds ratios for all three diseases.

Comment

This is the only study to date to have reported risks of cardiovascular disease among users of oral and injectable progestogen-only preparations. It demonstrates no significant increase in overall risk estimates for stroke, VTE, AMI or these three disorders combined with the use of any of these products.

A small, non-significant increase in odds ratio for VTE (1.74) was seen in association with the use of all oral progestogens, which is compatible with data on the progestogen type in combined pills and VTE risk. Odds ratios for stroke in women without a history of high blood pressure were not increased in users of all types of progestogen-only contraceptives. This is compatible with data from observational studies suggesting that POPs do not increase blood pressure. However, among hypertensive women the odds ratio for stroke compared with non-users of steroid contraceptive hormones with no history of hypertension rose from 7.21 (6.10–8.52) for non-users of steroid hormones to 12.4 (4.09–37.6) among users of all oral progestogens. In addition there were five cases of stroke among women with a history of hypertension using progestogen-only injectables with no control subjects who used these products. In view of the small number of cases and controls, the apparent interaction between use of progestogen-only contraceptives and a history of high blood pressure observed in this study should be interpreted with caution and requires further investigation. This is of particular importance as women with a history of hypertension are often given POPs in preference to combined pills.

The WHO Collaborative Study clearly has its limitations, but a more accurate classification of cases was achieved than in many studies and extreme care was taken to ensure the accuracy of the information obtained about the types and effects of steroid hormone contraceptives. The possibility of biased recall of steroid hormone contraceptive exposure due to the severity of the cases' diagnoses was not evaluated in this study. It is probably reasonable to assume that the cases recruited into the study were typical of the majority of women of reproductive age who experience stroke, VTE or AMI.

The major limitation of these data is the potential for false-negative findings as evidenced by the wide confidence intervals resulting from the small number of cases and controls using the products under investigation. However, the data suggest that there is little or no increased risk of stroke, VTE or AMI associated with the use of progestogen-only contraceptives. Further investigation into the use of progestogen-only products by women with a history of high blood pressure is indicated.

Implants

Subdermal implants provide long-acting, highly effective and reversible contraception by producing low and stable concentrations of synthetic progestogens. Because they require little compliance, user failure rates are very similar to method failure rates. Norplant® was licensed in the UK in 1993 and was the only subdermal contraceptive implant system in general use for 6 years. It is estimated that 55 000 women in the UK and approximately 6 million women world-wide have used Norplant®. The initial clinical experience with Norplant® was promising, but negative reports started to appear in both the medical and lay press, mostly related to problems with removal and unrealistic expectations of the method. The distributor discontinued marketing Norplant® in November 1999 for economic reasons soon after the launch of Implanon®.

A critical review of the efficacy and safety of Norplant® detailing 20 years of experience with the first licensed implant system can be found in the 1998 Norplant® consensus statement and background review (see Further reading).

Capsule implant contraceptives were developed in the 1970s and marketed formulations have comparable effectiveness to sterilization for up to 7 years, but with the advantage of reversibility.

During the 1980s the Population Council conducted trials using a prototype rod system (then known as Norplant®-2). Two 4 cm rod implants provided similar release rates and blood levels of levonorgestrel as six 3 cm capsule Norplant® implants for 3 years. Three-year pregnancy rates for women using the rods were equal or below those for women randomized to receive Norplant® |3|. After 3 years of use the annual pregnancy rate rose in heavier women, although not in Asian women, where contraceptive effectiveness was maintained for 5 years.

Norplant®-2 was not distributed widely because an elastomer used in its manufacture proved unavailable in commercial quantities. In the late 1980s new rod implants made with a substitute material were shown to have similar in vitro release rates of levonorgestrel as the prototype rods and Norplant®. Clinical trials using the reformulated rod implants were started in 1990. Evidence from blood level and in vitro release rate studies suggested that the new rod implants could deliver 25–30 µg levonorgestrel/day for 5 years—enough to protect women within the range of body weights found in developed countries from pregnancy.

The levonorgestrel rod (Jadelle®) consists of two individual implants each 4.3 cm in length and 2.5 mm in diameter. Encased within a thin wall of silicone rubber tubing is a drug-releasing core called a rod. The ends of each implant are sealed with medical-grade adhesive. Each rod is a cured mixture containing 75 mg of levonorgestrel and an equal weight of silicone elastomer. Each two-rod set thus contains 150 mg of levonorgestrel.

Rods differ from capsules. In rods, levonorgestrel is dispersed within a matrix of cured elastomer and then covered by tubing, whereas in capsules the drug is not dispersed, but lies contiguously within a thicker tubing.

In the first month the average daily release of levonorgestrel from a set of two-rod implants is approximately 80 µg, this declines to approximately 50 µg at 9 months and more gradually to 25–30 µg/day thereafter.

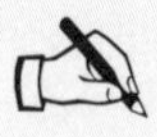

Contraception with two levonorgestrel rod implants. A five year study in the United States and Dominican Republic.

I Sivin, F Alvarez, DR Mishell, *et al. Contraception* 1998; **58**: 275–82.

BACKGROUND. Clinical trials of the levonorgestrel rod initiated in 1990 reached the end of the third year with exceptionally low pregnancy rates (cumulative rate below 1 per 100 women) and the subjects were asked for and gave informed consent to a study extension to 5 years. This paper reports the 5-year performance of the new levonorgestrel rod implants among 594 women attending four clinics in the USA and the Dominican Republic.

The enrolled subjects were aged 18–40 years, in good health, sexually active and with no known contraindications to levonorgestrel implants. Women were excluded if they had a history or current evidence of any kind of cancer, undiagnosed, abnormal vaginal bleeding, hyperprolactinaemia or bloody breast discharge, hyperlipidaemia, severe cardiovascular problems, mental illness, diabetes mellitus, epilepsy, severe or frequent headaches, pelvic inflammatory disease since the last pregnancy or ectopic pregnancy. These last two exclusions were designed to ensure that the participants had unimpaired fertility.

The implants were placed within 7 days of the onset of menses. At all scheduled visits a general physical examination was performed, together with an inspection of the implant site and a determination of pregnancy status. Scheduled visits were at 1, 3 and 6 months after insertion and 6-monthly thereafter. Pelvic examinations and cervical smears were performed annually. The subjects also visited clinics 2–3 months after implant removal to ensure that method failures occurring immediately before removal would be documented, as would any side-effects related to removal.

Each clinic enrolled between 145 and 150 women. The study participants were young and with few children; 49% were under 25 years at enrolment. The women in the Dominican Republic clinic were both younger and of higher parity than the US subjects. Mean body weight was markedly higher among women recruited at the US centres than in the Dominican Republic.

INTERPRETATION. Two women judged not pregnant at implant insertion proved to be pregnant at their first postadmission visit, but with estimated dates of conception before placement. These women were considered not to have entered the study and their data were not used. The effective study size became 592 women. A third women, who was found to be pregnant shortly after admission to the study, had apparently given incorrect dates for her last pre-insertion menses, with the result that the rods were inserted late in the follicular phase. This pregnancy was considered a first-month method failure. Two other method failures occurred during the 5-year course of the study, at 18 and 36 months of use. There were no pregnancies during the fourth and fifth years. The cumulative 5-year life-table pregnancy rate was 0.8 ± 0.5 per 100. Women pregnant in months 1, 18 and 36 weighed 63, 80 and 65 kg, respectively, and were aged 32, 23 and 28 years at admission. One woman delivered a healthy child at term, one had a miscarriage and one pregnancy was terminated.

Table 3.4 shows the gross cumulative rates of discontinuation per 100 continuing users of levonorgestrel rod implants by reason for discontinuation.

Progestogen-induced changes in menstrual pattern led 17.7% of participants to have their implants removed during the 5-year study period. Year to year variation in the discontinuation rate for removals for bleeding problems was not statistically significant, although removal because of bleeding problems in the fifth year was uncommon. There were significant differences between removal rates for bleeding problems between the US centres and the Dominican Republic clinic and between the US centres. Forty-seven per cent of all menstrual problem discontinuations were attributed to prolonged bleeding/spotting, 31% to frequent, irregular bleeding or spotting and a further 10% to amenorrhoea. Despite frequent reports of prolonged bleeding, mean haemoglobin levels increased by 1–2 g /litre in each of the first 3 years.

Medical problems other than menstrual cycle changes were the most frequent reasons for removal, with a 5-year gross cumulative removal rate of 30.5 ± 2.5 per 100 women. Headache and weight change were the most frequent reasons for medical removal and were cited by more than 4% of women enrolled, with little variation in rate year on year. None of the headaches was classified as migraine.

Among all study participants the mean weight change in the first year was a gain of 1.5 kg. Ten per cent of women experienced a first-year weight loss of ≥3.7 kg and 10% a weight gain of ≥7.8 kg. The annual average weight change for the 5-year period was a gain of 1.1 kg.

Mood changes and depression accounted for 1–2% of discontinuations, with half the removals for depression and 64% of those for mood change taking place in the first 12 months. Pain or numbness at the implant site was the primary complaint resulting in removal for 1.2% of the women. Excessive hair loss (or other hair problems) and acne were each named as the primary reason for removal by about 1% of the women.

Annual continuation rates were >80 per 100 women per year in the first two study years. Thereafter, when there were more removals for personal reasons, annual continuation rates ranged between 73.8 and 74.9 per 100 per year. The median duration of implant contraception was 2.96 years.

In three clinic sites <5% of women ever had observable reactions at the implant site, e.g. allergic reactions, haematoma, infection, expulsion of an implant, increased pigmentation, pain or tenderness and numbness or tingling. These events were transient; 90% of such reports were not repeated at the next visit. At the fourth site a large number of women had allergic reactions which were traced to a specific bandage type used immediately after implant insertion.

The presence or absence of removal complications was reported in 391 women and removal time recorded in 387 cases. Of the 391 characterized removals, 7% were noted to have some complication; 5.1% of events represented provider problems, such as broken implants or tough pericapsular tissue, 2.3% of cases were judged to have affected the subjects. These included two cases which required two incisions, three removals with incisions of 8, 9 and 30 mm (instead of 2–4 mm) and two cases of presumed tissue trauma in which problems of deep placement or poor alignment were noted.

Removal time averaged 5.9 ± 0.6 min. Duration of implant use did not affect removal times. The mean time for removals without complication was 5.1 min, whereas that of

Table 3.4 Gross cumulative rates of discontinuation per 100 continuing users of levonorgestrel rod implants by reason for discontinuation

Reason	Year 1		Year 2		Year 3		Year 4		Year 5	
	Rate	SE	Rate	SE	Rate	SE	Rate	SE	Rate	SE
Pregnancy	0.2	0.2	0.4	0.3	0.8	0.5	0.8	0.5	0.8	0.5
Menstrual problem	7.1	1.1	12.9	1.5	18.5	1.8	23.0	2.1	24.3	2.2
Medical problem	6.8	1.1	13.2	1.5	18.8	1.8	25.6	2.1	30.5	2.5
Used other contraception	0.4	0.3	1.2	0.5	1.8	0.7	3.9	1.1	7.6	1.8
Planning pregnancy	1.1	0.5	4.0	0.9	12.2	1.7	18.4	2.1	25.9	2.6
Other personal	2.8	0.7	7.4	1.2	12.4	1.6	17.8	2.0	23.4	2.5
Continuation	82.7	1.6	66.2	2.0	49.5	2.1	36.6	2.0	27.4	1.9
Percentage lost to follow-up	2.2		3.0		3.4		3.7		4.2	
No. starting year	594		478		378		281		205	
No. completing year	478		378		281		205		145	
Cumulative women-years	532		957		1290		1526		1700	

SE = standard error.
Source: Sivin *et al.* (1998).

complicated removals was 15.7 min. A total of 93% of removals was accomplished in <15 min.

Comment

Both the first-year pregnancy rate of 0.2 per 100 and the 5-year cumulative pregnancy rate of 0.8 per 100 are exceptionally low, whether compared with other reversible methods of contraception or with sterilization procedures. This level of effectiveness, and particularly the absence of pregnancies during years 4 and 5, was unexpected by the authors given the slowly declining release rates of levonorgestrel and the young age of the study participants (mean 25.5 years at entry) who are unlikely to have had any age-related decline in fertility.

More than one-quarter of the study participants weighed ≥70 kg and only one pregnancy occurred in this group. Levonorgestrel rod implants effectively protect women for 5 years regardless of weight.

Five-year pregnancy rates in this study are similar to those found in a large randomized 5-year study of levonorgestrel rod and capsule implants (see below). Jointly, these studies indicate that a two-rod levonorgestrel implant is as effective as the six-capsule implant for a 5-year period.

Reducing the number of implants has advantages in terms of removal, with lower rates of complications and speedy removals. Only 2.3% of removals were complicated, of which five were either second incisions or long incisions, but in only one case was the incision >1 cm.

Continuation rates averaged 77 per 100 per year. The continuation rate of 50 per 100 at 3 years is comparable with the 2-year continuation rate for the Copper T 380A in the two largest US studies of this intrauterine device, indicating that the overall acceptance of the two-rod levonorgestrel implant by users is similar to that of the intrauterine device.

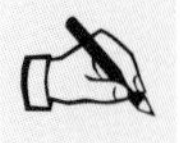

The performance of levonorgestrel rod and Norplant® contraceptive implants: a 5 year randomised study.

I Sivin, I Campodonico, O Kiriwat, *et al. Hum Reprod* 1998; **13**(12): 3371–8.

BACKGROUND. This study was designed to evaluate prospectively the new two-rod contraceptive implant Jadelle® in a randomized 5-year comparison with Norplant® capsule implants. The study involved 1198 women at seven centres in the USA, Chile, Bangkok, Finland, Singapore and Egypt.

The subjects were sexually active women aged 18–40 years with no contraindications to Norplant® use and willing to accept random assignment. The women agreed to clinic visits at 1, 3 and 6 months after insertion and 6-monthly thereafter. Women were excluded if they had a history or current evidence of any kind of cancer, undiagnosed, abnormal vaginal bleeding, hyperprolactinaemia or bloody

breast discharge, hyperlipidaemia, severe cardiovascular problems, mental illness, diabetes mellitus, epilepsy, severe or frequent headaches, pelvic inflammatory disease since the last pregnancy or ectopic pregnancy. These last two exclusions were designed to ensure that the participants had unimpaired fertility.

The volunteers initially signed a consent document for a 3-year study, but when cumulative pregnancy rates for each system were less than 1 per 100, the participants continuing at 36 months were invited to continue up to 5 years. At all scheduled visits a general physical examination was performed, together with an inspection of the implant site and a determination of pregnancy status. Pelvic examinations and cervical smears were performed annually. The subjects also visited the clinics 2–3 months after implant removal to ensure that method failures occurring immediately before removal would be documented, as would any side-effects related to removal.

A total of 600 women were scheduled for randomization to each implant regimen, but two sets of Norplant® became contaminated, limiting enrolment to 598 women. Women randomly assigned to the two implant systems did not differ in their distributions by age, parity, weight or desire for additional children.

INTERPRETATION. For 4 years after implant insertion no accidental pregnancies occurred. In the fifth year three women in the levonorgestrel rod group conceived, as did two Norplant® users. The corresponding fifth-year pregnancy rates were 1.0 and 0.7 per 100 continuing users of the levonorgestrel rod and Norplant®, respectively. Because of the previous lack of pregnancies, these figures are also the cumulative 5-year pregnancy rates. Pregnancy rates for the 5-year period were 0.13 and 0.09 per 100 woman-years of use for levonorgestrel rod and Norplant® users, respectively. Contraceptive failures occurred in levonorgestrel rod users weighing 48, 62 and 64 kg, indicating no significant effect of weight.

For women under 30 years at admission the pregnancy rate was 0.15 per 100 woman-years for the levonorgestrel rod and 0.16 for Norplant®. For women over 30 years the pregnancy rates were 0.11 and 0, respectively. One pregnancy in the levonorgestrel rod group was ectopic, giving an ectopic rate of 0.4 per 1000 users.

Most women reported menstrual disturbances during the study and these were the most frequent reasons for discontinuing use of the levonorgestrel rod. Five per cent of women had their rods removed for prolonged bleeding/spotting, 4% of women for irregular bleeding and 3% for perceived heavy bleeding. These removal rates were similar for Norplant®; an additional 1.8% of Norplant® users had their systems removed for amenorrhoea. There was no significant difference between the 5-year cumulative removal rates for menstrual disturbance of 16.4 per 100 for levonorgestrel rod users and 19.2 per 100 for Norplant® users.

Cumulative 5-year discontinuation rates for medical reasons were 15.0 and 12.0 per 100 for levonorgestrel rods and Norplant®, respectively (not a statistically significant difference). Headache, weight gain and acne represented >50% of removals for each implant type. Weight gain among continuing users averaged 0.7 kg per year for levonorgestrel rod users and 0.8 kg per year for Norplant® users. Whilst some women lost weight from baseline, many experienced more substantial weight gain, with 10% of women gaining 9–10 kg from admission to 5 years.

More than half the women using both levonorgestrel rods and Norplant® were still using their implants at 5 years; cumulative discontinuation rates were 55.1 and 53.0, respectively, among levonorgestrel rod users and Norplant® users. The mean duration of use was 3.74 years for levonorgestrel rod users and 3.70 years for Norplant® users.

At the cut-off date, removal times had been recorded for more than 260 women using each regimen. From incision to closure, the mean removal time for the levonorgestrel rod was 4.8 min, half of the 9.6 min mean for removing Norplant® ($P < 0.0001$). Two per cent of levonorgestrel rod removals took more than 15 min compared with 14% of Norplant® removals; 6.5% of Norplant® removals took longer than 20 min. Of the 524 removals, 9.9% were considered to have had complications; 6.9% of levonorgestrel rod removals and 14.8% of Norplant® removals ($P = 0.009$).

Comment

This study demonstrates that, as a result of implant redesign, fewer long-term removal complications occur with the levonorgestrel rod than with Norplant®. It also shows the levonorgestrel rod to have a pregnancy rate indistinguishable from that achieved with Norplant® at less than 1 per 100 continuing users. The single ectopic pregnancy produces a rate of 0.4 per 100 years of exposure and represents an 80–90% reduction in the risk of ectopic pregnancy compared with non-users of contraception.

The very high continuation rates achieved in this study undoubtedly reflect the good counselling received prior to insertion and at scheduled and unscheduled study visits. Most women experienced menstrual disturbances and without counselling the termination rates for menstrual problems would surely have been higher.

The reformulated levonorgestrel rods clearly provide removal advantages over Norplant®, with most removals taking under 5 min, only 2% taking more than 15 min and none more than 20 min. This represents a significant improvement over Norplant®. Ease of removal with identical efficacy and duration of action make levonorgestrel rod implants preferable to Norplant®.

Implanon® is a single-rod implant 4 cm long and with a diameter of 2 mm containing 68 mg of etonogestrel (ENG; 3-ketodesogestrel, the biologically active metabolite of desogestrel), in a core that is covered by an ethylene vinyl acetate membrane. A sterile, disposable applicator preloaded with an Implanon® is supplied for insertion (see Fig. 3.1). Implanon® is non-biodegradable and has a duration of action of 3 years.

Both POPs and progestogen-only implants inhibit FSH activity only partially, which allows follicular development and the secretion of endogenous oestrogen. The advantage is that exogenous oestrogens are not needed, but the disadvantage of an irregular, unpredictable vaginal bleeding pattern due to fluctuating oestradiol secretion and anovulation (resulting from inhibition of the LH surge by interference with the positive oestrogen feedback). The bleeding is primarily light and anaemia due to blood loss is very rare. Implanon®, unlike Norplant®, was spe-

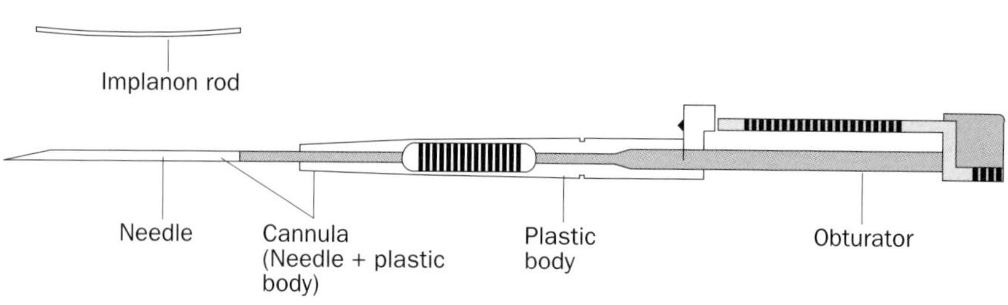

Fig. 3.1 Implanon and applicator. Source: Mascarenhas (1998).

cifically developed to inhibit ovulation during the entire treatment period. Because luteinizations/ovulations have been seen during months 30–36 of use, its duration of action has been restricted to 3 years.

Implanon® underwent pharmaceutical development between 1983 and 1988 and clinical development between 1988 and 1996. Registration was obtained in Indonesia in April 1997 and in all 15 member states of the European Union in December 1998.

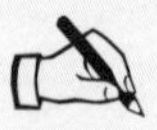

A multicentre efficacy and safety study of the single contraceptive implant Implanon®.

HB Croxatto, J Urbancsek, R Massai, H Coelingh Bennink, A van Beek and the Implanon® Study Group. *Hum Reprod* 1999; **14**(4): 976–81.

BACKGROUND. **The study was designed to determine the contraceptive reliability of Implanon® by means of pregnancy rate, its safety by means of regular medical examinations and assessment of adverse experiences and its acceptability by evaluation of vaginal bleeding patterns.**

Data were collected from 21 centres in nine European and South American countries. The study included sexually active women aged 18–40 years of child-bearing potential and requesting contraception. For inclusion, women needed menstrual cycles with a length of 24–35 days; pregnancy and breast feeding were exclusion criteria, as was weight outside 80–130% of ideal. Liver enzyme-inducing drugs were not allowed during the study. The implant was inserted in the inner aspect of the non-dominant upper arm between days 1 and 5 of a spontaneous menstrual period. The study started in November 1991 and was completed in December 1996. The study was originally designed to last for 2 years, but was extended to 3 years in two centres based on in vitro, ex vivo and non-human data and

human data from the use of an extracted implant tested in sterilized women. At baseline, medical and gynaecological histories were taken and physical and gynaecological examinations performed, including cervical cytology, blood pressure and weight and height measurements. Medical examinations were repeated annually or at the time of implant removal. Weight and blood pressure were recorded at 3, 6, 12, 18, 24, 27, 30, 33 and 36 months. Bleeding cards were checked every 3 months to check whether a pregnancy test was indicated in cases of amenorrhoea.

Analysis of the bleeding pattern was performed using standard 90-day reference periods.

INTERPRETATION. Implanon® was inserted in 635 women. The implant was inserted in four women who were later found to be pregnant at the time, nidation bleeding having been mistaken for menses. Other protocol violators were women aged >40 years, >130% above ideal body weight or having irregular menstrual cycles. Once entered into the study, a woman's data were included in the results. The centres varied in the number of women recruited from six to 114 volunteers; the centres in Budapest and Santiago contributed substantially more volunteers than the other centres. The safety and bleeding data from these two sites were compared with those from the remaining centres and no major differences were observed for bleeding data, although there were differences in the reporting of safety data.

The total exposure to Implanon® was 1200 woman-years (15 653 28-day cycles). No pregnancies occurred during treatment, resulting in a Pearl index of 0 (95% CI 0.0–0.2).

Of the 635 women, 436 completed 2 years of treatment. One hundred and sixty-two women were given the option to continue in the study for a third year; 147 decided to continue and 137 completed the extra year. At 6 months, 10% of women had discontinued, by 12 months this had risen to 20% and after 24 months 31% of women had discontinued. In the third year, 6% discontinued. During the first 2 years, 17.2% of women discontinued for bleeding irregularities, 8.5% for other adverse experiences, 1.7% for amenorrhoea and 3.5% for other reasons; 0.5% were lost to follow-up. During the third year, a further 0.7% of women discontinued because of an unacceptable bleeding pattern. Analysis of the bleeding pattern revealed that 17.2% of the discontinuations were due to irregular bleeding, 10.9% for frequent irregular bleeding, 3.3% for spotting, 2.4% for prolonged menstrual flow and 1.7% for amenorrhoea.

At the start of the study, 36% of women gave a history of dysmenorrhoea, by the end of the study 87% of these women said that their symptoms had improved. Four per cent of women reported dysmenorrhoea as a new symptom or as a worsening of an existing symptom; 12.8% of women experienced an improvement in their acne, whilst 12.6% of women described acne as a new symptom or a deterioration in the previous condition. In 10 women, clinically significant increases in blood pressure readings occurred; five (0.8%) had a clinically significant increase in systolic pressure and seven (1.1%) had a clinically significant increase in diastolic reading during or at the end of the study. The mean systolic and diastolic pressures showed a small increase over time.

There was a gradual mean increase in body mass index over the study period. The mean percentage increase in body mass index was 3.5%. In 20.2% of women there was an increase from baseline of >10% once or over several measurements; 2.4% of women gave weight gain as their reason for discontinuing treatment.

Swelling, redness, pain and or haematoma at the implant site were rarely reported.

Implanon® insertion took on average 2.2 min (SD 2.1) with a minimum of 0.03 min and a maximum of 10 min. In 1.3% of cases, some complication related to the insertion occurred. The average time needed for implant removal was 5.4 min (SD 5.4). The minimum time needed was 0.33 min and the maximum was 45 min. Removal was complicated in 3% of cases, usually as a result of the implant having been inserted too deeply.

Women were followed-up for 3 months after Implanon® removal. Of those using no method or a non-hormonal method of contraception, menses returned to normal in 90.9% within 3 months. This was not influenced by the length of time the implant had been in place.

Comment

This paper reports no pregnancies with Implanon® use for a total of more than 15 000 cycles of exposure, 2000 of which were in the third year of use, demonstrating that excellent contraceptive cover is provided for 3 years for women of all ages, weights and cultural backgrounds. Total protection from pregnancy in studies of this size is rarely seen.

Because of the many factors affecting contraceptive efficacy, comparisons between methods have limitations in the absence of a control group, but for implants the only objective measurement of clinical performance is the pregnancy rate which has been shown to be affected by age and body weight. The authors compared their results with reported results for other contraceptive implants (Norplant®, Norplant®-2, Uniplant and Nestorone) and found that in terms of contraceptive efficacy, Implanon® is as good or better than the only marketed implant.

This study confirms that progestogen-only methods are associated with a disturbed bleeding pattern in a high proportion of users and that many women discontinue use as a result. The bleeding pattern reported shows a shift towards amenorrhoea and infrequent bleeding. Amenorrhoea was an infrequent cause of discontinuation. There was great variation in the acceptance of irregular bleeding, discontinuation rates being a reflection of tolerance rather than safety.

The low incidence of adverse events at the implant site, together with the fast insertion and removal times, stand out as practical advantages over multiple-unit implants.

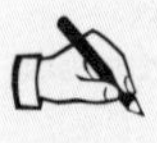

Bone mineral density during long-term use of the progestogen contraceptive implant Implanon® compared to a non-hormonal method of contraception.

R Beerthuizen, A van Beek, R Massai, L Makarainen, J in't Hout, H Coelingh Bennink. *Hum Reprod* 2000; **15**(1): 118–22.

BACKGROUND. Implanon® use results in the suppression of ovarian oestrogen production to early follicular phase concentrations, especially during the first

6 months of use. With prolonged use, oestrogen concentrations rise slightly, but with continuing ovulation inhibition oestrogen lacks cyclical peaks.

Oestrogen deficiency results in bone loss in premenopausal women or failure to reach the same peak bone mass as age-related peers with normal oestrogen status. During Implanon® use, amenorrhoea occurs in approximately 20% of women and therefore it is important to examine BMD and oestrogen concentrations of women using this implant for possible associations.

Whilst scientifically a randomized study design would be most desirable, the contraceptive choice of women being offered methods as diverse as intrauterine devices and implants has to be respected and does not allow randomization.

This study presents a 2-year prospective, comparative study of a progestogen-only contraceptive implant and a non-hormone medicated intrauterine device.

Women in the Netherlands, Chile and Finland interested in the study were offered the choice between Implanon® and a non-hormone intrauterine device and women already fitted with an intrauterine device were also allowed to be enrolled. The ratio of Implanon® to intrauterine device use was chosen to be 1.5:1. Women recruited had to be between 18 and 40 years old, in good physical and mental health and not suffering from a condition (present and history) affecting bone metabolism, not taking medication affecting bone metabolism and a weight between 80 and 130% of ideal. Women with significant scoliosis prohibiting accurate BMD measurements were also excluded. Current intake of more than 2 units per day of alcohol and smoking more than 10 cigarettes per day were exclusion criteria. Women engaging in rigorous exercise were also excluded. At enrolment the participating centres aimed to balance age and weight categories per centre.

During four successive weeks, oestradiol was measured twice weekly to obtain a baseline oestrogen status. This was repeated at months 12 and 24 or when women decided to discontinue the study. The study centres comprised one rural area, one urban area and one suburban area; the women were of Latin-American and European ethnicity.

The Lunar company's female USA/Europe data set was used and for comparison average BMD values for women 20–29 years and 30–39 years were used. Z scores were calculated. BMD measurements were taken at the lumbar spine, proximal femur (femoral neck, Ward's triangle, trochanter) and the distal radius. Measurements were taken at baseline and after 6, 12 and 24 months of treatment. If a woman wished to discontinue participation in the study she had a 'final' BMD measurement performed if this had last been done more than 6 months earlier. Changes in the Z score of the BMD were compared between treatment groups, using analysis of covariance, with centre, age, weight at baseline and treatment as covariates. The primary parameter was the change in BMD Z score at 'last measurement' (month 24 or on discontinuation). The study had adequate power to detect a treatment difference in change in Z score of 0.30 between Implanon® users and intrauterine device users. The DEXA instruments at the three different centres were calibrated at the start of the study and at the end of the study.

INTERPRETATION. Seventy-six women received treatment, 46 received Implanon® and 30 an intrauterine device or were already intrauterine device users. The intention-to-treat group consisted of 44 implant and 29 intrauterine device users, as at least one postbaseline measurement was needed. Overall, the two groups were well balanced with respect to age, height, weight and body mass index. The treatment groups differed with respect to smoking; 41.3% of the Implanon® group were smokers compared with 23.3% of intrauterine device users. Smokers were evenly distributed over the three centres.

At baseline, oestradiol concentrations between the two groups were comparable. There was no correlation between oestradiol concentrations and BMD at baseline. Women with the lower BMD did not necessarily have a low oestrogen status and vice versa.

The 'last' BMD measurement was considered to be the most important single measurement as it included all participants and was not influenced by discontinuers. In the Implanon® group, approximately 20% of volunteers discontinued during the 2 years; only 7% of intrauterine device users left the study. At the 'last measurement' the mean number of days of exposure to Implanon® was 642 (SD 198.9), whereas the intrauterine device group participated for 700.3 (SD 157.5) days.

The clinically significant mean decrease of one standard deviation (Z score -1) was not nearly reached at any point. Generally mean increases from baseline were seen except for the femoral neck in the Implanon® group and Ward's triangle in the intrauterine device group, where small decreases were seen. The covariance analysis at the last measurement showed that the increase in BMD adjusted for centre, weight and age at baseline was slightly greater in the Implanon® group than the intrauterine device group. At none of the anatomical sites was the difference between the intrauterine device and Implanon® groups statistically significant. There was no progression of bone loss in those women who had the lowest BMD at baseline.

During the study the Implanon® users experienced a small increase in weight, whilst there was no change in weight among the intrauterine device users. In those in whom there was an increase in BMD, weight both increased and decreased and the same applied to those with reductions in BMD. There was also no relationship between oestradiol at baseline and change in Z score of the BMD, nor was there a relationship between change in oestradiol and change in BMD Z score.

Comment

The results of this comparative study show that long-term use of Implanon® does not adversely affect BMD. Between 5 and 17% of women were amenorrhoeic during the study and the amenorrhoea was associated with constant oestradiol concentrations compatible with the ranges seen in the early or late follicular phases. Use of Norplant® has also been shown to have no effect on BMD.

Trabecular bone is most sensitive to oestrogen deficiency and this study included extensive measuring of anatomical sites with high trabecular bone content (lumbar spine, trochanter and Ward's triangle). Although there was a slight reduction in BMD at the femoral neck among Implanon® users, this did not approach the clinically significant magnitude of one standard deviation. Lumbar spine and femoral neck results show that there was no accelerated loss among women with low BMD at baseline. The lumbar spine and femoral neck are the best predictors of fracture risk.

The authors concluded that the results indicate that young women who have not yet achieved peak bone mass can safely use Implanon®. Whilst I think this is likely, this study included only one woman under 20 years of age and a total of seven women under 25 years. Implanon® is a very suitable method for sexually active young women, as contraceptive efficacy is achieved independently of user compliance, and personally I would like to see more data from those under 20 years of age.

The next five papers are meta-analyses of the full database of Implanon® in 1997, excluding data from the USA. Meta-analyses have been performed on pharmacokinetics, pharmacodynamics, efficacy, bleeding pattern, side-effects and insertion and removal of Implanon®.

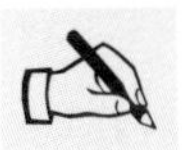

Insertion and removal of Implanon®.

L Mascarenhas. *Contraception* 1998; **58**: 79S–83S.

BACKGROUND. Implants require insertion and removal by medical professionals. Prior to insertion, detailed counselling is essential and should include information about contraceptive efficacy, insertion and removal procedures and possible adverse events.

The Implanon® rod is inserted into the inside of the non-dominant upper arm, 6–8 cm above the elbow, under aseptic conditions. The procedure should be performed by a medical professional familiar with the technique. A preloaded sterile applicator containing a single rod is used for insertion. The needle is introduced directly under the skin, the obturator is then turned through 90°. The cannula is pulled out of the arm slowly whilst keeping the obturator tightly fixed in place (see Fig. 3.1). After correct insertion, Implanon® remains invisible for most women, but palpable in the sulcus between the biceps and triceps. Ease of removal of Implanon® is determined by its correct and careful insertion. For this reason it is imperative that medical professionals familiarize themselves with the correct technique. Implanon® is removed using the 'pop-out' technique; this involves locating the rod, making a vertical 2-mm incision at the distal tip of the implant, pushing the rod towards the incision until it pops out and then grasping the implant with forceps. If the implant cannot be palpated then ultrasonography can be used.

INTERPRETATION. The analysis included data from 13 different trials conducted according to good clinical practice and performed in Europe, North and South America and Southeast Asia between 1989 and 1997. Six studies were open, non-comparative trials and seven were open, randomized comparative trials; Norplant® was the reference product. Combining the studies gave a total of 1716 Implanon® users and 689 Norplant® users.

The study participants were between 18 and 40 years of age, sexually active and of child-bearing potential. They were in good mental and physical health, had regular menstrual cycles, accepted the implant as the sole method of contraception and gave informed, written consent. Implanon® was inserted between days 1 and 5 of their menstrual cycle and Norplant® between days 1 and 7. The volunteers used their implant for between 1 and 5 years.

In comparative studies the time needed for insertion of Implanon® or Norplant® was assessed in 670 and 665 women, respectively. As Table 3.5 shows, the mean time needed to insert Implanon® was 1.1 min compared with 4.3 min for Norplant®. For Implanon®, 98% of insertions were completed within 3 min, whereas this was the case for only 37% of Norplant® insertions. The mean time for Implanon® removal was 2.6 min versus 10.2 min for Norplant®. Implanon® was removed within 5 min in 87% of women, whereas this was the case for only 35% of Norplant® users.

Complications with insertion were assessed in 689 women and problems with removal in 644 women using Implanon® and 145 women using Norplant® in comparative studies. Two Implanon® insertions were associated with complications (0.3%); one case of bleeding and one case where the rod followed the cannula out of the skin. No insertion complications were reported with Norplant®. The incidence of removal complications was statistically significantly lower for Implanon® compared with Norplant® (0.2 versus 4.8%; $P < 0.001$). The only problem reported with Implanon® was one case of significant fibrosis at the implant site; there were seven complications with Norplant®—broken capsules and difficulties locating capsules.

During implant use problems at the insertion site were found more often with Norplant® (2.6%) than Implanon® (1.3%). Pain was the most frequently reported symptom with an incidence of 0.9% for Implanon® and 1.9% for Norplant®.

Comment

These studies indicate that insertion and removal of Implanon® are relatively uncomplicated procedures. There was a four-fold difference in insertion and removal times compared with Norplant®; the mean insertion time for Implanon® being 1.1 min and for Norplant® being 4.3 min and the mean removal times being 2.6 and 10.2 min, respectively. Implanon® consists of one semirigid rod whereas Norplant® consists of six soft capsules.

In studies of more than 1700 women, only minor complications have been reported with Implanon® insertion and removal and only rarely. In experienced hands insertion and removal are easy, quick and uncomplicated.

Table 3.5 Implant insertion and removal times (minutes)

	All trials	**All comparative trials**	
Insertion times	Implanon (n = 1466)	Implanon (n = 670)	Norplant (n=665)
Mean	1.5	1.1	4.3
SD	1.6	0.9	2.1
Range	0.03–10.00	0.03–5.00	0.83–18.00
Removal times	Implanon (n = 1561)	Implanon (n = 633)	Norplant (n = 137)
Mean	3.6	2.6	10.2
SD	3.9	2.0	8.2
Range	0.2–45.0	0.2–20.0	1.3–50.0

SD = standard deviation.
Source: Mascarenhas (1998).

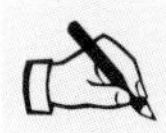

Pharmacokinetics of Implanon®. An integrated analysis.

J Huber. *Contraception* 1998; **58**: 85S–90S.

BACKGROUND. This meta-analysis aimed to present data on the pharmacokinetics, clearance, bioavailability and in vitro absorption of ENG and to present the results of a longitudinal analysis of the plasma concentration–time curves of ENG and the results of a cross-sectional analysis on the association of body weight with serum ENG concentrations.

The in vitro release profile of Implanon® is characterized by an initial release rate of 60–70 μg/day, followed by a gradual decline to about 40, 34 and 25–30 μg/day at the end of the first, second and third years, respectively. The mean in vitro release over 3 years approximates to 40 μg/day.

To assess the bioavailability of ENG, eight women participating in a Swedish and Finnish study of Implanon® use received an intravenous bolus of ENG before, during (after 1 year) and after Implanon® use. One hundred and fifty micrograms of ENG was administered as an intravenous bolus and frequent sampling took place over the next 96 h and at 3 ,6, 9, 15, 18 and 21 months after implant insertion and just prior to removal of the implant. A similar dose of 150 μg of ENG was injected at month 12 of Implanon® use and after implant removal.

Sixty-two women participating in four trials in Finland, Indonesia, Sweden and Thailand had ENG levels measured at regular intervals. The time periods immediately following implant insertion and removal were closely monitored in Scandinavian women and measurements were made monthly and twice weekly during intensive monitoring periods. In the other studies levels were measured every 3 months.

For the cross-sectional analysis, blood samples were taken just prior to implant removal in 11 studies of the core data set and four additional studies. A total of 1872 women were recruited and data from women participating for at least 6 months were included in this analysis. Descriptive statistics of serum ENG concentrations extrapolated to 3 years of use were calculated for four body weight categories (<50, 50–59.9, 60–69.9 and ≥70 kg). The effect of body weight changes during Implanon® use was also investigated.

INTERPRETATION. The results of the intravenous administration study showed that Implanon® had an absorption rate of almost 60 μg/day after 3 months, which slowly decreased to 30 μg/day at the end of 2 years. The bioavailability over this period was constant and close to 100%. Clearance remained around 7.5 litres/h. With constant bioavailability and clearance it was concluded that accumulation of ENG does not take place.

The longitudinal analyses showed that after Implanon® insertion, serum ENG concentrations reached levels associated with ovulation inhibition within 8 h. At 8 and 24 h after insertion, the respective mean concentrations of ENG were 266 pg/ml (range 114–340 pg/ml) and 526 pg/ml (range 364–1020 pg/ml). Maximum serum concentrations amounted to 813 pg/ml on average (range 472–1270 pg/ml) and the time to reach maximum concentration was 4 days (range 1–13 days). After reaching the maximum serum concentration, ENG serum concentrations declined to about 196 pg/ml (range 150–261 pg/ml) at 12 months and 156 pg/ml (range 111–202 pg/ml) by 36 months. Within 1 week after Implanon® removal, serum ENG concentrations declined to less than 20 pg/ml (the detection limit of the assay). Body weight was the only significant determinant of ENG serum concentrations.

A total of 1063 blood samples taken just prior to Implanon® removal provided the data for the cross-sectional analysis. The analysis was based on a continuous time profile, which assumed a log linear relationship between serum ENG concentration and duration of use. Individual serum ENG concentrations were adjusted for duration of use and extrapolated to 3 years of use. A body weight trend was apparent; the highest levels of ENG were found in women weighing <50 kg and the lowest levels in women ≥70 kg, with intermediate levels for the women in the two intermediate weight categories. An increase in body weight during Implanon® use was not shown to have an additional effect on ENG serum levels.

Comment

These studies show that, as with other implants, serum concentrations of ENG exhibit a gradual decrease over time after an initial period of higher levels. The constant bioavailability, remaining close to 100%, and clearance of 7.5 litres/h indicate that there is no accumulation and that the decrease in serum concentration is caused by the slightly lowering release rate over time.

The half-life of elimination of ENG is around 25 h and much lower than the 41.7 h seen for levonorgestrel with Norplant®. Implanon® also showed less variation in half-life of elimination and serum concentration than Norplant®. ENG is mainly bound to albumin, which is not affected by changes in oestrogen concentration. The type of carrier in which the contraceptive steroid is presented also affects variation in serum concentration. The ethylene vinyl acetate co-polymer of Implanon® provides controlled release over 3 years in a single-rod implant and this formulation allows a total dose of 68 mg ENG to provide contraception for 3 years.

From a contraceptive efficacy viewpoint, the relationship between serum steroid concentration and body weight is important. The absence of pregnancies precludes any prediction about the serum concentration of ENG at which an individual might theoretically run a higher risk of pregnancy. The primary mechanism of action of Implanon® is ovulation inhibition and this is maintained in the majority of women for 3 years. The authors therefore concluded that Implanon® provides a contraceptive life span of 3 years for women of all weights.

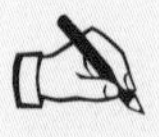

The pharmacodynamics and efficacy of Implanon®. An overview of the data.

HB Croxatto, L Makarainen. *Contraception* 1998; **58**: 91S–7S.

BACKGROUND. The objective of this meta-analysis was to evaluate the contraceptive efficacy of Implanon® in terms of its mechanism of action and capacity to prevent pregnancy.

The women recruited to the trials were between 18 and 40 years of age, sexually active and of child-bearing potential. They were in good mental and physical health, had no contraindications to the use of contraceptive steroids, had regular menstrual cycles and gave written informed consent. Implanon® was inserted between days 1 and 5 of a menstrual period. Eighteen clinical trials studied the effects of Implanon®, five of which were excluded from this analysis—one US study to be reported elsewhere, three studies were considered not compliant with good clinical practice as full verification with source data was not possible and one study was performed using a leached implant to obtain a release rate similar to the second year of use and the study was performed in sterilized women. A total of 2362 women participated in the 13 studies, contributing 73 429 cycles (5629 woman-years of use). A small amount of 4- and 5-year Implanon® data was obtained in Thailand and Indonesia.

Pharmacodynamic analysis was based on the assessment of ovarian activity/ ovulation, gonadotrophin estimation, analysis of cervical mucus and ultrasound and histological assessment of the endometrium. Contraceptive efficacy analysis was assessed by the occurrence of in-treatment pregnancies. A pregnancy test was always performed if there was any suspicion of pregnancy, e.g. amenorrhoea >6 weeks. Return of ovulation was assessed in four studies during the first 3 months after Implanon® removal using either progesterone estimation or ovarian ultrasound.

INTERPRETATION. Table 3.6 shows the proportion of cycles with ovulation and the footnotes give details about the subjects in whom ovulation was judged to have occurred. The high serum progesterone levels seen with both Implanon® (4/244 cycles) and Norplant® (2/164 cycles) in the first year were either from ovulation in the cycle before insertion or were single isolated observations. In the second year, all high serum progesterones with Implanon® were single isolated observations. With Implanon®, the first ovulation occurred in the third year in two of 46 women, in one subject at month 30 and in the other repeatedly at months 30, 33 and 36. Although Implanon® effectively inhibited ovulation, ovarian follicular activity was not completely suppressed. Ultrasound

Table 3.6 Proportion of Implanon® cycles with high progesterone values and ovulation

Year	Number of subjects	Proportion of cycles * with High progesterone, n1/n (%)	Ovulation, n2/n (%)
≤1	62	4/244 (1.6)	0/244 (0)
1–2	54	1/148 (0.7)	0/148 (0)
2–3	46	4/131 (3.1)	4/131[a] (3.1)
3–4	32	2/115 (1.7)	1/115[b] (0.9)
4–5	27	1/82 (1.2)	1/82[c] (1.2)

*Treatment duration was divided into cycles (28 days) to facilitate interpretation.
n1 = number of cycles with progesterone values >16 nmol/litre; n2 = number of cycles with ovulation; n = total number of cycles assessed.
Relevant characteristics of women in whom ovulation was judged to have occurred:
[a]Subject 1 weighed 57.5 kg, ovulation confirmed by ultrasound at 30, 33 and 36 months and subject 2 weighed 69.5 kg, ovulation confirmed by ultrasound at 30 months.
[b]Subject weighed 59.0 kg, ovulation possible at 39 months (limited progesterone data and no ultrasound).
[c]Subject weighed 47.0 kg, ovulation possible at 42 months (limited progesterone data and no ultrasound).
Source: Croxatto *et al.* (1998).

data showed follicular development, with pre-ovulatory sized follicles, in most women after 1 year of Implanon® use.

In one study, serum oestradiol measurements were made concomitantly with ovarian ultrasound. Prior to insertion, normal pre-ovulatory serum oestradiol levels were recorded, after insertion mean levels decreased initially and then rose gradually. There was considerable variation in individual serum oestradiol levels and neither consistently low nor high levels were recorded. In another study, serum LH and FSH levels were measured; the main effect seen was the prevention of LH surges. Serum FSH levels were all within the follicular phase range.

The possibility of increased cervical mucus viscosity contributing to the contraceptive efficacy of Implanon® was investigated in the leached implant study. Mean Insler scores decreased from 12.8 prior to insertion to 0.8–4.2 during Implanon® use. Sperm penetration tests were negative throughout except in one case at the equivalent of 30 months when ultrasound and serum progesterone levels still indicated ovulation inhibition.

Ultrasound measurement of endometrial thickness showed a mean double wall thickness of 4 mm. Endometrial biopsies showed primarily inactive or weakly proliferative endometrium; no hyperplasia or endometrial carcinoma was observed with Implanon® use.

The efficacy core data set includes 1716 women treated with Implanon® for 53 530 cycles (4103 woman-years). No in-treatment pregnancies were observed, giving a Pearl index of 0.0 (95% CI 0.00–0.09). If the US study and those not fully compliant with good clinical practice are included, then the total exposure to Implanon® amounts to 2362 women providing 73 429 cycles (5629 woman-years). The resulting Pearl index is 0.0 (95% CI 0.00–0.07). One hundred and two women weighing more than 70 kg used Implanon® between 2 and 3 years.

Four studies assessed return of ovulation after Implanon® removal. Postremoval serum progesterone concentrations and/or ultrasound findings consistent with ovulation were observed in 94% of women, usually within 3 weeks after implant removal.

Comment

The contraceptive efficacy of Implanon® is optimal with a Pearl index of 0.0 (95% CI 0.00–0.09) during 53 530 cycles. This is higher than reported for any other method of contraception.

This optimal efficacy is explained by effective inhibition of ovulation combined with independence from user compliance. It seems that ENG exerts a negative feedback on the hypothalamic–pituitary axis resulting in inadequate LH surges. This results in ovulation inhibition with normal endogenous oestradiol synthesis.

In two women (4%) ovulation started to occur after 2.5 years; this confirms the 3-year duration of ovulation inhibition in most women. Those who ovulate in the third year can rely on the other contraceptive effects of the progestogen, primarily the increased viscosity of cervical mucus.

The data presented provide reassurance for women weighing more than 70 kg and suggest that the high efficacy will probably not be altered when Implanon® is used by heavier women. Because Implanon® both inhibits ovulation and is independent of user compliance it should protect users from ectopic pregnancy.

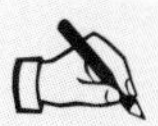

An integrated analysis of vaginal bleeding patterns in clinical trials of Implanon®.

B Affandi. *Contraception* 1998; **58**: 99S–107S.

BACKGROUND. Bleeding disturbance is the main reason why women stop using Norplant® and similar patterns are evident in the individual studies of Implanon®, although wide variation in discontinuation rates is seen. Careful assessment of bleeding patterns is needed to provide a sound basis for counselling.

The objective of this meta-analysis was to evaluate the bleeding patterns seen during the use of Implanon® and to make a comparison with Norplant® use. The acceptability of these bleeding patterns, as indicated by discontinuation rates, was also assessed, as were the effects of Implanon® on dysmenorrhoea and anaemia.

To permit comparison of menstrual bleeding patterns from different studies, this meta-analysis used a standardized approach known as reference period analysis. Data from daily menstrual diaries are analysed on the basis of reference periods, usually 90 days. The extent of deviation from a normal menstrual bleeding pattern is defined by WHO bleeding pattern indices which include amenorrhoea, infrequent bleeding, frequent bleeding and prolonged bleeding.

The data from 13 different trials performed in Europe, North and South America and Southeast Asia were used to provide an overview of the menstrual effects of Implanon®. Women recorded their vaginal bleeding patterns daily on diary cards, recording 'none', 'spotting' (less than one sanitary pad/tampon used), or 'bleeding' (more than two sanitary pads/tampons used). The cards were checked and collected at each clinic visit.

To assess the discontinuation rate due to the vaginal bleeding pattern, women were included for whom one of the following predefined menstrual problems was indicated as the primary reason for study discontinuation: frequent irregular bleeding, heavy menstrual flow, prolonged menstrual flow, dysmenorrhoea, amenorrhoea, spotting and other bleeding problems. Whilst these terms are not identical to those used in the reference period analysis, they describe the subjective experience of the women.

The individual studies demonstrated a geographical difference between acceptance of bleeding patterns so the authors chose to present data separately for two regions, Europe with Canada and Southeast Asia with Chile.

Because most studies had bleeding pattern data for 2 years, the main analysis was based on all subjects completing 2 years. Some data were also presented for women completing 3 years of Implanon® use.

INTERPRETATION. Data relating to vaginal bleeding were available for 1716 women using Implanon®, providing 13 888 reference periods or 4103 woman-years of exposure, as well as for 689 women using Norplant®, providing 6315 reference periods or 1826 woman-years of use.

Bleeding irregularities constituted the main reason for early discontinuation with Implanon®. There were dramatic differences in discontinuation rates due to bleeding pattern between the two geographical regions. The overall discontinuation rate for disturbance of bleeding pattern with Implanon® was 23% for Europe and Canada compared with only 1.8% in Southeast Asia and Chile. Amenorrhoea was common, but was rarely a reason for discontinuation. Frequent irregular bleeding was the least acceptable pattern of bleeding and was responsible for approximately 50% of bleeding-related discontinuations. The discontinuation rates for bleeding pattern disturbances were not significantly different between Implanon® and Norplant®.

The bleeding patterns of those who discontinued use during the first 2 years were compared with the patterns of those completing 2 years. Those discontinuing both Implanon® and Norplant® displayed more bleeding than those completing 2 years. Among the Implanon® users, those who discontinued showed about twice as many bleeding and bleeding/spotting days and three times as many cases of frequent and prolonged bleeding/spotting as those who completed 2 years. The incidence of amenorrhoea among those completing 2 years was five times as high as that seen in those discontinuing, indicating that amenorrhoea is perceived as an acceptable bleeding disturbance.

There was no consistent change in bleeding seen in either Implanon® or Norplant® users over time. The incidence of amenorrhoea with Implanon® was higher than with Norplant® (17.9–24.8% compared with 2.0–7.0%, $P < 0.0001$). The incidences of infrequent bleeding, frequent bleeding and prolonged bleeding were higher among Implanon® users, but the differences were not statistically significant. A shift analysis performed on the consistency of bleeding pattern within an individual woman revealed that the bleeding pattern is not really predictable.

Dysmenorrhoea was present in 40% of women at baseline and in 9% of women on removal of Implanon®. In 82% of women with pre-existing dysmenorrhoea symptoms improved or disappeared. In 2% of women the symptoms worsened and 4% of women developed dysmenorrhoea whilst using Implanon®. The mean value of haemoglobin increased slightly in all studies of Implanon® use.

Comment

Implanon® users reported less bleeding than Norplant® users, but the patterns seem to be more variable. The differences seem to be without consequence for acceptability as there were no statistically significant differences between discontinuation rates.

This analysis suggests that women find amenorrhoea acceptable in contrast to prolonged and frequent bleeding/spotting. There were marked regional differences in discontinuation rates for bleeding problems, indicating that the acceptability of bleeding patterns is influenced by factors other than the bleeding patterns themselves, e.g. personal, social or cultural.

The outcome of this integrated analysis is important for adequate counselling, which is known to improve the acceptability of disturbances in vaginal bleeding patterns. These data indicate that initial bleeding patterns, during the early months of exposure, are not necessarily predictive of later bleeding patterns. However, women without bleeding or with infrequent bleeding have a small chance of becoming frequent bleeders and vice versa.

There was an overall improvement in dysmenorrhoea among both Implanon® and Norplant® users.

In summary, Implanon® users had, on average, less vaginal bleeding and fewer bleeding/spotting episodes than untreated women or Norplant® users, but they were more likely to experience irregular bleeding patterns.

An integrated analysis of nonmenstrual adverse events with Implanon®.

J Urbancsek. *Contraception* 1998; **58**: 109S–15S.

BACKGROUND. In addition to bleeding irregularities, progestogen-only contraceptives are associated with a variety of adverse events; there may be an increase in the prevalence of headaches, breast tenderness, nausea and dizziness. The androgenic activity of progestogens is also said to lead to acne, hirsutism and weight gain. Between 21 and 45% of POP users report non-menstrual adverse events and up to 10% of women discontinue use because of symptoms. The most commonly reported reasons for removal of Norplant® are headaches, weight gain, depression, anxiety and mood changes; loss of libido, acne, breast tenderness, dizziness and nausea are also reported frequently.

The aim of this meta-analysis was to evaluate non-menstrual adverse events, to look at the effect of Implanon® on blood pressure and body weight and to compare the profile of Implanon® with that of Norplant®.

This meta-analysis included data from 13 different clinical trials performed in Europe, North and South America and Southeast Asia between 1989 and 1997. Six were open, non-comparative trials and seven were open, randomized comparative trials. Norplant® was used as the reference product. The definitions and the methods used to record adverse events were the same for all the trials included in this analysis.

All women enrolled in the trials were between 18 and 40 years of age, sexually active, and of child-bearing potential; they were in good mental and physical health, had no contraindications to the use of contraceptive steroids, had regular menstrual cycles and gave written informed consent.

The participants visited the trial clinics at least once every 3 months. At each visit the implant site was examined, diary cards were checked and collected and possible signs of pregnancy, occurrence of adverse events and use of concomitant medication were assessed by open questioning. Blood pressure and weight were recorded at insertion, after 3 and 6 months and every 6 months thereafter. A pelvic examination was performed annually.

All adverse events and serious adverse events were recorded according to terminology defined by the WHO. The drug relatedness of serious adverse events was judged both by the investigator and by Organon's Serious Adverse Events Committee. Serious adverse events thought to be possibly, probably or definitely related to the study drug administration were classified as drug related; those that were thought to be unlikely or not related were classed as not related.

From individual study data regional differences in the reporting of adverse events were apparent, so a preliminary analysis of these differences was performed to determine whether data from any region should be excluded from the data set.

Acne intensity was assessed before implant insertion and at removal in four studies. A systolic blood pressure of >140 mmHg and an increase of >20 mmHg from

baseline on at least two visits or at last assessment were considered clinically significant. The diastolic readings considered significant were >90 mmHg and an increase of >10 mmHg from baseline. An increase in body weight of >10% from baseline at least once during treatment was considered clinically significant.

INTERPRETATION. The preliminary adverse events analysis indicated that there were no consistent differences between countries, although far fewer adverse events were reported in Indonesia and many more were reported in Chile than in the other regions. The results for the other countries were presented together and those for Indonesia and Chile were presented separately.

The total exposure was 4103 woman-years for Implanon® and 1826 woman-years for Norplant®. There were no deaths reported among the study populations. In total, 61 serious adverse events were reported with Implanon®. Overall, 0.7% of women receiving Implanon® had serious adverse events that were considered to be possibly or probably drug related; none was considered to be definitely drug related. The conditions reported included breast fibroadenosis, headache, uterine fibroids, ovarian cyst, cervical dysplasia, teratoma and asthma.

The overall incidence of adverse events in Implanon® studies was 72%; the figures for Chile and Indonesia were 99 and 5%, respectively. In all Implanon® studies, 47% of women reported adverse events that were considered to be drug related. In comparative studies, 61% of Implanon® users reported adverse events compared with 69% of Norplant® users; the difference was not statistically significant.

In the Implanon® studies the most frequently reported drug-related adverse events were acne (15.3%), breast pain (9.1%), headache (8.5%) and weight gain (6.4%). Adverse events of severe intensity were experienced by 10.1% of Implanon® users; in Chile and Indonesia the incidences were 29.0 and 0.0%, respectively.

Overall, 7.3% of Implanon® acceptors discontinued use, citing an adverse event other than bleeding irregularities as the primary reason. The most frequently occurring reasons for discontinuation in all Implanon® studies were weight gain and acne. In comparative studies the reasons for discontinuation were the same for Implanon® and Norplant® users.

Acne was present in 24% of women at baseline and in 21% of women at Implanon® removal. In 59% of the women with pre-existing acne the condition disappeared or improved, in 10% the condition worsened during treatment and 14% of women unaffected at baseline developed acne.

Clinically significant increases in blood pressure with Implanon® use were very rare, with 0.4% of women experiencing a clinically significant increase in systolic blood pressure and 0.7% of women experiencing a clinically significant increase in diastolic blood pressure. The median systolic and diastolic pressures were unchanged in both treatment groups.

Weight gain was reported as a drug-related adverse event in 6.4% of all Implanon® users and in 7.1% of Norplant® users in comparative studies. Clinically significant increases in body weight (>10% from baseline) were seen in 20.7% of all Implanon® users. A gradual mean increase in body weight over time (1.5–2% per year) was seen in both Implanon® and Norplant® users. In one study which included users of non-medicated intrauterine devices, mean body weight increases were 2.6, 2.9 and 2.4% over 2 years for Implanon®, Norplant® and intrauterine devices, respectively.

Comment

Overall, 47% of Implanon® users had drug-related non-menstrual adverse events during their participation in the studies. Acne, breast pain, headache and weight gain were the most frequent drug-related adverse events, with acne and weight gain most commonly leading to discontinuation of Implanon® use. Similar incidences were reported for Norplant®.

Large regional differences in both the levels and distribution of adverse events have also been seen in studies with Norplant® and probably represent differences in cultural, social and environmental factors; there may also be a contribution from differences in the basic rates of symptoms and in the interpretation of protocols.

The adverse events seen most frequently in this meta-analysis are typical of the spectrum of adverse events seen with progestogen-only contraceptives and with Norplant® in particular.

Acne was frequently reported as an adverse event with both implant systems. However, in the Implanon® studies, where acne was looked at closely, those with acne at baseline largely improved whereas the condition appeared in 14% of users and worsened in 10%. Acne probably presents less of a problem for implant users than the adverse event data indicate and illustrates the negative bias which can be introduced by presenting only adverse events and not highlighting improvements in pre-existing conditions.

Small, but steady increases in weight were seen with both Implanon® and Norplant® use, but the comparative study including a reference group of intrauterine device users indicates that weight gain with implant use is largely attributable to a normal increase over time and only partly due to the implant.

With the refinement of implant technology culminating in the development of Implanon® and Jadelle® and the production of a POP which inhibits ovulation, progestogen-only methods are now able to take their rightful place as first-choice methods for all women, not only those with contraindications to the use of synthetic oestrogens. Implanon® in particular provides a combination of efficacy and compliance acceptable to both users and health care providers.

References

1. Cundy T, Evans M, Roberts H, Wattie D, Ames R, Reid IR. Bone density in women receiving depot medroxyprogesterone acetate for contraception. *Br Med J* 1991; **303**: 13–6.

2. Naessen T, Olsson SE, Gudmundson J. Differential effects on bond density of progestogen-only methods for contraception in premenopausal women. *Contraception* 1995; **52:** 35–39.

3. Sivin I. International experience with Norplant® and Norplant®-2 contraceptives. *Stud Fam Plann* 1988; **19:** 81–94.

Further reading

Fraser IS, Tiitinen A, Brache V, *et al.* Norplant® consensus statement and background review. *Contraception* 1998; **57:** 1–9.

Edwards JE, Moore A. Implanon®, a review of clinical studies. *Br J Fam Plann* 1999; **24:** 3–16.

4

Emergency contraception

Introduction

World-wide, about 50 million pregnancies are terminated each year |1|. These pregnancies result from contraceptive failure, inadequate contraceptive technique, failure to use any type of contraception because of unanticipated and thus unprotected sexual intercourse, or as a result of sexual assault or coercion.

Given this large number of unintended pregnancies, emergency contraception remains highly underused. The term refers to contraceptive methods used as an emergency measure to prevent an unwanted pregnancy after unprotected sexual intercourse. They are simple to use and are safe and effective for the majority of women who may need them. It has been calculated that each year the widespread use of emergency contraception in the USA could prevent over 1 million abortions and 2 million unintended pregnancies that end in childbirth |2|. However, despite its availability for at least three decades, many practitioners and patients have inadequate information about its use.

In recent years, emergency contraception has emerged from the shadows to the forefront of reproductive health care. Research in the 1990s concentrated on: (1) developing hormonal methods of emergency contraception that are more effective and better tolerated; (2) determining effectiveness and mechanisms of action; and (3) improving availability |3|.

In 1995, an international consortium for emergency contraception comprising seven organizations involved in health and family planning was established to increase its availability through global information campaigns and model introduction programmes in a number of countries |4|.

Methods of emergency contraception

Following the introduction of high-dose oestrogens in the 1960s, the so-called Yuzpe regimen, involving the combined use of oestrogen (100 μg ethinyloestradiol) and progestogen (0.5 mg levonorgestrel or 1 mg DL-norgestrel) repeated twice 12 h apart with the first dose given within 72 h of unprotected intercourse, became popular in the late 1970s to early 1980s |5|. A combined oestrogen and progestogen emergency contraception pill formulation, Schering, PC4, became available in the UK in 1984. Subsequently, other drugs were tried, including Danazol, progestogens and the antiprogestogen, Mifepristone. A progestogen-only emergency contraception pill formulation, Levonelle-2®, has been licensed for use in the UK since 1999. More recently, it has been licensed for sale by pharmacists and has a 'P' status.

The insertion of an intrauterine device (IUD) postcoitally is the most contraceptively effective option which can be used within 5 days of the earliest episode of intercourse within a cycle. The IUD also has the advantage that it can provide ongoing contraception which hormonal methods cannot.

The Faculty of Family Planning and Reproductive Health Care, Royal College of Obstetricians and Gynaecologists, Guidance April 2000; Emergency Contraception: Recommendations for Clinical Practice (see Appendix) provides information about the currently licensed emergency contraceptive methods available in the UK. Subsequent to the release of this document, the progestogen-only emergency contraceptive pill, Levonelle-2®, has acquired a change of legal status from a prescription-only medicine to pharmacy status as Levonelle®.

Recent clinical trials

Two recent multicentre studies conducted by the United Nations Development Programme (UNDP)/United Nations Family Planning Association (UNFPA)/ World Health Organization (WHO) /World Bank Special Programme of Research have looked at finding effective and acceptable methods of emergency contraception. One study examined the effectiveness of levonorgestrel in comparison with the Yuzpe regimen and the other assessed treatment with three different doses of mifepristone.

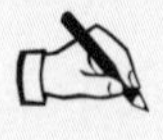

Randomised controlled trial of levonorgestrel versus the Yuzpe regimen of combined oral contraceptives for emergency contraception.

WHO Task Force on Postovulatory Methods of Fertility Regulation. *Lancet* 1998; **352**: 428–33.

BACKGROUND. A previous randomized study |6| had suggested that levonorgestrel given alone in two separate doses each of 0.75 mg within 48 h of unprotected intercourse, caused nausea and vomiting in fewer women and might be more effective than the Yuzpe regimen of combined oral contraceptives for emergency contraception, although the difference was not significant. The present study set out to confirm these findings in research on a larger scale, including women from different populations. This compared the two regimens when started within 72 h of unprotected coitus.

METHODS. A total of 1998 women were enrolled in this double-blind randomized trial at 21 centres world-wide. Women with regular periods not using hormonal contraception and requesting emergency contraception after one episode of unprotected coitus received levonorgestrel (0.75 mg repeated 12 h later) or the Yuzpe regimen.

RESULTS. Outcome was unknown for 43 women (25 assigned levonorgestrel, 18 assigned the Yuzpe regimen). The proportion of pregnancies prevented compared with the expected number without treatment was 85% (95% CI 74–93) with the levonorgestrel regimen and 57% (95% CI 39–71) with the Yuzpe regimen. Nausea (23.15 versus 50.5%) and vomiting (5.6 versus 18.8%) were significantly less frequent with the levonorgestrel regimen than with the Yuzpe regimen (*P* < 0.01). The efficacy of both treatments declined with increasing time following unprotected coitus (*P* < 0.01).

INTERPRETATION. The levonorgestrel regimen was better tolerated and more effective than the Yuzpe regimen. With both, earlier treatment resulted in greater effectiveness. When treatment was initiated within 24, 48 and 72 h of unprotected sex, the levonorgestrel regimen prevented 95, 85 and 58% of expected pregnancies, respectively. With the Yuzpe regimen, the figures for prevented expected pregnancies were 77, 36 and 31%, respectively, when treatment was initiated within 24, 48 and 72 h of unprotected sex.

Comment

Retrospective urine tests had shown that four women had already been pregnant at enrolment; the pregnancy status at admission to the study of a further five women could not be determined. Thus, the figures of prevented pregnancies are underestimates because these women had been included.

The findings of this study are of significant public health importance. Based on this evidence, the Faculty of Family Planning and Reproductive Health Care

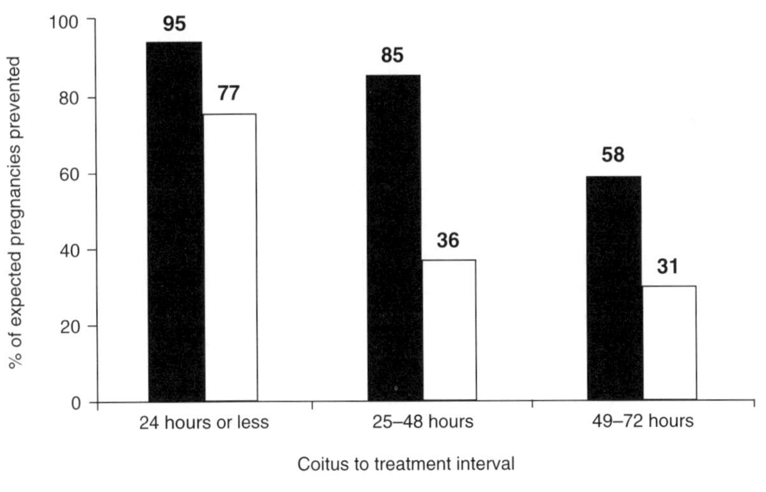

Fig. 4.1 Efficacy of oral emergency contraception. Source: WHO (1998).

recommends that all contraceptive service providers should now offer levonor-gestrel-only emergency hormonal contraception as a first-line treatment. The other important message from this study is that women should receive treatment as soon as practicable, preferably within 24 h.

Fig. 4.1 shows the efficacy of oral emergency contraception with interval from coitus.

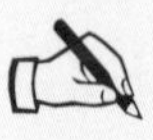

Comparison of three single doses of mifepristone as emergency contraception: a randomised trial.
WHO Task Force on Postovulatory Methods of Fertility Regulation. *Lancet* 1999; **353**: 697–702.

BACKGROUND. Mifepristone is a highly effective and well tolerated emergency contraceptive when given in a dose of 600 mg within 72 h of unprotected coitus. This study assessed whether the same effectiveness can be achieved with lower doses (50 and 10 mg) and a longer postcoital treatment period (120 h).

METHODS. A total of 1717 healthy women with regular menstrual cycles who requested emergency contraception within 120 h of unprotected coitus were randomly assigned to three treatment groups in this multicentre single-masked randomized trial.

RESULTS. The 600, 50 and 10 mg groups did not differ in the proportion of pregnancies: 7/559 (1.3%), 6/560 (1.1%) and 7/565 (1.2%), respectively; with the expected number of pregnancies based on recognizable conceptions, the prevented fractions for the 600, 50 and 10 mg groups were 84, 86 and 85%, respectively. Thus, overall, mifepristone prevented 85% of the pregnancies that would have occurred without treatment. Among women without further acts of intercourse, treatment delay did not appear to influence the effectiveness. No major side-effects occurred except a delay in the onset of the next menses, significantly ($P < 0.01$) related to the mifepristone dose.

INTERPRETATION. Lowering the dose of mifepristone 60-fold did not decrease its effectiveness as an emergency contraceptive under typical use, although a study of this size could not exclude differences in effectiveness up to almost three-fold. Lower doses of mifepristone were associated with less disturbance of the menstrual cycle. Lowering the mifepristone dose from 600 to 10 mg has important advantages without significantly compromising effectiveness: (1) it would be substantially cheaper; (2) it avoids problems with delay in the onset of the next menses, and women worrying about unintended pregnancies; (3) it avoids the risk of delayed ovulation most commonly associated with higher doses. This potentially minimizes the risk of pregnancy should the woman have further acts of unprotected intercourse in that cycle.

Comment

As mifepristone seems to be an effective emergency contraceptive at doses much lower than those required to induce abortion, it may prove valuable in preventing unwanted pregnancies and recourse to abortion. Whether mifepristone is a better choice than levonorgestrel awaits the results of a randomized trial comparing them. Although possibly the best method tested so far, mifepristone is unlikely to become widely available as emergency contraception in the foreseeable future because it is known to be an abortifacient |3|.

The use of IUDs for emergency contraception

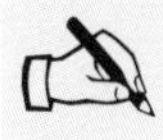

Preliminary analysis of a multicenter clinical trial using Multiload® Cu 375SL for emergency contraception.
L Zhou, B Xiao. *Adv Contracept* 1998; **14**: 161–70.

BACKGROUND. IUDs are used for emergency contraception as an alternative to hormonal methods. More than 8400 postcoital IUD insertions have been reported in the literature, with a failure rate that does not exceed 0.1% |7|. This study was conducted in China to evaluate the efficacy, side-effects and acceptability of the Multiload® Cu 375SL IUD used as emergency contraception.

METHOD. Women who attended the clinic within 120 h (5 days) after unprotected coitus and gave informed consent had a Multiload® Cu 375SL IUD inserted at admission. The inclusion criteria for these women were: good general health, history of regular menstrual cycles (24–42 days), at least one spontaneous cycle of normal length after discontinued hormonal contraception or a recent abortion or delivery. Women with genital tract infections, tumours, abnormality, vaginal bleeding of unknown aetiology, systemic disease or suspected pregnancy were excluded. A urine pregnancy test was performed on admission to exclude those women who were already pregnant. The study subjects were given a prophylactic dose (600 mg/day) of metronidazole for 3 days after the IUD insertion. They were followed-up at the end of the first postinsertion menstruation.

The efficacy rate was defined as the success at preventing pregnancy, which would have occurred if no emergency contraception was used. The probabilities of pregnancy on different menstrual days were weighted figures drawn from several studies |8|. The number of expected pregnancies was calculated from the estimates of the probability given and the efficacy rate was calculated according to the formula: efficacy rate = [(number of expected pregnancies − number of actual pregnancies)/number of pregnancies] × 100%.

User failure was defined as the failure due to non-compliance of the subject to the study protocol, e.g. unprotected intercourse taking place more than 120 h before treatment.

RESULTS. Of the 633 women who were recruited between March 1997 and March 1998 and had a Multiload® Cu 375SL IUD inserted, a preliminary analysis was performed on 515 subjects who completed the follow-up. The majority were parous women (428; 83.1%). The efficacy rate was 92.40%. Two pregnancies were detected at follow-up visits. One of them was considered to be a user failure. There were no failures in insertion procedure and no pelvic infections. The removal rate in the nulliparous group (14.9%) was significantly higher than in the parous group (3.5%).

The reasons for removal were mostly pain and bleeding. Approximately 40% of the women in the nulliparous group experienced some change in menstrual cycle, either shortening (20.7%) or prolonging (16.1%), which was significantly different from the experience in the parous group ($P < 0.01$).

INTERPRETATION. Based on this study, the authors concluded that insertion of a copper IUD is a very effective and safe method for emergency contraception. It is more acceptable to parous women who wish to continue using an IUD for long-term contraception. Pre-insertion counselling about the insertion procedure and possible side-effects such as pain and menstrual disturbances, should be carried out carefully, particularly with nulliparous women.

Comment

Insertion of an IUD for emergency contraception has some advantages and also limitations. The advantages are: the IUD can be inserted up to the time of implantation, i.e. 5 days following the estimated day of ovulation; some IUDs can provide up to 10 years of contraceptive protection once in place, if longer use is desired. Pregnancy due to further acts of unprotected intercourse after treatment can be avoided, as the IUD is highly effective once inserted. The limitations are that any IUD insertion is an invasive procedure, which requires aseptic clinic facilities and insertion skills. There may be pain and difficulty in insertion in nulliparous women.

No pelvic infections were reported in the study subjects, perhaps due to the policy of administering prophylactic antibiotics after IUD insertion. The paper alludes to laboratory tests that were performed at the time of IUD insertion, although it does not make it explicit that these were to screen for infection.

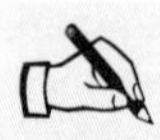

Interventions for emergency contraception.

L Cheng, AM Gulmezoglu, E Ezcurra, PFA Van Look. *The Cochrane Library*, Issue 3, 2000.

BACKGROUND. **The objective of this review was to determine which emergency contraceptive method following unprotected intercourse is the most effective, safe and convenient for use in preventing pregnancy. Randomized or quasi-randomized studies including women attending services for emergency contraception following a single act of unprotected intercourse were eligible.**

RESULTS. **Fifteen trials were included in the review. The majority (eight) of the trials were conducted in China. Levonorgestrel appears to be more effective than the Yuzpe regimen (two trials |6, 9|; relative risk 0.51, 95% CI 0.31–0.84) and causes less side-effects (relative risk 0.80, 95% CI 0.74–0.86). Levonorgestrel was less effective than locally manufactured mifepristone in a single, large Chinese study (relative risk 2.17, 95% CI 1.00–4.77). This trial has not yet been published in full and the wide confidence intervals mitigate against drawing a firm conclusion. The effectiveness of different doses of mifepristone seems to be similar, but the frequency of delay in onset**

of the subsequent menstrual period increases with increased dose. Three cases of ectopic pregnancy (two after 50 mg of mifepristone and one after 10 mg of mifepristone) were identified among the 15 trials reviewed.

Comment

Of the hormonal methods, levonorgestrel and mifepristone seem to offer the highest efficacy with an acceptable side-effect profile. One disadvantage of mifepristone is that it causes delays in the onset of subsequent menses, which may induce anxiety. However, this seems to be dose related and low doses of mifepristone minimize this side-effect without compromising effectiveness. The sooner emergency contraception is started, the higher its efficacy. IUD insertion can be offered to women who present too late for oral hormonal interventions, are not at risk of sexually transmitted diseases and who would like this method for long-term contraception.

Future research should focus on determining the optimal dose of mifepristone and whether this is superior to levonorgestrel in the doses tested so far. Particular attention in these studies will need to be paid to the risk of ectopic pregnancy in association with mifepristone use. The comparative effectiveness of IUD insertion has not been investigated adequately. Although it may be difficult to conduct randomized controlled trials comparing IUDs with other interventions with the woman as the unit of randomization, cluster randomization may overcome this problem and allow a randomized comparison of IUD insertion with an oral drug regimen.

Ongoing studies [4]

A large double-blind randomized study involving 10 centres is underway in China to compare the efficacy and side-effects of the 10 and 25 mg doses of Chinese mifepristone. The Special Programme of Research, UNDP, has developed the study protocol and forms for data collection in collaboration with the National Research Institute for Family Planning, Beijing. A total of 3000 women will be recruited for this study.

The programme as above is also currently carrying out a large multinational randomized double-blind study to compare the efficacy and side-effects of 10 mg of mifepristone and two different regimens of levonorgestrel (i.e. two doses of 0.75 mg administered with a 12-hour interval, or one dose of 1.5 mg) in emergency contraception up to 120 h after unprotected intercourse. This study began in mid-1998 with a target of recruitment of 4200 women.

A prospective study is ongoing at 18 centres in China to study the efficacy, acceptability, side-effects and possible complications of postcoital insertion of copper IUDs as emergency contraception and aims to recruit 2000 women. The study protocol includes follow-up until 1 year after IUD insertion to observe the continuation rate and observe late side-effects.

Studies looking at the mechanism of action of levonorgestrel are underway.

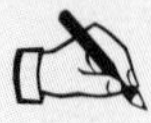

Efficacy and side effects of immediate post coital levonorgestrel used repeatedly for contraception.

United Nations Development Programme/United Nations Population Fund/World Health Organization/World Bank Special Programme of Research, Development and Research Training in Human Reproduction, Task Force on Post-ovulatory Methods for Fertility Regulation. *Contraception* 2000; **61**: 303–8.

BACKGROUND. This study evaluated the efficacy and side-effects of immediate postcoital administration of levonorgestrel 0.75 mg used repeatedly as the only method of contraception.

METHOD. A total of 295 healthy women with infrequent coitus were enrolled at six study sites in five countries (China, Cuba, Pakistan, Russia and Slovenia). The women had to be older than the legal age for consent, to have regular menstrual cycles and of proven fertility with their present partner. Each woman took 0.75 mg of levonorgestrel by mouth immediately after intercourse for 6 months as the only method of contraception.

Data on side-effects and acceptability and the Pearl index failure rates over 133 women-years of use were calculated.

RESULTS. The Pearl index failure rate was 6.8 (95% CI 3.1–12.9) pregnancies per 100 woman-years of use. The overall probability of pregnancy per treated coital act was 1.4 per 1000. Menstrual complaints were reported by 70% of women.

INTERPRETATION. Postcoital levonorgestrel is not suitable for regular contraception. Existing hormonal contraceptives are much more effective for long-term use with fewer side-effects. Thus, postcoital levonorgestrel appears to have its place only as a back up method in a contraceptive emergency.

Safety

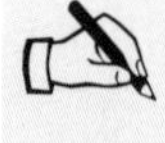

Risk of venous thromboembolism in users of post-coital contraceptive pills.

C Vasilakis, SS Jick, H Jick. *Contraception* 1999; **59**: 79–83.

BACKGROUND. A population-based cohort study with a nested case–control analysis was conducted using women from the UK General Practice Research Database to assess the risk of idiopathic venous thromboembolism in relation to the Yuzpe regimen of postcoital pill.

METHOD. This study reviewed the incidence of deep vein thrombosis and pulmonary embolism in a cohort of 73 302 women less than 50 years of age who collectively received 100 615 prescriptions for postcoital pills as per the Yuzpe regimen at some time between 1 January 1989 and 31 October 1996.

RESULTS. There were no women with idiopathic venous thromboembolism within current exposure to postcoital pills, i.e. within 45 days of using Schering, PC4. The incidence rates for venous thromboembolism were 0/100 000 person-years (95% CI 0–30.9) for current postcoital pill users, 5.3/100 000 person-years (95% CI 1.4–19.2) for second generation oral contraceptive pill users, 10.7/100 000 person-years (95% CI 4.9–23.3) for third generation oral contraceptive users, and 15.5/100 000 person-years (95% CI 6.6–36.3) for women who were pregnant or postpartum. The incidence rate of venous thromboembolism in unexposed women was 3.0/100 000 person-years (95% CI 1.4–6.6).

INTERPRETATION. Short-term use of postcoital pills is not associated with an increased risk of venous thromboembolism.

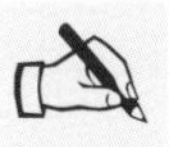

Meclizine for prevention of nausea associated with use of emergency contraceptive pills—a randomised trial.

EG Raymond, MD Creinin, KT Barnhart, AE Lovvorn, RW Rountree, J Trussell. *Obstet Gynecol* 2000; **95**(2): 271–7.

BACKGROUND. The Yuzpe regimen is associated with a high incidence of nausea and vomiting. Pretreatment with an anti-emetic may help prevent these problems. This randomized controlled trial was conducted to determine whether pretreatment with meclizine reduced the incidence of nausea and vomiting associated with the Yuzpe regimen.

METHOD. A total of 343 women aged 18–45 years who were not at risk of pregnancy were randomly assigned to pretreatment with 50 mg of meclizine, placebo or no drug 1 h before the first two doses of emergency contraceptive pills. The participants were asked to complete a questionnaire at 12, 24 and 48 h after the first dose of emergency contraceptive pills.

RESULTS. The incidence of nausea was 47% in the group pretreated with meclizine and 64% in the other two groups (relative risk adjusted for centre 0.7, 95% CI 0.6–0.9 for comparison of meclizine with both placebo and no drug). The severity of the nausea and the incidence of vomiting were also significantly lower in the meclizine pretreatment group than in the other two groups. Drowsiness was twice as common in this group (31%) compared with the other groups (13% in the placebo group, 16% in the no pretreatment group; *P* < 0.01 for both comparisons).

INTERPRETATION. Meclizine is effective for the prevention of nausea and vomiting associated with the Yuzpe regimen. Women using this drug should be cautioned to anticipate drowsiness.

Summary

The main concern with the issue of the safety of the Yuzpe regimen is in relation to cardiovascular disease, particularly venous thromboembolism, because of a tendency to extrapolate from data associated with the combined pill, as the total dose of ethinyloestradiol is six times that of a single low-dose combined oral contraceptive pill |**3**|. This risk is not borne out in studies. Similarly, there have been no serious adverse effects with levonorgestrel in the two published studies |**6, 9**|. Mifepristone too has an extremely reassuring safety profile with no serious risks associated with its use |**3**|.

Awareness and accessibility

The UK has been a leader in the provision of emergency contraception with exponential growth in prescriptions since the mid-1980s |**10**|. Emergency contraception was prescribed by National Health Service clinics on 240 000 occasions in 1999–2000, an increase of 10% over 1998–1999 |**11**|, indicating increasing awareness.

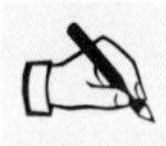

Emergency contraception: change in knowledge of women attending for termination of pregnancy from 1984 to 1996.

AF Gordon, P Owen. *Br J Fam Plann* 1999; **24**: 121–2.

B ACKGROUND. **The objective of this study was to compare the knowledge of emergency contraception in women attending a hospital for termination of pregnancy in 1984 and 1996.**

M ETHOD. **The knowledge of emergency contraception of cohorts of 100 consecutive women undergoing termination of pregnancy in 1984 and 1996 at the Ninewells Hospital, Dundee, UK was evaluated via a questionnaire.**

R ESULTS. **Over this 12-year period, there was a significant improvement in the knowledge of emergency contraception. Seventy-three per cent had a good knowledge of the postcoital pill in 1996 compared with 12% in 1984 ($P < 0.0001$). Although most women in the 1996 cohort recognized a reason for contraceptive failure and had adequate knowledge of emergency contraception, only 17% considered the possibility of pregnancy.**

I NTERPRETATION. Poor knowledge of postcoital contraception is no longer a major factor leading to the failure of women to obtain emergency contraception. Improved uptake in the use of emergency contraception is likely to result from a greater awareness of the possibility of condom failure and easier availability of the emergency methods.

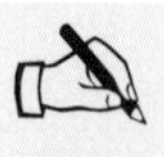

Access to emergency contraception.

J Trussell, V Duran, T Schochet, K Moore. *Obstet Gynecol* 2000; **95**(2): 267–70.

B ACKGROUND. **The objective of this study was to evaluate access to emergency contraception among women seeking help from clinicians who registered to be listed**

on the toll-free Emergency Contraception Hotline and the Website operated by the Reproductive Health Technologies Project and the Office of Population Research at Princeton University, USA.

METHOD. Two investigators posing as women who had a condom break the previous night called 200 providers to seek help.

RESULTS. Only 76% of attempts resulted in an appointment or telephone prescription from a hotline provider within 72 h, 14% were failures, and 11% resulted in referrals to other providers not listed on the hotline or Website.

INTERPRETATION. Even under ideal conditions, access to emergency contraception is constrained. The potential for emergency contraception to reduce the incidence of unintended pregnancies will not be realized unless women have better access to emergency contraceptive pills.

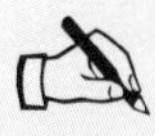

Concerns and cautions about prescribing and deregulating emergency contraception: a qualitative study of GPs using telephone interviews.

S Ziebland, A Graham, A McPherson. *Fam Pract* 1998; **15**(5): 449–56.

BACKGROUND. The objective of this study was to describe general practitioners' responses to a clinical scenario of a request for a repeat prescription for hormonal emergency contraception, their views about over the counter availability and beliefs about absolute contraindications.

METHOD. Semi-structured tape-recorded telephone interviews were conducted with 76 general practitioners randomly selected from three Health Authorities which were chosen for high, medium and low prescribing rates for emergency contraception.

RESULTS. The response rate was 71–76%. There was a wide variation in the number of times that general practitioners would be happy to prescribe emergency contraception to the same woman in a year. The content of the consultations appeared patchy. While 77.6% of the general practitioners said that they would discuss future contraception with the woman, only 21.1% said they would talk about possible side-effects and 36.3% would discuss the timing of the next menstrual period and the possibility of method failure. Fifty-two of the practices had a family planning-trained practice nurse, yet only four (7.7%) had arrangements whereby the nurse could provide emergency contraception. Unqualified enthusiasm for deregulation was rare. Concerns included that women would lose out on the benefits of the consultation; worries about the safety of the method; that some women might 'abuse' it by using it frequently; and that certain characteristics of the pharmacy might make it an unsuitable setting for the provision of emergency contraception.

INTERPRETATION. This study revealed concerns about repeated use of emergency contraception and caution about the prospects of deregulation. Family planning-trained nurses are an under-utilized resource in the provision of emergency contraception.

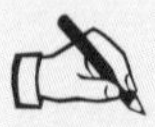

Repeated use of hormonal emergency contraception by younger women in the UK.

S Rowlands, L Ross, J Logie, B Ineichen. *Br J Fam Plann* 2000; **26**(3): 138–43.

BACKGROUND. The objectives of this study were to establish how common repeated use of emergency contraception is in younger women in general practice and to relate this to subsequent establishment of regular contraception.

METHOD. A cohort of women aged 14–29 years in 1993 was identified from the UK General Practice Research Database and followed-up for a period of 4 years. Patient files were searched for evidence of use of emergency and regular contraception.

RESULTS. Of the 95 007 women, 15 105 (16%) had received emergency contraception during the study period (average 5% per year). There was a small year on year increase in uptake of emergency contraception between 1994 and 1997. Only 4% of emergency contraception users received emergency contraception more than twice in any year. More than 70% of those who had no previous record of use of regular contraception used regular contraception within 1 year of using emergency contraception. Teenagers were more likely than other age groups to use emergency contraception, to be repeat users of emergency contraception and to fail to start regular contraception after first use of emergency contraception until later in the study period.

INTERPRETATION. These results disprove the notion of widespread repeated use of emergency contraception. They show that the provision of emergency contraception does not result in failure to initiate regular contraception or abandonment of regular contraception; rather, they show many women using regular contraception for the first time after use of emergency contraception.

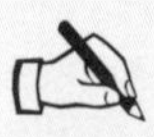

Questionnaire study of use of emergency contraception among teenagers.

E Kosunen, A Vikat, M Rimpela, A Rimpela, H Huhtala. *Br Med J* 1999; **319**: 91.

BACKGROUND. The objective of this study was to determine the knowledge of emergency contraception and frequency of its use among teenage school pupils in 96 municipalities in Finland using a structured questionnaire survey.

RESULTS. There were 52 700 respondents. Only 3% of the 14–15 year olds and 1.5% of the 17 year olds did not know what emergency contraception was. The proportion of girls between 14 and 17 years who had used emergency contraception increased with age from 2.1 to 15.1%. Over two-thirds of all girls who had used emergency contraception had done so only once.

INTERPRETATION. The adolescent girls were widely aware of emergency contraception, although this may not indicate their knowledge of details of its use. Emergency contraception had not become a contraceptive choice replacing conventional methods among adolescents. Only a small proportion had used it repeatedly. These results suggest that easy access to contraceptive services (including emergency contraception) and intensive sex education did not increase adolescent sexual activity.

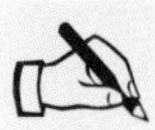

Barriers to the use of IUDs as emergency contraception.

S Reuter. *Br J Fam Plann* 1999; **25**: 63–8.

BACKGROUND. This study was conducted to evaluate potential barriers to the use of the IUD as emergency contraception.

METHOD. A postal survey of 100 family planning doctors and 100 general practitioners was conducted in the Trent Region, UK, during March 1998.

RESULTS. The response rate was 70%. Lack of time was the most important factor that influenced doctors' decisions not to offer IUDs to the majority of women requesting emergency contraception. Most doctors registered concern about the risk of pelvic inflammatory disease. Other barriers identified were cost, lack of swab-taking facilities and instruments, need for a chaperone, training issues, misconceptions and a lack of accurate information.

INTERPRETATION. Considerable effort would be required to increase doctors' knowledge and willingness to offer IUDs routinely to women requesting emergency contraception.

Summary

An important component of programmes promoting emergency contraception is providing women with information about this option before they need it, because the time-frame for seeking treatment is short. Women need to know where to seek services and understand that it must be started within 3 days of unprotected sexual intercourse. Women in most developed countries have heard about a morning after pill, but most know little more. Many health care providers are themselves poorly informed on this issue. Lack of knowledge among women and difficulties in access contribute to a great extent to the widespread underuse of emergency contraception.

Health professionals' concerns about safety of repeated use are not justified.

Self-administration of emergency contraception

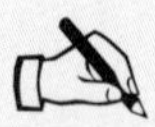

The effects of self-administering emergency contraception.

A Glasier, D Baird. *New Eng J Med* 1998; **339**(1): 1–4.

BACKGROUND. This study was conducted to learn how women might behave if given a supply of emergency contraceptive pills to keep at home.

METHOD. This study was set in a family planning clinic and a large hospital in Edinburgh, UK and was conducted between January 1994 and December 1996. Five hundred and fifty-three women were assigned to be given a replaceable supply of hormonal emergency contraceptive pills to take home (the treatment group) and 530 women were assigned to use emergency contraception obtained by visiting a doctor (the control group). The women were assigned to the treatment or control groups on the basis of their dates of birth (women whose birthdays fell on even-numbered days were assigned to the treatment group). The frequency of use of emergency contraception, the use of other contraceptives, and the incidence of unwanted pregnancy were determined in both groups of women 1 year later.

RESULTS. Results were available for 549 women in the treatment group and 522 women in the control group. A total of 180 of the women in the treatment group (47%) used emergency contraception at least once. Among those who returned the questionnaire, 98% used it correctly. Eighty-seven of the women in the control group (27%) used emergency contraception at least once. Statistically this difference was highly significant ($P < 0.001$). The women in the treatment group were not more likely to use emergency contraception repeatedly. Their use of other methods of contraception was no different from that of the women in the control group. There were 18 unintended pregnancies in the treatment group and 25 in the control group (relative risk 0.7, 95% CI 0.4–1.2).

INTERPRETATION. The findings suggest that making emergency contraception more easily obtainable does no harm and may reduce the rate of unwanted pregnancies. A criticism of over the counter emergency contraception is that women will use it instead of more reliable methods. However, that concern was not borne out in this study. The results show that women can use the medication correctly without untoward effects.

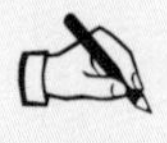

Emergency contraception: advance provision in a young, high-risk clinic population.

T Raine, C Harper, K Leon, P Darney. *Obstet Gynaecol* 2000; **96**(1): 1–7.

BACKGROUND. The aims of this study were to assess whether advance provision of emergency contraception increases its use and whether it has secondary effects on regular contraceptive use.

METHOD. This was a controlled trial involving a culturally diverse group of adolescents and high-risk young women aged 16–24 years attending the family planning clinic in San Francisco between June and November 1998, who were systematically assigned to receive an advance provision of emergency contraception and education (treatment) or education only (control). The main outcome measures were emergency contraception knowledge and use, frequency of unprotected sex, and pattern of contraceptive use in the past 4 months.

RESULTS. Among the 263 participants enrolled, follow-up was completed in 213. The participants were aware of emergency contraception at follow-up, but the treatment group was three times more likely to use it ($P = 0.006$). Although the treatment group did not report higher frequencies of unprotected sex than the control group, women in the treatment group (28%) were more likely than those in the control group (17%) to report using less effective contraception at follow-up compared with enrolment ($P = 0.05$). The proportion of women in both groups who reported consistent pill use increased from enrolment to follow-up (34 versus 45%). However, the control group (58%) was more likely than the treatment group (32%) to report consistent pill use at follow-up ($P = 0.03$).

INTERPRETATION. The authors concluded that use of emergency contraception was increased by providing it in advance, but not by education alone. Of concern, however, is the finding that significantly more women in the treatment group reported using less effective contraceptive methods at follow-up. A positive finding was that there was no significant increase in the proportion of women in the treatment group who reported unprotected sex or a decrease in consistent condom use at follow-up.

Ongoing study

A much larger 2-year research project in which all women between the ages of 16 and 29 years living in one health board area of Scotland (over 85 000 women) are being offered supplies of emergency contraception to keep at home, is ongoing to see if improving the availability of emergency contraception will reduce unplanned pregnancies and lower the abortion rate |12|.

Changes in legislation—wider availability of emergency contraception |13|

Recognizing that emergency contraception is safe and that the benefits of easier access almost certainly outweigh the risks |3|, the beginning of the 21st century has witnessed a change in legislation making hormonal emergency contraception available for women aged 16 years and above in the UK to buy from pharmacists without a prescription. This is the result of an application to the Medicines Control Agency to change the legal status of levonorgestrel 0.75 mg from a prescription-only medicine to a pharmacy medicine. The Committee on Safety of Medicines and the Medicines Commission had advised in favour of the application. This advice and the result of a public consultation exercise were put to UK ministers who approved the change.

The order came into effect on 1 January 2001. It reclassified progestogen-only emergency contraception to pharmacy availability for women aged 16 years and over.

Pharmacists are required to develop links into existing networks for family planning services so that under 16s and other women that need to see a doctor can be referred on quickly. Up to date information on these services including location, hours of opening and services provided must be made available in every pharmacy.

In some areas, pharmacies are already supplying emergency contraception free of charge under the National Health Service using a patient group direction. Although pharmacy supply will require women to pay, it will provide an additional point of access to emergency contraception. This will be particularly useful at weekends and evenings when other services might not be available. However, the cost of the emergency hormonal contraceptive is too high at £19.99 and this may deter those who would most benefit from it. Hormonal emergency contraception will remain free of charge on prescription for women of all ages including under 16s, from general practitioners, family planning clinics, youth clinics and some genito-urinary medicine and accident and emergency departments.

Summary

Major shifts in emergency contraception service provision in the UK, such as access via nurses |**14**|, pharmacists |**15**| working to protocols, prescribing emergency contraception in advance |**12, 16**| and pharmacist availability status will hopefully increase accessibility of emergency contraception. Strategies to increase awareness about emergency contraception should focus on health professionals, encouraging them to discuss emergency contraception as part of routine contraceptive counselling |**17**|. A consistent approach to the provision of postcoital contraception by different health professionals would enable more women to prevent unplanned pregnancies |**18**|.

References

1. Van Look PFA, Von Hertzen H. Induced abortion: a global perspective. In: Baird DT, Grimes DA, Van Look PFA (eds): *Modern Methods of Inducing Abortion*. Blackwell Science, Oxford, 1995, pp. 1–24.

2. Trussell J, Stewart F. The effectiveness of postcoital contraception. *Fam Plann Perspect* 1992; **24**: 262–4.

3. Glasier A. Emergency contraception. *Br Med Bull* 2000; **56**(3): 729–38.

4. UNDP/UNFPA/WHO/World Bank Special Programme of Research, Development and Research Training in Human Reproduction (HRP). Improving methods of emergency contraception. *Prog Hum Reprod Res* 1999; **51**: 1–8.

5. Yuzpe AA, Lancee WJ. Ethinylestradiol and DL-norgestrel as a postcoital contraceptive. *Fertil Steril* 1977; **28**: 932–6.

6. Ho PC, Kwan MSW. A prospective randomised comparison of levonorgestrel with the Yuzpe regimen in post-coital contraception. *Hum Reprod* 1993; **8**: 389–92.

7. Trussell J, Ellertson C. Efficacy of emergency contraception. *Fertil Contr Rev* 1995; **4**: 8–11.

8. Dixon GW, Schlesselman JJ, Ory HW, *et al.* Ethinyl estradiol and conjugated oestrogens as post-coital contraceptives. *J Am Med Assoc* 1980; **244**(12): 1336–9.

9. WHO Task Force on Postovulatory Methods of Fertility Regulation. Randomised controlled trial of levonorgestrel versus the Yuzpe regimen of combined oral contraceptives for emergency contraception. *Lancet* 1998; **352**: 428–33.

10. O'Brien PA. Emergency contraception with levonorgestrel: one hormone better than two. *Br J Fam Plann* 2000; **26**(2): 67–9.

11. Department of Health Statistical Bulletin, October 2000, p. 27. HM Government Statistical Service.

12. Christie B. Project makes emergency pill more available. *Br Med J* 1999; **319**: 661.

13. Duncan A, Howe J, Smith C. Improving access to emergency contraception. *Br Med J* 2001; **322**: 186–7.

14. Brittain D. Establishing an educational programme for nurses to supply emergency hormonal contraception (combined method) to protocol. *Br J Fam Plann* 1999; **25**: 118–21.

15. O'Brien K, Gray N. Supplying emergency hormonal contraception in Manchester under a group prescribing protocol. *Pharm J* 2000; **264**: 518–9.

16. BPAS Press Release. Emergency contraception: before the emergency, 8 July 1999.

17. Delbanco SF, Mauldon J, Smith MD. Little knowledge and limited practice: emergency contraceptive pills, the public, and the obstetrician-gynaecologist. *Obstet Gynaecol* 1997; **89**(6): 1006–11.

18. Walsh J. Policies and practices in postcoital contraceptive provision: a survey of general practitioners and hospital A&E departments. *Br J Fam Plann* 1995; **20**: 121–5.

Appendix

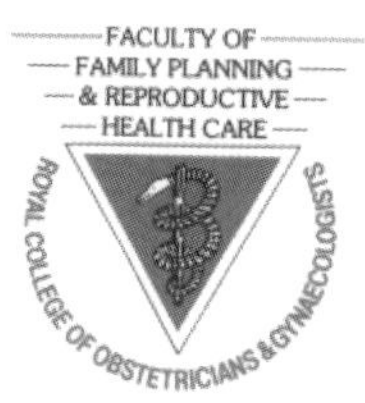

Faculty of Family Planning and Reproductive Health Care, Royal College of Obstetricians and Gynaecologists, Guidance April 2000, Emergency Contraception: Recommendations for Clinical Practice

This document is based on previous recommendations for practice issued by the Faculty of Family Planning and Reproductive Health Care [1, 2].

This document has been published to disseminate information about currently licensed emergency contraceptive methods and about research findings that are immediately relevant to professional practice in the UK. Fully revised recommendations for clinical practice will be available from the faculty in 2001.

Methods currently licensed in the UK: progestogen-only (Levonelle-2™), combined oestrogen–progestogen (Schering® PC4) and the copper IUD

Emergency contraception (also called postcoital contraception) is a safe and effective way of preventing an accidental pregnancy after unprotected sex. There are three emergency contraceptive methods licensed for use in the UK: two oral hormonal preparations and the postcoital insertion of a copper-containing IUD.

Efficacy of emergency contraceptive methods

Because many women treated with emergency contraception would not have become pregnant even without treatment, describing the overall effectiveness of the method is complex.

The overall risk of pregnancy after a single act of unprotected sex on any day in the menstrual cycle is 2–4%. The pregnancy risk from a single act of intercourse is highest (between 20–30%) in the days before and just after ovulation. Counting the first day of menstrual bleeding as day 1, the pregnancy risk is low before day 7 and after day 17 inclusive in a 28-day cycle. Adjusting for shorter and longer cycles displaces these estimated fertile days earlier and later, respectively, within the cycle.

The efficacy of emergency contraceptive methods as demonstrated in clinical trials can be described in two ways:

(a) Expressed as a failure rate, i.e. citing the proportion of women who become pregnant despite using the method. This approach includes as treatment successes all women who had treatment and did not become pregnant in that cycle, many of whom would not have become pregnant even without treatment.

(b) Expressed as the ratio of observed to expected pregnancies, i.e. estimating the number of pregnancies expected without treatment from the menstrual and coital histories of all women in the trial, and comparing this number with the actual number of pregnancies occurring after treatment.

Both of these approaches obviously rely on accurate recollection of the date of the last menstrual period and coital history.

Oral hormonal emergency contraception

There are two different types of emergency contraceptive pill, progestogen-only and combined oestrogen–progestogen. Both are currently prescription-only medicines, licensed solely for emergency contraceptive use within 72 h of exposure to risk of pregnancy.

While emergency contraceptive pills are effective when treatment is started within 72 h, available evidence from a WHO trial strongly suggests that hormonal emergency contraceptive regimens are most effective in preventing pregnancy when the first dose is taken within 24 h of unprotected sex. As the coitus to treatment interval increases (towards the 72 h limit), the failure rate increases [3, 4]. Calculation of the coitus to treatment interval starts from the time of the first episode of unprotected sex in the current menstrual cycle.

Emergency contraceptive pills do not protect against pregnancy for the remainder of the menstrual cycle. Women who use emergency contraceptive pills must use an effective method of contraception, or abstain from sex, for the remainder of the menstrual cycle after using emergency contraception. For women using regular combined or progestogen-only pills, contraceptive cover is restored when seven pills have been taken on consecutive days after using emergency contraception. Women who have used emergency contraception because of missed pills should continue to take their regular contraceptive pills as usual, and must use an additional (i.e. barrier) method of contraception if they have sex within 7 days of the first dose of emergency contraception.

Timing of the next menses after treatment

Research has demonstrated a range of disturbances in the timing of the next reported menses after both types of oral hormonal emergency contraception. A recent study found that most women (57%) started their next period within 3 days of their expected date, some (15%) started early, some (15%) were up to 7 days late and the remainder (13%) were more than 7 days late |3|. It is important to advise women to return for a pregnancy test if they are more than 7 days late with their expected next period. Some intermenstrual bleeding may occur before the next menses after hormonal emergency contraception |5|.

Some bleeding between menses is common after IUD insertion. There is no evidence that the timing of the next menses is altered after postcoital insertion.

Principal indications for emergency contraception

There is no day of the menstrual cycle when a clinician can be certain that unprotected sex would not result in pregnancy, particularly if the woman reports having irregular periods or is unsure of her dates. Where there is anxiety, consider treating rather than waiting to see what happens.

Unprotected sex

- Consensual sex, no contraceptive method used.
- Rape or sexual assault with risk of pregnancy.
- Coitus interruptus/failed coitus interruptus.
- Ejaculation on external genitalia.

Potential barrier method failures

- Condom rupture, dislodgement or misuse.
- Diaphragm/cap inserted incorrectly, torn, dislodged during intercourse, removed too early.

Potential pill failure when alternative methods not used/failed

Efficacy of regular (non-emergency) combined or progestogen-only contraceptive pills compromised, e.g. unprotected sex/failure of barrier method within 7 days after:

Combined pills:

- two or more pills missed from the first seven pills in a packet, or
- four or more pills missed mid-packet.

If two or more combined pills are missed from the last seven pills in a packet, emergency contraception is not necessary provided that the pill-free break is omitted, i.e. the woman starts her next packet of pills the day after finishing the current packet.

Progestogen-only pills:

- one or more pills taken more than 3 h after the usual pill-taking time, or missed.

Potential IUD failure

- Complete or partial expulsion of an IUD.
- Mid-cycle IUD removal considered absolutely necessary.

Risk of conception while advised to avoid pregnancy

- Following administration of cytotoxic drugs or potentially teratogenic agents.

Progestogen-only emergency contraceptive pills

The Committee on Safety of Medicines approved the progestogen-only emergency contraceptive pill formulation Levonelle-2™ (Schering Health Care Ltd) for use in the UK in 1999. One pack of Levonelle-2™ consists of two tablets, each containing a 750 µg dose of levonorgestrel. The first dose (one tablet) must be taken within 72 h of unprotected intercourse, and within 24 h for best effect. The second dose is taken 12 h after the first.

Efficacy [3]

The 1998 WHO trial demonstrated that this progestogen-only emergency contraceptive regimen prevented 86% of expected pregnancies when treatment was initiated within 72 h of unprotected sex.

Effect of coitus to treatment interval [3, 4]

Coitus to treatment interval	Percentage of expected pregnancies prevented
24 h or less	95
25–48 h	85
49–72 h	58

The pregnancy rate found for women who reported no further intercourse between treatment and next menses (0.8%; 5/602) was considerably lower than for those who had further unprotected intercourse or used barriers (1.6%; 6/372).

Commonly reported side-effects—nausea and vomiting [3]

The WHO trial found that 23.1% of women who used the progestogen-only regimen experienced nausea, and 5.6% reported vomiting.

Eligibility criteria for use [6, 7]

Established pregnancy contraindicates use. The WHO considers that, on currently available evidence, there are no other medical contraindications to the use of emergency contraceptive pills and that, because the dose of hormones is relatively small and the pills are used for a short period of time, the contraindications associated with regular use of progestogen-only pills do not apply to progestogen-only emergency contraceptive pills.

While provision of contraceptive steroids to some women (i.e. those with particular medical conditions or risk factors) requires careful consideration and precautionary measures, the benefits of using progestogen-only emergency contraception will generally outweigh the risks. The summary of product characteristics for Levonelle-2™ includes severe hypertension, diabetes mellitus associated with vascular complications or neuropathy, ischaemic heart disease, stroke or a past history of breast cancer as relative contraindications.

It is highly unlikely that progestogen-only emergency contraceptive pills would have an adverse effect on a continuing pregnancy. However, a normal outcome to any pregnancy cannot be guaranteed.

Combined oestrogen–progestogen emergency contraceptive pills

The Committee on Safety of Medicines approved the combined oestrogen–progestogen emergency contraceptive pill formulation Schering® PC4 (Schering Health Care Ltd) in 1984.

One pack of Schering® PC4 consists of four tablets, each containing 50 μg of ethinylestradiol plus 500 μg of norgestrel (equivalent to 250 μg of levonorgestrel). The first dose (two tablets taken together) must be taken within 72 h of unprotected intercourse, and within 24 h for best effect. The second dose of two tablets is taken 12 h after the first.

Efficacy |3, 8|

A 1999 review of efficacy studies estimated that the combined oestrogen–progestogen regimen prevents at least 74% of expected pregnancies when treatment is initiated within 72 h |8|, whereas the 1998 WHO trial found that the combined oestrogen–progestogen regimen prevented 57% of expected pregnancies when treatment was initiated within 72 h |3|. This difference is probably due to slightly different methodologies being used in the calculation of conception probabilities, and is being investigated.

Effect of coitus to treatment interval |3, 4|

The 1998 WHO trial found that the combined oestrogen–progestogen regimen was more effective when treatment was initiated within 24 h of unprotected sex.

Coitus to treatment interval	Percentage of expected pregnancies prevented
24 h or less	77
25–48 h	36
49–72 h	31

The pregnancy rate found for women who reported no further intercourse between treatment and next menses (1.9%; 12/619) was considerably lower than for those who had further unprotected intercourse or used barriers (5.3%; 19/360).

Commonly reported side-effects—nausea and vomiting |3|

The WHO trial found that 50.5% of women who used the combined oestrogen–progestogen regimen experienced nausea, and 18.8% reported vomiting.

Eligibility criteria for use |6, 7|

Established pregnancy contraindicates use. The WHO considers that, on currently available evidence, there are no other medical contraindications to the use of emergency contraceptive pills and that, because the dose of hormones is relatively small and the pills are used for a short period of time, the contraindications associated with regular use of combined oral contraceptives do not apply to combined emergency contraceptive pills. No evidence was found that this method increases the risk of ectopic pregnancy above the woman's pre-existing risk.

The current summary of product characteristics for Schering® PC4 includes a history of severe cardiovascular complications, acute focal migraine, severe liver disease and a possible relative increase in ectopic pregnancy amongst other conditions as contraindications or precautions for use.

It is highly unlikely that combined oestrogen–progestogen emergency contraceptive pills would have an adverse effect on a continuing pregnancy. However, a normal outcome to any pregnancy cannot be guaranteed.

Intrauterine emergency contraception

A copper-containing IUD is inserted in the usual way within 5 days (120 h) of unprotected sex, at any time in the menstrual cycle. Where the earliest episode of unprotected sex was more than 5 days previously an IUD can be fitted, in good faith, up to 5 days after the calculated earliest day of ovulation (i.e. up to day 19 of a 28-day shortest cycle by history, counting the first day of menstrual bleeding as day 1).

Providers should be aware of the risk of postinsertion pelvic infection, and must consider testing women for sexually transmitted infection, particularly *Chlamydia trachomatis*. If positive, appropriate follow-up and contact tracing should be arranged. Antibiotic cover is advisable where a sexually transmitted infection risk is identified and where testing is unavailable or not practical.

The levonorgestrel-releasing intrauterine system, Mirena®, is not recommended for postcoital use.

Efficacy

The copper IUD has the highest efficacy of any currently available emergency contraceptive, and is the method of choice where efficacy is the priority. From the number of reported pregnancies following postcoital copper IUD insertion, the failure rate has been estimated to be no higher than 0.1% |**9**|.

Side-effects

As associated with IUDs fitted for ongoing contraception. An IUD fitted post-coitally can be removed at the beginning of menstruation if the woman does not wish to continue to use it.

Eligibility criteria for use |**6, 7**|

Established pregnancy contraindicates use. The WHO considers that the same eligibility criteria that apply to insertion of a copper IUD in routine circumstances should be applied for insertion as an emergency contraceptive. Providers should be aware of the contraindications and precautions listed by the manufacturer in the data sheet/summary of product characteristics, including known hypersensitivity to product components.

Failure of a postcoital IUD is highly unlikely |**9**|. The risks and benefits of gently removing the device (if easily accessible) should be discussed if a woman who is pregnant despite postcoital IUD fitting chooses to continue her pregnancy |**10**|.

The management of a request for emergency contraception

1. Estimate likely date of ovulation and risk of pregnancy by recording

- usual length of menstrual cycle;
- did the last period start at the expected time and was it shorter or lighter than usual?
- timing of all inadequately protected intercourse (including any missed pill history and intercourse during a lengthened pill-free interval)—which day(s) of the current cycle?

2. Calculate the number of hours since the first episode of unprotected intercourse

3. Identify any contraindications to emergency contraceptive methods and conditions which require consideration and/or precautionary measures

Note: Pelvic examination cannot be justified routinely to exclude pregnancy. If the date or character of the last menstrual period and recent coital history give cause for concern, urine hCG estimation will give a more sensitive and specific diagnosis.

4. Explain method options

If less than 72 h since unprotected sex, offer emergency contraceptive pills or copper IUD. Explain:

- mode of action;
- efficacy;
- risks and side-effects;
- possible effect on menstrual cycle;
- if emergency contraceptive pills are used, need to abstain from sex or use a barrier method correctly and consistently for the remainder of the current menstrual cycle;
- the importance of follow-up if next period does not start within 7 days of the expected date;
- that, while there is no evidence that emergency contraceptive methods carry any risk of teratogenicity, a normal outcome to any pregnancy cannot be guaranteed.

If oral hormonal emergency contraception chosen, advise:

- when pills should be taken;
- what to do if either dose of pills is vomited within 2 h.

Domperidone maleate 10 mg may be prescribed to counter acute nausea and vomiting. This preparation does not readily cross the blood–brain barrier and is less likely to cause extra-pyramidal side-effects than metoclopramide or the phenothiazines.

If more than 72 h since unprotected sex, explain and offer copper IUD.

5. Document, sign and date an accurate record

Document the consultation and the woman's decision regarding emergency contraception after full discussion backed by written information such as the Family Planning Association leaflet.

6. Discuss ongoing contraception and offer follow-up

Future contraception must be discussed sympathetically, and preferably arranged for the time until the next menses if an IUD has not been used, and for the next cycles as appropriate. Women who have taken emergency hormonal contraception because of missed pills should discard any missed tablets and the tablet for the day of postcoital treatment. They should then continue to take their pills as usual, and be warned that they will not be contraceptively covered until they have taken seven tablets on consecutive days at the correct time. If women wish to start using the combined or progestogen-only pill, these may be started on the first day of the subsequent period without additional precautions. Depot medroxyprogesterone acetate can be started up to day 5 of the next menstrual cycle without additional precautions.

- Advise when she can expect her next period. Advise her to seek immediate help if the bleeding is significantly different from her usual period, especially if the period is exceptionally short or light (i.e. possible failed treatment) and how to contact such help.

- Offer appointment/explain arrangements for seeking advice if she experiences any other problems or concerns about treatment.

- Offer appointment/explain arrangements for ongoing contraceptive information/supply as necessary.

- Offer appointment/make arrangements for communication of infection screen results and IUD removal if not required for ongoing contraception.

References

1. Kubba A, Wilkinson C. Recommendations for clinical practice: emergency contraception. Clinical and Scientific Committee, Faculty of Family Planning and Reproductive Health Care. November 1998 update.

2. Recommendations for clinical practice: emergency contraception. Faculty of Family Planning and Reproductive Health Care. October 1999 update.

3. Randomised controlled trial of levonorgestrel versus the Yuzpe regimen of combined oral contraceptives for emergency contraception. Task Force on Postovulatory Methods of Fertility Regulation. *Lancet* 1998; **352**: 428–33.

4. Piaggio G, von Hertzen H, Grimes DA, Van Look PF. Timing of emergency contraception with levonorgestrel or the Yuzpe regimen. Task Force on Postovulatory Methods of Fertility Regulation. *Lancet* 1999; **353**: 721.

5. He CH, Shi YE, Xu JQ Van Look PF. A multicenter clinical study on two types of levonorgestrel tablets administered for post-coital contraception. *Int J Gynaecol Obstet* 1991; **36**(1): 43–8.

6. World Health Organization. *Emergency Contraception: a Guide to Service Delivery.* WHO, Geneva, 1998.

7. World Health Organization. *Improving Access to Quality Care in Family Planning: Medical Eligibility Criteria for Contraceptive Use.* WHO, Geneva, 1996.

8. Trussell J, *et al.* Updated estimates of the effectiveness of the Yuzpe regimen of emergency contraception. *Contraception* 1999; **59**: 147–51.

9. Van Look P, Stewart F. Emergency contraception. In: Hatcher R, *et al.* (eds): *Contraceptive Technology*, 17th revised edn. Ardent Media, New York, 1998.

10. World Health Organization. *Mechanism of Action, Safety and Efficacy of Intrauterine Devices.* WHO, Geneva, 1987.

Part II

The menopause

5

New developments in osteoporosis

Introduction

Osteoporosis is a major cause of morbidity and mortality in the Western world. As women are living longer, it has become more common to make a diagnosis of osteoporosis in postmenopausal women. One in three women surviving to the age of 80 years will suffer a hip fracture. Following a hip fracture there is a 5–20% mortality within 1 year, 20% have severely impaired mobility after 12 months which requires long-term nursing care and 50% never regain their previous mobility. The cost to the National Health Service has been estimated to be £700 million per year [1].

The incidence of osteoporotic fractures increases with age. As life expectancy increases, the incidence of osteoporosis will increase; this will obviously have major implications for health care provision and funding in the future.

There have been several improvements in the treatment of osteoporosis in recent years which have enhanced the range of therapeutic options available to the clinician.

However, there has been a shift in emphasis in the treatment and prevention of osteoporosis. Prevention of fracture is now considered the gold standard, and raises the question of how increasing bone mineral density (BMD) correlates with a reduction in fracture risk.

Definition

Osteoporosis is currently defined as a 'progressive systemic skeletal disease characterized by low bone mass and microarchitectural deterioration of bone tissue, with a consequent increase in bone fragility and susceptibility to fracture' [2]. The World Health Organization (WHO) has defined thresholds for diagnostic purposes in women based on BMD (T scores) [3].

A 'T score' is the number of standard deviations (SD) the bone mineral content (BMC) or BMD is below the young adult mean reference.

Normal	BMC or BMD < 1 SD below the young adult mean reference
Low bone mass	BMC or BMD 1–2.5 SD below the young adult mean reference
Osteoporosis	BMC or BMD > 2.5 SD below the young adult mean reference
Severe osteoporosis	BMC or BMD > 2.5 SD below the young adult mean reference and the presence of one or more fragility fractures

The risk of fracture increases approximately two-fold for each standard deviation decrease in BMD. However, in addition to BMD, there are other considerations to be made when assessing a person's risk of developing osteoporosis, such as diet, family history, concurrent medication and likelihood of falls.

Pathology

The most important predisposing factor for the development of osteoporosis is low bone mass. This depends upon the peak bone mass achieved between the ages of 20 and 30 years and upon the rate of subsequent loss. Bone is continually undergoing change. In normal circumstances each remodelling cycle is balanced so that resorption of bone occurs at the same rate as formation of bone. Bone resorption always precedes bone formation. This remodelling cycle usually takes between 90 and 130 days.

There are two mechanisms of bone loss:

(1) An increase in activation frequency results in increased bone turnover as a result of a greater number of bone remodelling units on the bone surface. This is the most important mechanism of bone loss in osteoporosis, but it is potentially reversible.

(2) A change within individual bone remodelling units is called remodelling imbalance and this occurs when the amount of bone formed is less than the amount of bone resorbed. This can be due to an increase in the amount of bone resorbed, or a decrease in the amount of bone formed, or a combination of the two. This is an irreversible form of bone loss.

In osteoporosis, these two mechanisms of bone loss co-exist. This ultimately leads to thinning of the bone and an increase in susceptibility to fracture.

Risk factors

Factors affecting peak bone mass include:

- genetic determinants (the most important factor);
- hormonal influences, such as adequate and timely secretion of sex steroids or amenorrhoea during reproductive age;
- diet (adequate calcium);
- exercise (balanced physical activity can optimize BMD).

Factors affecting bone loss:

- premature menopause/amenorrhoea during reproductive age;
- family history (genetic component);

- steroid therapy;
- thyrotoxicosis;
- low body weight;
- cigarette smoking;
- excess alcohol intake;
- dietary factors, e.g. low intake of calcium or vitamin D;
- physical inactivity;
- high caffeine intake.

Oestrogen deficiency is a major cause of bone loss in women during the peri- and postmenopausal period. Osteoporosis is a much more common disease in women and in the past prevention and treatment strategies have concentrated on women.

Diagnosis

In 1999 The Royal College of Physicians produced a document |4| which is a comprehensive detailed account of osteoporosis (diagnosis and definition), and an up to date review of all available evidence for the prevention and treatment of osteoporosis. This is an invaluable aid to all clinicians working in this field. A supplement was published in 2001. It suggests that at present there are insufficient data to support a population-based screening strategy to decrease fracture risk. There is, however, evidence that by targeting people at high risk of developing osteoporosis ('the high-risk strategy') bone mass can be modulated to reduce fracture risk. The gold standard method for diagnosing osteoporosis is dual-energy X-ray absorptiometry (DEXA) to assess BMD. BMD assessment can also be used to monitor responses to treatment.

BMD measurements are recommended for the following indications where assessment would influence management |4|:

- radiographic evidence of osteopenia and/or vertebral deformity;
- loss of height, thoracic deformity (after radiographic confirmation of vertebral deformity);
- previous fragility fracture;
- prolonged corticosteroid therapy (prednisolone >7.5 mg daily for 6 months or more);
- premature menopause (age <45 years);
- prolonged secondary amenorrhoea (>1 year);
- primary hypogonadism;
- chronic disorders associated with osteoporosis;
- maternal history of hip fracture;
- low body mass index ($<19 \, kg/m^2$).

BMD assessment is usually performed at the hip and lumbar spine (L2-4). For diagnostic purposes, DEXA at the hip is the preferred site, particularly in the elderly, because of its higher predictive value for fracture risk. The spine is not a suitable site for diagnosis in the elderly because of the high prevalence of arthrosis and arthritis, but it is the preferred site for assessing response to treatment |4|.

However, in the majority of health authorities in the UK, DEXA is a limited resource. There is increasing interest in using peripheral ultrasound techniques to assess the skeleton to predict fracture risk |5, 6|. This method could be used to identify a population at high risk of developing osteoporosis. A pilot study has been performed in a general practice which suggests that this could be used in primary care to identify women at high risk of developing osteoporosis and therefore could improve the cost-effectiveness of referral for DEXA |7|. However, further studies are needed, and it is not recommended by The Royal College of Physicians for the diagnosis of osteoporosis at present.

In addition, diagnostic assessment of individuals with osteoporosis should include not only the assessment of BMD when indicated, but also the exclusion of diseases that mimic osteoporosis, elucidation of the cause of the osteoporosis and the management of any associated morbidity |4|.

Genetics

We know that a large proportion (up to 80%) of the differences seen in individual BMD could be attributable to genetic factors. Epidemiological studies have shown that the risk of fractures is doubled in the daughters of women with fractures independent of BMD |8|. There is still a lot to be learnt in this area, but the identification of the genes involved in the development of osteoporosis could help the understanding of the disease greatly and lead to huge advances in diagnosis, risk prediction, and preventative and therapeutic measures.

Biochemical markers

Biochemical markers of bone turnover can essentially be divided into resorption and formation markers. These can be measured in urine or serum and could provide information about the rate of bone loss or formation. Unfortunately at present the use of these markers in clinical situations is limited. Most are not sufficiently discriminatory to be used as a diagnostic test for osteoporosis and their values vary on a daily basis which means that several samples need to be taken before a clinical decision can be made. Another possible application of biochemical markers is to monitor therapy. However, until all these applications have been put to the test in randomized clinical studies, their use will still be limited. This is an area that The Royal College of Physicians has highlighted as a field that requires more research.

Lifestyle changes

For anyone who is at risk of developing osteoporosis or who has osteoporosis, lifestyle habits should be reviewed. These can help in the prevention as well as the treatment of osteoporosis. These include increasing physical activity (especially weight-bearing activities), reducing alcohol and caffeine intake, stopping smoking and ensuring calcium intake is adequate. There are several options that can be applied to help reduce the likelihood of falling and these can include careful monitoring of concomitant medication, e.g. sedatives. Hip protectors can also be of use in the frail and elderly, and a study by Lauritzen *et al.* |9| published in 1993 showed that use of a padded polypropylene external hip protector significantly reduced the incidence of hip fractures. However, they are not popular as they are cosmetically unattractive and compliance with these protectors is poor |9|.

Therapeutic options

There have been improvements in this area, which has meant that there is now a greater choice of therapeutic options available for the treatment and prevention of osteoporosis. Below is a summary of the recent studies that have been performed in this area, what is known on this subject and present thinking regarding their use. The majority of therapeutic options available to prevent or treat osteoporosis are antiresorptive drugs, i.e. they inhibit bone resorption. This group includes oestrogens, selective oestrogen receptor modulators (SERMs), bisphosphonates and calcitonin. Other drugs, such as fluoride and parathyroid hormone (PTH), increase bone formation that can also lead to an increase in bone density, although this does not necessarily translate into a reduction in fracture risk as it depends upon the quality of the new bone formed.

Hormone replacement therapy (HRT)

It is now well established that oestrogen replacement therapy has beneficial effects on the female skeleton and it remains the first choice for the prevention of post-menopausal bone loss in women with a low bone density. There is a role for HRT in the treatment of osteoporosis as well as the prevention. However, the exact mechanisms whereby oestrogen exerts its effect are still only partially understood. Oestrogen receptors have been shown to be present on osteoblasts |10|, osteoclasts |11| and marrow stromal cells (osteoblast precursors) |12|. It is generally thought that oestrogen largely exerts its effect by reducing bone turnover |13| as it has not been shown as yet to improve remodelling balance.

The type of preparation and the route are largely dependent on patient preference, as there is no evidence to suggest that they vary in their effectiveness in maintaining BMD. Studies have shown that oestrogen is effective at reducing bone loss at the hip and at the spine, although prevention of fracture data are still largely observational |14|.

As women who take HRT tend to be healthier, 'the healthy user effect', the observed 50% reduction in fracture risk associated with HRT is likely to be an over-estimate of fracture reduction. However, a study comparing 1 year of transdermal oestrogen with placebo in postmenopausal women with osteoporosis showed that the risk of developing a vertebral fracture in the treatment group was significantly lower than in the placebo group [15].

Komulainen *et al.* [16] published the results of a 5-year trial comparing HRT, vitamin D, HRT and vitamin D and placebo and found that there was a significant decrease in non-vertebral fractures in women in the HRT alone group and in the HRT and vitamin D group compared with vitamin D alone or placebo. Further studies are still needed in this area.

However, it has been shown that there is an optimum length of treatment required—at least 7 years, preferably longer—and that the benefits only last for the duration of treatment [17]. The major problem with HRT is that long-term adherence is poor. The main reason cited by patients for non-continuation with treatment is bleeding problems. This has improved since the introduction of period-free forms of therapy, which have been shown to be as effective at reducing post-menopausal bone loss in a 2-year prospective study [18], but poor adherence still remains a big problem, as women are scared of HRT being 'unnatural' and the risk of developing cancer, especially of the breast. The collaborative re-analysis of 51 epidemiological studies published in the *Lancet* in 1997 concluded that the relative risk of having breast cancer diagnosed increased by a factor of 1.023 for each year of HRT use [19]. However, when looking at mortality statistics for women, cardio-vascular disease kills 12 times as many women as breast cancer. Women tend to fear developing breast cancer much more than cardiovascular disease and this is why adequate and thorough counselling by the doctor at the initial consultation is imperative to ensure that patient concerns regarding long-term HRT use are addressed, as in the majority of women the benefits of taking HRT outweigh the potential risks. Careful monitoring of treatment to observe the therapeutic effect is also useful in improving adherence to therapy.

There is unfortunately no consensus regarding the optimum time to start and to stop oestrogen replacement therapy in postmenopausal women. What is known is that bone loss is a continuous process after the menopause and oestrogen is effective at preventing this loss in the younger as well as the older postmenopausal woman. It has been suggested that to help overcome the issue of poor long-term adherence, the timing of therapeutic intervention could shift from the immediate postmenopause, to later life when the risk of osteoporotic-related fracture is higher, and the rewards in preventing them are much higher [20].

However, older women who have not been exposed to oestrogen for many years may experience significant side-effects, so one could consider lower dose preparations that have been shown to cause fewer side-effects, yet attain the same protective effect on BMD [21].

Tibolone

Tibolone is a synthetic nor-steroid with oestrogenic, progestogenic and weak androgenic properties. It is metabolized in the human body into three major metabolites: 3α and 3β hydroxytibolone and Δ4 tibolone. Each has different binding affinities for the oestrogen, progestogen and androgen receptors. The 3α and 3β hydroxytibolone metabolites bind preferentially to the oestrogen receptors, whereas the Δ4 tibolone metabolite binds to the progestogenic and androgenic receptors and has no affinity for oestrogen receptors. At the level of the endometrium, tibolone is exclusively metabolized to the Δ4 tibolone metabolite by the enzyme 3β hydroxysteroid dehydrogenase. As this does not stimulate the oestrogen receptors, the endometrium remains atrophic and there is no cyclical bleeding.

It is becoming increasingly popular as an HRT option in the treatment of menopausal symptoms and in the prevention of osteoporosis. An open non-randomized study |**22**| has demonstrated that over 8 years bone density loss is prevented at all sites with tibolone. However, the exact mechanism of tibolone at the level of the bone has not yet been defined. However, the fact that the effects of tibolone on bone metabolism are blocked by the synthetic anti-oestrogen (ICI 164.384) but not by an anti-androgen (flutamide) or an antiprogestogen (Org 31710) |**23**| suggests that the mechanism is akin to that of the action of oestrogens on bone. It should only be used in women who are definitely postmenopausal, i.e. at least 1 year since their last menstrual period, follicle stimulating hormone (FSH)/luteinizing hormone (LH) levels consistent with postmenopause or >53 years of age. As with continuous combined therapies, earlier administration will not induce abnormal endometrial pathology, but the breakthrough bleeding rate will be increased and this will adversely affect adherence. Although the UK recommended dose is 2.5 mg, lower doses of 1.25 mg have proven to be bone protective in older women |**24**|.

Bisphosphonates

These are a large group of compounds that are stable analogues of pryrophosphate. In vitro, they prevent the precipitation of calcium and phosphorus in solution, block transformation of amorphous calcium phosphates in hydroxyapatite and inhibit aggregation of hydroxyapatite crystals |**25**|. Bisphosphonates are potent selective inhibitors of osteoclastic bone resorption. As postmenopausal osteoporosis is characterized by an increase in bone turnover, it is logical to consider this group of compounds for the prevention of postmenopausal osteoporosis. They are not well absorbed from the intestine and must not be given with food. There are now three licensed for use in both postmenopausal osteoporosis and glucocorticoid-induced osteoporosis in the UK. These are cyclical etidronate (Didronel), alendronate (Fosamax), and risedronate (Actonel).

Etidronate (Didronel)

Etidronate has been extensively studied in postmenopausal women. Cyclical etidronate has also been shown to increase bone mass and reduce fracture risk in postmenopausal women |26|. It is suggested that it works by decreasing both bone turnover and the remodelling space. This preparation cannot, however, be given on a continuous basis as it can adversely affect the mineralization of bone. It is therefore prescribed in a cyclical manner over 90 days: 400 mg is given for 2 weeks followed by 11 weeks of calcium (500 mg).

Alendronate (Fosamax)

The results from the Fosamax international trial were published in 1996 |27|. It was a placebo-controlled, double-blind trial in postmenopausal women with established osteoporosis which demonstrated that alendronate treatment significantly increased BMD in the lumbar spine, the femoral neck, the trochanter and Ward's triangle and total hip compared with placebo. It also demonstrated that alendronate reduced the incidence of clinical fractures at the spine and the hip.

Cummings *et al.* |28| have published the results of the second arm of this study which looked at postmenopausal women with a low femoral neck BMD, but no vertebral fracture at baseline. Their conclusions were that alendronate significantly increased BMD when compared with placebo at the femoral neck, total hip and lumbar spine and there was a non-significant reduction in all clinical fractures. This can be given on a continuous basis. The recommended dose is 5 mg for the prevention of postmenopausal osteoporosis and for the prevention and treatment of glucocorticoid-induced osteoporosis and 10 mg for the treatment of postmenopausal osteoporosis. There is some evidence to suggest that intermittent administration produces similar effects to daily administration of alendronate |29|.

Risedronate (Actonel)

Risedronate has recently received a licence for the prevention and treatment of osteoporosis in postmenopausal women and for the prevention and treatment of glucocorticoid-induced osteoporosis in the UK. It has been shown in two randomized controlled trials |30, 31| to reverse bone loss at the lumbar spine, femoral neck and trochanter in postmenopausal women with established osteoporosis. It was also shown that risedronate significantly reduced the relative risk of developing both vertebral and non-vertebral fractures. It was well tolerated with no increase in the incidence of gastrointestinal side-effects compared with the placebo group. The 5 mg dose was shown to be the more effective dosage regimen than the 2.5 mg dose.

SERMs

SERMs represent a structurally diverse group of compounds which interact with the oestrogen receptor, but they elicit different responses (agonist or antagonist) depending on the organ system. They have the potential to address the long-term needs of postmenopausal women, while overcoming some of the limitations of HRT. This group of compounds includes tamoxifen, clomiphene, droloxifene and raloxifene. Clomiphene and tamoxifen are in widespread clinical use. Raloxifene is a benzothiophene derivative that was originally investigated as therapy for breast cancer. In human studies it has been shown to bind to the oestrogen receptor and inhibit bone resorption (like oestrogen), but without stimulating the endometrium in postmenopausal women. A multicentre, randomized, blind, placebo-controlled study |32| to determine the effect of raloxifene therapy on the risk of vertebral and non-vertebral fractures concluded that in women with osteoporosis, raloxifene increases BMD in the spine and the femoral neck. When compared with placebo, raloxifene increases BMD in the femoral neck by 2.1% (60 mg dose), and in the spine by 2.6%. There were significant reductions in vertebral fracture risk in women with or without a history of one or more vertebral fractures at baseline. The risk of non-vertebral fracture did not differ significantly between the two groups.

A recent study |33| compared raloxifene with oestrogen and found that although overall raloxifene does reduce bone turnover and increase bone density, it is to a lesser extent than with oestrogen. Raloxifene also has an oestrogenic effect on serum lipids and coagulation/fibrinolysis. There has been no increase in the incidence of vaginal bleeding observed with raloxifene and no increased risk of developing endometrial cancer. Cummings *et al.* |34| reported that the relative risk of developing breast cancer after a median follow-up of 40 months of raloxifene treatment was significantly reduced. However, this effect was only apparent with oestrogen receptor-positive tumours, as no reduction was seen in oestrogen receptor-negative tumours.

Possible side-effects include hot flushes, leg cramps and peripheral oedema, and an increase in the incidence of venous thromboembolism has been observed which is similar in magnitude to that observed with HRT use. It is therefore considered to be an alternative when HRT is contraindicated for the prevention and treatment of osteoporosis in postmenopausal women. At present the dose of 60 mg daily is licensed in the UK.

Calcium

There is considerable evidence that calcium supplementation can improve bone health. It has been shown that supplements of calcium are capable of slowing the rate of bone loss in postmenopausal women with or without osteoporotic fractures at a variety of skeletal sites, and Kanis |35| published a review of the evidence for this. The effect of calcium salts in the treatment of osteoporosis appears to be due to a decrease in bone turnover |36|. This is translated into small increments induced in serum calcium levels, and the resulting decrease in PTH and the activation of bone turnover, in a similar way to that seen in younger individuals |37|. The majority of studies have been performed in women and so evidence for its use in men is scant. A recent review published in 1999 showed that there is a protective effect of calcium on fracture risk irrespective of the concurrent use of vitamin D when all randomized controlled trials were analysed |38|. The recommended dose is 700 mg daily.

Vitamin D

The use of appropriate doses of vitamin D can lead to the suppression of PTH and thus lead to a decrease in bone loss |39|. The active metabolite of vitamin D, calcitriol, and the related alphacalcidol, increase calcium absorption and may have direct effects on bone cells. It should be considered in elderly patients who are at higher risk of vitamin D deficiency, especially if they are housebound (lack of sunlight) or live in institutions. A large epidemiological study has demonstrated that use of vitamin D can reduce fracture risk in elderly women with a low body mass index |40|. The risks from taking vitamin D are very small and the potential benefits usually outweigh these. The optimum dose is 400 IU daily.

Other possible options

Increasing exercise can be very helpful in the management of established osteoporosis. It can help skeletal bone mass to a limited extent, but it is important to consider the other benefits. Exercise can have huge benefits on self-confidence, increase muscle strength, postural stability and sense of well-being which can all lead to a reduction in the incidence of falls.

PTH stimulates bone formation by an unknown mechanism but results in an increase in BMD. It also stimulates synthesis of 1,25-dihydroxyvitamin D3 which increases intestinal absorption of calcium and phosphorus. There is as yet no information on its effect on fracture rate. PTH could be a promising treatment for osteoporosis in the future. The main problem with PTH at present is that it is only available as intramuscular injections, which may not be well tolerated by patients.

Calcitonin is a 32 amino acid peptide that is normally produced by the thyroid C cells and results in decreased bone resorption. Osteoclasts have calcitonin receptors and calcitonin rapidly inhibits the action of osteoclasts. It has to be administered by subcutaneous or intramuscular injection at present, although an intranasal spray may make therapy more acceptable. The dose can be up to 100 IU per day and it is very expensive. It does appear to increase BMD, but it is more effective at preventing cancellous bone loss in postmenopausal women than cortical bone loss |41|. It is not widely used in the UK for the prevention or treatment of osteoporosis. Side-effects include an analgesic effect that can be beneficial, but nausea, flushing and diarrhoea can cause problems. In addition, resistance can occur in some patients with long-term use.

Fluoride stimulates osteoblasts. However, although it does appear to increase bone density this does not appear to translate into a reduction in fracture risk. It is not licensed for use in the UK and is given under specialist supervision.

A potential beneficial treatment that has been suggested is the use of UVB radiation to increase vitamin D production, which could be beneficial in the treatment of osteoporosis. However, this theory has not been supported in clinical evidence to date.

There is increased interest in phyto-oestrogens and natural progestogens as alternative therapies for postmenopausal women for the alleviation of oestrogen-deficient symptoms and preventing bone loss. The theory behind this is that women who have a diet rich in phyto-oestrogens, such as Japanese women, seem to have fewer problems with oestrogen deficiency. Some work has been performed in this area suggesting that phyto-oestrogens can reduce bone loss in postmenopausal women, but they may work via a different mechanism to oestrogen |**42**|. Further studies are required to evaluate their clinical use.

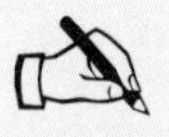

HRT and vitamin D in prevention of non-vertebral fractures in postmenopausal women; a 5 year randomized trial.

MH Komulainen, H Kroger, MT Tuppurainen, *et al. Maturitas* 1998; **31**: 45–54.

BACKGROUND. For many years, oestrogen has been considered the primary therapeutic choice for the prevention of postmenopausal bone loss in women with a low BMD. The type of preparation and the route are largely dependent on patient preference, as there is no evidence to suggest that they vary in their effectiveness in maintaining BMD. Recent data have questioned this standard. This is largely due to the fact that until recently there have been limited data from randomized controlled trials on the role of HRT and the prevention of fractures. Oestrogen has been shown to reduce bone remodelling and prevent bone loss and recent evidence has shown that it does reduce fracture risk at the level of the vertebral spine. However, until now, the evidence for the prevention of hip fractures has come mainly from observational studies. This study was the first prospective randomized study to investigate the effects of HRT on the prevention of peripheral fractures in non-osteoporotic postmenopausal women.

INTERPRETATION. This 5-year prospective trial randomized a total of 464 early postmenopausal women into four groups: HRT alone, vitamin D alone, HRT and vitamin D, and placebo. It was the first study to confirm the beneficial effect of HRT on the prevention of peripheral fractures in non-osteoporotic postmenopausal women.

There was a significant reduction in the incidence of new non-vertebral fractures in women taking HRT when compared with the placebo group. In the women taking vitamin D alone, there was a non-significant decrease in fracture incidence when compared with the placebo group. The addition of vitamin D to HRT did not appear to confer any additional benefit.

Comment

Although this was the first study to look prospectively at HRT and non-vertebral fracture risk, the results are promising. There is an obvious need for more studies to be performed in this area, looking at the older postmenopausal woman, women who are already osteoporotic and lower dosage HRT.

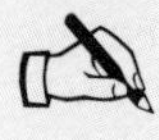

Tibolone: prevention of bone loss in late postmenopausal women.

NH Bjarnason, K Bjarnason, J Haarbo, C Rosenquist, C Christiansen.
J Clin Endocrinol Metab 1996; **81**(7): 2419–22.

B A C K G R O U N D . Tibolone is a synthetic nor-steroid with oestrogenic, progestogenic and weak androgenic properties. It is becoming increasingly popular as an HRT option in the treatment of menopausal symptoms and in the prevention of osteoporosis, with the additional benefit of no cyclical bleeding, as it does not stimulate the endometrium. It has also been shown to improve mood and libido. It should only be used in women who are definitely postmenopausal, i.e. at least 1 year since their last menstrual period, FSH/LH levels consistent with postmenopause or >53 years of age. As with continuous combined therapies, earlier administration will not induce abnormal endometrial pathology, but the breakthrough bleeding rate will be increased and this will adversely affect adherence. Recent studies have shown that tibolone is effective at increasing spine BMD and an open non-randomized study |16| has shown beneficial effects on BMD at the hip as well as the spine. However, prevention of fracture data are not available at any skeletal site.

This recent study investigated the effects of two dose regimens of tibolone on BMD in late postmenopausal women.

I N T E R P R E T A T I O N . This was a 2-year, double-blind, randomized, placebo-controlled study of 91 healthy women, who were all more than 10 years postmenopause, comparing the effects of two dosage regimens of tibolone (1.25 and 2.5 mg) with placebo. This study showed that a steady and equal rise in BMD occurred in both of the two tibolone groups at both the level of the spine and in the forearm. Increases in BMD at the spine of $5.9 \pm 0.9\%$ in the 1.25 mg group, $5.1 \pm 0.9\%$ in the 2.5 mg group and $0.4 \pm 1.1\%$ in the placebo group were observed. In the forearm, increases of $2.2 \pm 0.7\%$ in the 1.25 mg group and $1.9 \pm 1.1\%$ in the 2.5 mg group were seen, whereas the placebo group lost $2.1 \pm 1\%$. This was supported by changes in biochemical markers of bone resorption and bone formation.

Comment

The authors concluded that tibolone at two different doses had similar effects on BMD at the spine and the forearm and suggested that lower doses of tibolone may be effective at reducing bone loss.

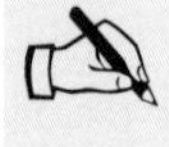

Reduction of vertebral fracture risk in post-menopausal women with osteoporosis treated with raloxifene: results from a three-year randomized clinical trial.

MORE Investigators. *J Am Med Assoc* 1999; **282**(7): 637–45.

B A C K G R O U N D . As an alternative to hormone or oestrogen replacement therapy for the prevention and treatment of osteoporosis, there has been enormous interest in the

development of SERMs. Raloxifene, which is a benzothiophene derivative, is the first of these agents to be licensed for use at present. The concept is to provide oestrogen-like effects in tissues such as bone, but anti-oestrogen effects at other tissues such as the endometrium and the breast. Raloxifene binds to the oestrogen receptor and inhibits bone resorption without stimulating the endometrium in postmenopausal women.

INTERPRETATION. This study was a multicentre, randomized, blind, placebo-controlled study to determine the effect of raloxifene therapy on the risk of vertebral and non-vertebral fractures in 7705 women aged between 31 and 80 years with osteoporosis. All women had been menopausal for at least 2 years and fulfilled the WHO criteria for osteoporosis. The study was performed in 25 countries, and the participants were randomized to 60 or 120 mg/day of raloxifene or a placebo. All participants also received calcium and vitamin D. At 3 years, when compared with placebo, raloxifene increased BMD in the femoral neck by 2.1% (60 mg dose) and 2.4% (120 mg dose), and in the spine by 2.6% (60 mg dose) and 2.7% (120 mg dose) ($P < 0.001$ for all comparisons). There were significant reductions in vertebral fracture risk in all women receiving raloxifene with or without a history of one or more vertebral fractures at baseline. The relative risk of vertebral fracture was 0.7 (95% CI 0.5–0.8) for the 60 mg group and 0.5 (95% CI 0.4–0.7) for the 120 mg group. The risk of non-vertebral fracture for raloxifene versus placebo did not differ significantly (relative risk 0.9, 95% CI 0.8–1.1). However, these studies are ongoing and further information will be available in the near future.

Comment

The conclusion from this study was that raloxifene, the first SERM to be developed, prevents bone loss at the spine and the femoral neck and reduces the incidence of vertebral fracture risk in postmenopausal women with osteoporosis. These effects are, however, less marked than those seen with oestrogens. There was no increase in incidence of vaginal bleeding with raloxifene or risk of developing endometrial cancer. There was a lower incidence of breast pain with raloxifene and a lower incidence of breast cancer. However, this effect appears to be only apparent with oestrogen receptor-positive tumours, as no effect was seen in the reduction of oestrogen receptor-negative tumours. Possible side-effects include hot flushes, leg cramps and peripheral oedema; an increase in the incidence of venous thrombo-embolism has been observed which is similar in magnitude to that observed with HRT use. There are other SERMs under development (droloxifene, idoxifene and levormeloxifene) which could further expand the therapeutic options available for the treatment and prevention of osteoporosis.

Raloxifene can therefore be considered as an alternative to HRT when contra-indications to oestrogen exist. At present, raloxifene 60 mg daily is licensed in the UK for the prevention and treatment of osteoporosis in postmenopausal women.

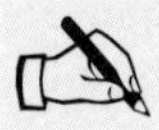

Effects of risedronate treatment on vertebral and non-vertebral fractures in women with postmenopausal osteoporosis.

ST Harris, NB Watts, HK Genant, *et al. J Am Med Assoc* 1999; **282**: 1344–52.

BACKGROUND. Bisphosphonates are a large group of compounds which are stable analogues of pryrophosphate and work by reducing bone turnover. They have been developed over the last 10–15 years and represent another treatment option for osteoporosis. There are now three licensed for use in both postmenopausal and glucocorticoid-induced osteoporosis in the UK: cyclical etidronate (Didronel), alendronate (Fosamax) and risedronate (Actonel).

Cyclical etidronate has also been shown to increase bone mass and reduce vertebral fracture risk |6|. There is currently no evidence for a beneficial effect on other fractures. This preparation cannot, however, be given on a continuous basis as it can adversely affect the mineralization of bone. It is therefore prescribed in a cyclical manner over 90 days; 400 mg is given for 2 weeks followed by 11 weeks of calcium (500 mg).

The results from the Fosamax international trial were published in 1996 |7|. It was a placebo-controlled, double-blind trial in postmenopausal women with established osteoporosis which demonstrated that alendronate treatment significantly increased BMD in the lumbar spine and the femoral neck of the femur compared with placebo. It also demonstrated that alendronate reduced the incidence of clinical fractures at the spine and the hip by 50% compared with placebo-treated women. This can be given on a continuous basis, and the recommended dose is 5 mg for the prevention of postmenopausal osteoporosis and 10 mg for the treatment of postmenopausal osteoporosis. There is some evidence to suggest that intermittent administration produces similar effects to daily administration of alendronate |21|.

Risedronate is the most recently developed bisphosphonate.

INTERPRETATION. This was a randomized, double-blind, placebo-controlled study of 2458 ambulatory postmenopausal women less than 85 years of age with at least one vertebral fracture at baseline performed in North America. The subjects were allocated to one of three treatment groups: risedronate 2.5 mg, risedronate 5 mg or placebo. All subjects received calcium and vitamin D if required. The 2.5 mg risedronate arm was discontinued after 1 year. In the placebo and the 5 mg risedronate arms, 450 and 489 subjects, respectively, completed all 3 years of the trial. Treatment with 5 mg/day of risedronate, when compared with the placebo group, reduced the incidence of new vertebral fractures by 41% over 3 years. A fracture reduction of 65% was seen in the first year. The cumulative incidence of non-vertebral fractures over 3 years was reduced by 39%. BMD increased significantly compared with the placebo group at the lumbar spine, femoral trochanter and the mid-shaft of the radius.

Comment

This was the first study to investigate the effects of risedronate in postmenopausal women. It has been previously shown that it is effective and well tolerated in the treatment of Paget's disease of bone and other metabolic bone diseases. The study suggests that risedronate is effective at increasing BMD and reducing vertebral and non-vertebral fracture risk significantly in postmenopausal women with established osteoporosis. It was also shown to be well tolerated, with no increase in the incidence of gastrointestinal side-effects compared with the placebo group. The 5 mg dose was shown to be the more effective dosage regimen than the 2.5 mg dose.

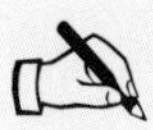

Fluoride salts are no better at preventing new vertebral fractures than calcium–vitamin D in postmenopausal osteoporosis: the FAVO Study.

PJ Meunier, JL Sebert, JY Reginster, *et al. Osteoporosis Int* 1998; **8**(1): 4–11.

BACKGROUND. Sodium fluoride stimulates bone formation by an unknown mechanism. However, although fluoride has been shown to increase spinal BMD linearly, the effects of this gain in BMD on fracture rate remains controversial. Fluoride salts are not licensed for use in the UK and are only given under specialist supervision.

INTERPRETATION. This 2-year, multicentre, prospective, randomized, double-blind clinical trial was conducted in 354 osteoporotic women with vertebral fractures. They either received sodium fluoride 50 mg/day or monofluorophosphate at one of two doses (200 or 150 mg/day). All patients received calcium and vitamin D. At 2 years the fluoride group had increased their lumbar spine BMD by 10.8% compared with 2.4% in the placebo group. There were no differences in new fracture rate between the groups.

Comment

The conclusion of this study was that fluoride with calcium and vitamin D supplementation was no more effective than calcium and vitamin D alone at the prevention of new vertebral fractures in postmenopausal women with osteoporosis. This shows that huge increases in BMD do not necessarily translate into fracture reduction.

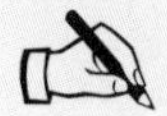

Randomized controlled trial to compare the efficacy of cyclical parathyroid hormone versus cyclical parathyroid hormone and sequential calcitonin to improve bone mass in postmenopausal women with osteoporosis.

AB Hodsman, LJ Fraher, PH Watson, *et al. J Clin Endocrinol Metab* 1997; **82**(2): 620–8.

BACKGROUND. PTH increases bone remodelling and may also stimulate bone formation directly and therefore increase BMD. It also stimulates synthesis of 1,25-dihydroxyvitamin D3 which increases intestinal absorption of calcium and phosphorus.

At present, data available from small clinical trials using PTH suggest that increases in BMD have been observed of greater magnitude than those seen with agents such as bisphosphonates. This study's aim was to investigate bone mineral mass and fracture incidence in postmenopausal women with osteoporosis.

INTERPRETATION. This 2-year randomized controlled trial was to compare the efficacy of cyclical PTH versus cyclical PTH and sequential calcitonin to improve bone mass in postmenopausal women with osteoporosis. It was a relatively small study of 30 women aged 67 ± 8 years. At the end of 2 years, the lumbar spine BMD had increased by 10.2% in the PTH group and by 7.9% in the PTH and sequential calcitonin group. These values both reached statistical significance. Changes in femoral neck BMD did not reach statistical significance. Very low incident vertebral fracture rates were observed over the study period.

Comment

This was a small study, and larger studies are needed to confirm the effects of PTH on femoral neck BMD and fracture reduction. The main problem with PTH at present is that it is only available as intramuscular injections, which may not be well tolerated by patients.

This could be a promising therapeutic option for the treatment of osteoporosis in the future, if the results of this study are confirmed in larger randomized controlled trials.

Low and conventional dose transdermal oestradiol are equally effective at preventing bone loss in spine and femur at all post-menopausal ages.

SF Evans, MWJ Davie. *Clin Endocrinol* 1996; **44**: 79–84.

BACKGROUND. **It is known that HRT is a well-established and effective treatment of postmenopausal bone loss. However, little is known about the minimum dose of oestrogen required to prevent bone loss. The general opinion is that a minimum dose of 0.625 mg of conjugated equine oestrogen (CEE) or 0.05 mg of transdermal oestrogen is required to prevent bone loss in the perimenopausal period. HRT can cause side-effects that will obviously be less marked with a lower dose of oestrogen. It is important for long-term adherence to minimize side-effects, especially in the older age group where side-effects can be more problematic.**

INTERPRETATION. This paper reports the results of an open, rather than a placebo-controlled, study investigating the efficacy of two different doses of transdermal oestrogen [a lower dose preparation Estraderm 25 (E25) versus a conventional dose Estraderm 50 (E50)] in Caucasian postmenopausal women. If a woman still had an intact uterus, 700 μg of norethisterone was given orally for the last 14 days of each 28-day cycle with E25 and 1 mg was given for the last 12 days of each cycle with E50. A total of 196 women were studied over 1–2 years, with 80 women reaching 3 years of treatment. All patients were offered HRT if their BMD at the lumbar spine was below

0.8 g/m^2, or if their present BMD value would suggest that they might fall below this value before the age of 80 years. They were informed about the two different doses available within the study. If they wished to use HRT, allocation of the dose was made randomly unless there were specific contraindications, such as side-effects with the combined oral contraceptive pill or migraine associated with periods premenopausally. The results were then divided into those women who were under the age of 67 years and those who were above 67 years of age at the start of treatment.

BMD was measured with DEXA at the lumbar spine (L2-4 inclusive) and at the femoral neck at baseline (196 women), at 1 year (169 women), at 2 years (139 women) and at 3 years (80 women). In the lumbar spine, BMD increased maximally in the first year in all groups and the gain was maintained after 3 years. The change was similar whether age or dosage divided the patients. For those women on E25, the mean change in BMD at the lumbar spine after 3 years of treatment was 8.1 ± 6.8% and on E50 it was 9.0 ± 8.3%. At the femoral neck, significant changes were only observed after 3 years of therapy, and only in the >67 year age group taking E25 and in the <67 year age group taking E50. This averaged 2.3 ± 5.4% for all patients.

Comment

The authors of this study concluded that transdermal oestrogen is effective at preventing bone loss in the spine at all postmenopausal ages and is capable of doing this even at lower doses. The effect in the dose range used was most marked at the level of the spine, but at neither the spine nor the femoral neck was there an obvious increase in the response with higher dosage/kg. This study also shows that age is not a barrier to bone response to oestrogen and also that use of E25 may be valuable because the lower dose of oestrogen is less likely to cause side-effects. However, there were no comments about compliance to medication or to the side-effects experienced by the women on the different doses of oestrogen participating in this study. This information would have been a useful addition to the promising results of this study.

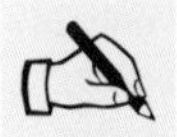

The effect of different doses of calcitonin on bone mineral density and fracture risk in postmenopausal osteoporosis.

S Hizmetli, H Elden, E Kaptanoglu, V Nacitarhan, S Kocagil. *Int J Clin Prac* 1998; **52**(7): 453–5.

BACKGROUND. Calcitonin decreases bone resorption via a direct inhibitory effect on osteoclasts. It can be given subcutaneously or intranasally. It has been reported that calcitonin can decrease further loss of bone and may even cause an increase in BMD in established osteoporosis. The intranasal preparation has fewer side-effects than the subcutaneous preparation.

INTERPRETATION. This paper reports the results of a prospective, open-label study of 107 women to determine the effects of different doses of intranasal calcitonin on BMD and fracture risk in postmenopausal osteoporosis. The women were recruited over a period of 11 months. Entry criteria included a bone density of 2.5 SD of that found in normal adolescents. Once any secondary cause of osteoporosis was ruled out, the patients were enrolled into the study. The patients were randomly divided into three groups. Thirty-five were given 50 IU/day of intranasal salmon calcitonin and 41 were given 100 IU/day. The remaining 31 patients comprised the control group. All three groups were given 1000 mg/day of elementary calcium and vitamin D according to the levels of 24-hour urinary calcium excretion. The women were followed for 2 years and lumbar and femoral neck BMD were assessed at 6, 12 and 24 months of treatment. The relative risk of developing a vertebral fracture was also assessed at 6, 12 and 24 months.

At 6 months 98 women remained in the study, at 12 and 24 months, 91 and 87 women remained, respectively. Twenty women were excluded for various reasons, 12 from the active groups due to side-effects. Compliance with medication was assessed at each visit and no problems were detected. The results showed significant increases in BMD at both measured sites with both doses of calcitonin. The increase in BMD was greater in those women on the higher 100 IU/day dose of calcitonin. There was a decrease in fracture risk in both calcitonin groups, but this reduction did not reach statistical significance.

Comment

The conclusions of this study were that intranasal salmon calcitonin treatment increases BMD when compared with treatment with calcium and vitamin D alone, and that although the increase in BMD varies depending upon the dosage used, the lower dose of 50 IU/day seems to be effective in the treatment of postmenopausal osteoporosis.

A comparison of the effects of raloxifene and estrogen on bone in postmenopausal women.

KM Prestwood, M Gunness, DB Muchmore, Y Lu, M Wong, LG Raisz.
J Clin Endocrinol Metab 2000; **85**: 2197–2202.

BACKGROUND. Oestrogen replacement therapy is the mainstay of treatment for menopausal symptoms, as well as for the prevention and treatment of osteoporosis in postmenopausal women. However, oestrogen use is associated with unwanted side-effects. Uterine bleeding, breast tenderness and fear of breast cancer are frequently cited as reasons for women to refuse initial therapy or to discontinue HRT early. Thus, for many women, the long-term skeletal benefits of HRT are not realized. Raloxifene is a benzothiophene-derived SERM with oestrogen agonist effects on the skeleton and serum lipids and oestrogen antagonist activity on endometrial and breast tissue. It has been shown in clinical studies of postmenopausal women that raloxifene has beneficial effects on bone and lipid metabolism without adversely affecting the endometrial tissue. It has not been previously shown how raloxifene compares with oestrogen at the level of the bone.

INTERPRETATION. This paper reports the results of a phase II randomized double-blind study to compare the effects of raloxifene (Evista 60 mg/day) with conjugated equine oestrogen (CEE) (Premarin 0.625 mg/day) on bone architecture, bone turnover and BMD. All women who participated in this study were Caucasian and at least 5 years postmenopausal, between the ages of 55 and 85 years inclusive, with lumbar spine BMD between 1 SD above and 3 SD below peak bone mass. Fifty-one women participated in the study and were randomly assigned to 6 months of treatment with either raloxifene or CEE. Women with an intact uterus were given 5 mg/day medroxyprogesterone acetate (MPA; Provera) for 14 days at the end of the 6-month treatment phase. Anterior iliac crest bone biopsies were performed at baseline and at the end of the study period and were analysed after double tetracycline labelling for standard histomorphic indices. Serum and urinary biochemical markers of bone turnover were measured at baseline and at 4, 10, 18 and 24 weeks of treatment. Total body, lumbar spine and hip BMD were measured at baseline and at the end of the study using DEXA.

The results show that there were no statistically significant differences between the two groups in baseline characteristics. The rate of compliance was measured by pill counts and ranged from 94 to 97% for both treatment groups. The incidence of discontinuations due to adverse events was significantly higher in the CEE group than in the raloxifene group. Forty-four women completed the study, and activation frequency and bone formation rate/bone volume were significantly decreased from baseline in the CEE group, but not in the raloxifene group. Bone mineralization did not change in either group. Most markers of bone resorption and formation decreased in both groups, but to a greater degree in the CEE group ($P < 0.05$). Total body and lumbar spine BMD increased from baseline in both groups, with a greater increase in the CEE group ($P < 0.05$). Hip BMD significantly increased from baseline in the raloxifene group, but the change was not that different from that in the CEE group.

Comment

This study concluded that raloxifene has smaller effects on bone turnover and bone density than CEE. However, raloxifene therapy was associated with fewer side-effects than CEE. Thus, raloxifene is an alternative to CEE for the prevention and treatment of osteoporosis in postmenopausal women.

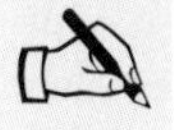

Prevention of postmenopausal bone loss with minimal uterine bleeding using a low dose continuous estrogen/progestin therapy: a 2-year prospective study.

H Mizunuma, H Okano, M Soda, *et al. Maturitas* 1997; **27**: 69–76.

BACKGROUND. Since Genant *et al.* |42| suggested that a daily dose of less than 0.6 mg of CEE was ineffective in reducing vertebral bone loss assessed using computed tomography, a daily dose of 0.625 mg of CEE is the standard for the prevention of postmenopausal bone loss. However, recent biochemical evidence has suggested that a lower dose of 0.31 mg/day may be effective if BMD changes are measured with a more accurate instrument such as DEXA. This study was designed to clarify whether HRT using less than 0.625 mg/day of CEE can be an appropriate option for treating postmenopausal bone loss in Japanese women wishing to eliminate withdrawal bleeding.

INTERPRETATION. This paper describes the methods and results from a 2-year prospective open-label randomized study to compare three different treatment groups with an untreated control group. The three treatment groups included CEE 0.625 mg/day; CEE 0.625 mg/day plus MPA 2.5 mg/day; CEE 0.31 mg/day plus MPA 2.5 mg/day. Fifty-two postmenopausal women were recruited into the study. Forty-eight had undergone a natural menopause and four had undergone a bilateral oophorectomy at least 1 year prior to the study. All patients were randomly assigned to one of the four groups. The women were assessed every 2 months to determine medication adherence and to assess the incidence of vaginal bleeding. Forty-nine women completed 1 year of the study, and 36 women completed 2 years. BMD at the L2-4 region of the lumbar spine and four areas of the femoral neck were measured by DEXA at baseline, and after 6, 12 and 24 months of treatment. Blood samples were collected for biochemical analysis every 6 months. There were no statistically significant differences between the four groups for baseline demographic data or baseline BMD measurements.

At the lumbar spine, at the end of the first and second years of treatment, significant increases in BMD were seen in all treatment groups, but the control group showed a significant decrease. The percentage changes in BMD in the first year for CEE alone, CEE 0.625 + MPA and CEE 0.31 + MPA were 5.42, 6.13 and 2.9%, respectively, and those in the second year were 6.85, 7.4 and 3.2%, respectively. BMD of the treated groups were significantly higher than their pretreatment values and the control group at each point.

The femoral BMD showed a decline in the control group, but the difference was not significant. There were no significant differences between the treatment groups in any part of the femur. The incidence of bleeding was significantly lower in women taking CEE 0.31 + MPA. No significant changes in lipid profile were seen in the control group or in the group of women taking CEE 0.31 + MPA, although increases in high-density lipoprotein cholesterol were observed in the other two treatment groups.

Comment

The authors concluded that continuous HRT using 0.31 mg of CEE and 2.5 mg of MPA daily is effective in increasing lumbar BMD in postmenopausal women and could be an appropriate treatment for women wishing to eliminate unscheduled vaginal bleeding and reduce both hormonal side-effects and menopausal symptoms. However, a daily dose of 0.3 mg of CEE has no beneficial effects on the serum lipid profile. It could therefore be appropriate to use this dosage in women who have a normal lipid profile. This study has shown that although a lower dose of oestrogen can still increase BMD, it does not exhibit the same extent of benefit as higher doses.

Summary

If we are to manage osteoporosis effectively, we need to maintain BMD and prevent fractures. In addition to therapeutic options, a full assessment of a woman's risk for developing osteoporosis should be undertaken, with considerations made for family history, concomitant medication and lifestyle habits. Prevention of osteoporosis is of utmost importance, as well as the treatment of this disease once it has been diagnosed. There are several options that can be applied to help reduce the likelihood of falling and these can include careful monitoring of concomitant medication, e.g. sedatives. Hip protectors can also be of use in the frail and elderly, and use of a padded polypropylene external hip protector has been shown to reduce significantly the incidence of hip fractures. However, they are not popular as they are cosmetically unattractive and compliance with these protectors is poor.

The gold standard for assessing BMD and diagnosing osteoporosis is DEXA and this can also be used to monitor response to treatment and encourage adherence to therapy. For diagnostic purposes, DEXA at the hip is the preferred site, particularly in the elderly, because of its higher predictive value for fracture risk.

Regarding therapeutic options, increasing BMD is now not considered to be the main factor in efficacy; fracture reduction must be the ultimate goal. We therefore need more information regarding the effectiveness of hormone/oestrogen replacement therapy at preventing non-vertebral fractures, and also we need data for tibolone and fracture reduction. Newer and safer bisphosphonates have been introduced and the SERMs will definitely become a more attractive option in the future. However, for the moment, for the prevention of osteoporosis in postmenopausal women at the time of ovarian failure, HRT is still the most logical and appropriate first-line treatment of choice. In addition to the beneficial effects that HRT has on bone, there are other benefits, which have to be weighed against the potential risks of long-term therapy.

Interesting concepts are appearing for the future, including low-dose HRT which could minimize side-effects, especially for the older postmenopausal woman |21|. Period-free forms of therapy, including tibolone, have already been shown to improve long-term adherence to therapy, which is essential if we are to obtain the long-term benefits for the female skeleton. To help overcome the issue of poor long-term adherence, the ideal timing of therapeutic intervention could shift from the immediate postmenopause to later life when the risk of osteoporotic-related fracture is higher and the rewards in preventing them are much higher |20|. Raloxifene (a SERM) can be considered if oestrogen is contraindicated and has been shown to decrease vertebral fracture risk. Although raloxifene appears to decrease the risk of developing breast cancer, it still increases the risk of venous thrombo-embolic events to the same extent as oestrogen. Bisphosphonates are widely available and are being used increasingly in the prevention and treatment of osteoporosis. For women with existing fractures, the first line of treatment is a bisphosphonate, followed by raloxifene or HRT.

There is considerable evidence that calcium supplementation can improve bone health. The recommended dose is 700 mg daily. Vitamin D should be considered in elderly patients who are at higher risk of vitamin D deficiency, especially if they are housebound (lack of sunlight) or live in institutions. A large epidemiological study has demonstrated that use of vitamin D can reduce fracture risk in elderly women with a low body mass index |40|. The risks from taking vitamin D are very small and potential benefits usually outweigh these. The optimum dose is 400 IU daily.

There is increased interest in phyto-oestrogens and natural progestagens as alternative therapies for postmenopausal women for the alleviation of oestrogen-deficiency symptoms and preventing bone loss. Some work has been done in this area to suggest that they can reduce bone loss in postmenopausal women, but they may have a different mechanism to oestrogen |**43**|. Further studies are required to evaluate their clinical use.

References

1. Dolan P, Torgerson DJ. The cost of treating osteoporotic fractures in the United Kingdom female population. *Osteoporosis Int* 1998; **8**: 611–7.

2. Who are candidates for prevention and treatment for osteoporosis? *Osteoporosis Int* 1997; **7**: 1–6.

3. Kanis JA, Melton LJ III, Christiansen C, Johnstone CC, Khaltaev N. The diagnosis of osteoporosis. *J Bone Miner Res* 1994; **9**: 1137–41.

4. The Consensus Workshop Group. The Royal College of Physicians. *Osteoporosis—Clinical Guidelines for the Prevention and Treatment.* The Lavenham Press, Sudbury, Suffolk, 1999.

5. Thompson P, Taylor J, Oliver R, Fisher A. Quantitative ultrasound (QUS) of the heel predicts wrist and osteoporotic fractures in women aged 45–75 years. *J Clin Dens* 1998; **1**: 219–25.

6. Hans D, Dargent-Molina P, Schoti AM, *et al.* Ultrasonographic heel measurements to predict hip fracture in elderly women: the EPIDOS prospective study. *Lancet* 1996; **348**: 511–4.

7. Hodson J, Pearson D. Identification of women at high risk of osteoporosis in primary care. *J British Menopause Society* 2000; **6**(2): 73–4.

8. Eisman JA. Genetics of osteoporosis. *Endocrine Rev* 1999; **20**(6): 788–804.

9. Lauritzen JB, Peterson MM, Lund B. Effect of external hip protectors on hip fractures. *Lancet* 1993; **341**: 11–13.

10. Erikson EF, Colvard DS, Berg NJ, *et al.* Evidence of estrogen receptors in normal human osteoblast-like cells. *Science* 1988; **241**: 84–6.

11. Oursler MJ, Pederson L, Fitzpatrick L, *et al.* Human giant cell tumours of the bone (osteoclastomas) as estrogen target cells. *Proc Natl Acad Sci USA* 1994; **91**: 5227–31.

12. Girasole G, Jilka RL, Passeri G, *et al.* 17 beta-estradiol inhibits interleukin-6 production by bone marrow-derived stromal cells and osteoblasts *in vitro*: a potential mechanism for the antiosteoporotic effect of estrogens. *J Clin Invest* 1992; **89**: 883–91.

13. Steiniche T, Hasling C, Charles P, *et al.* A randomized study on the effects of oestrogen/gestagen or high dose calcium on trabecular bone remodeling in postmenopausal osteoporosis. *Bone* 1989; **10**: 313–20.

14. Naessen T, Persson I, Adami HO, Bergstrom R, Bergkvist L. Hormone replacement therapy and the risk for first hip fracture: a prospective, population based cohort study. *Ann Intern Med* 1990; **113**: 95–103.

15. Lufkin EG, Wahner HW, O'Fallon WM, *et al.* Treatment of postmenopausal osteoporosis with transdermal estrogen. *Ann Intern Med* 1992; **117**: 1–9.

16. Komulainen MH, Kroger H, Tuppurainen MT, *et al.* HRT and Vitamin D in prevention of non-vertebral fractures in postmenopausal women; a 5 year randomised trial. *Maturitas* 1998; **31**: 45–54.

17. Felson DT, Zang Y, Hannan MT, Kiel DP, Wilson PWF, Anderson JJ. The effect of postmenopausal estrogen therapy on bone density in elderly women. *New Engl J Med* 1993; **329**: 1141–6.

18. Mizunuma H, Okano H, Soda M, *et al.* Prevention of postmenopausal bone loss with minimal uterine bleeding using a low dose continuous combined estrogen/progestin therapy: a 2-year prospective study. *Maturitas* 1997; **27**: 69–76.

19. Collaborative Group on Hormonal Factors in Breast Cancer. Breast cancer and hormone replacement therapy: collaborative reanalysis of data from 51 epidemiological studies of 52 705 women with breast cancer and 108 411 women without breast cancer. *Lancet* 1997; **350**: 1047–59.

20. Kanis J. Treatment strategies in osteoporosis. *J BMS* 2000; **6**(S2): 17–19.

21. Gallager JC. Moderation of the daily dose of HRT: prevention of osteoporosis. *Maturitas* 1999; **33**(S1): S57–63.

22. Rymer J, Robinson J, Fogelman I. Effects of 8 years of treatment with Tibolone 2.5 mg daily on postmenopausal bone loss. *Osteoporosis International* 2001; **12**(6): 478–83.

23. Ederveen AGH, Kloosterboer HJ. Tibolone exerts an estrogenic effect on bone leading to prevention of bone loss and reduction in bone resorption in ovariectomised rats. *Osteoporosis Int* 1998; **8**(S3): 95.

24. Bjarnason NH, Bjarnason K, Haarbo J, Rosenquist C, Christiansen C. Tibolone: prevention of bone loss in late postmenopausal women. *J Clin Endocrinol Metab* 1996; **81**(7): 2419–22.

25. Fleisch H. Diphosphonates: history and mechanisms of action. *Metab Bone Dis Rel Res* 1981; **3**: 279–88.

26. Storm T, Harris ST, Genant HK, *et al.* Intermittent cyclical etidronate therapy on bone mass and fracture rate in women with post-menopausal osteoporosis. *New Engl J Med* 1990; **322**: 1265–71.

27. Black DM, Cummings SR, Karpf DB, *et al.* Randomised trial of effect of alendronate on risk of fracture in women with existing vertebral fractures. *Lancet* 1996; **348**: 1535–41.

28. Cummings SR, Black DM, Thompson DE, *et al.* Effect of alendronate on risk of fracture in women with low bone density but without vertebral fractures—results from the Fracture Intervention Trial. *J Am Med Assoc* 1998; **280**: 2077–82.

29. Schnitzer T, Bone HG, Crepaldi G, *et al.* Therapeutic equivalence of alendronate 70mg once weekly and alendronate 10mg daily in the treatment of osteoporosis. *Aging Clin Exp Res* 1998; **12**: 1–12.

30. Harris ST, Watts NB, Genant HK, *et al.* Effects of risedronate treatment on vertebral and non-vertebral fractures in women with postmenopausal osteoporosis. *J Am Med Assoc* 1999; **282**: 1344–52.

31. Reginster J-Y, Minne HW, Sorenson OH, *et al.* Randomized trial of the effects of risedronate on vertebral fractures in women with established postmenopausal osteoporosis. *Osteoporosis Int* 2000; **11**: 83–91.

32. MORE Investigators. Reduction of vertebral fracture risk in post-menopausal women with osteoporosis treated with raloxifene. Results from a three-year randomized clinical trial. *J Am Med Assoc* 1999; **282**(7): 637–45.

33. Prestwood KM, Gunness M, Muchmore DB, Lu Y, Wong M, Raisz LG. A comparison of the effects of raloxifene and estrogen on bone in post menopausal women. *J Clin Endocrinol Metab* 2000; **85**(6): 2197–202.

34. Cummings SR, Eckert S, Krueger KA, *et al.* The effect of raloxifene on risk of breast cancer in postmenopausal women. *J Am Med Assoc* 1999; **261**: 2189–97.

35. Kanis JA. Calcium nutrition and its implications for osteoporosis. Parts I and II. *Eur J Clin Nutr* 1994; **48**: 757–67, 833–41.

36. Nordin BEC, Need AG. The rationale for calcium therapy in the prevention and treatment of osteoporosis. *Triangle* 1989; **28**(S1): 49–56.

37. Reid IR, Ames RW, Evans MC, Gamble GD, Sharpe SJ. Effect of calcium supplementation on bone loss in postmenopausal women. *New Engl J Med* 1993; **328**: 460–4.

38. Kanis JA. The use of calcium in the management of osteoporosis. *Bone* 1999; **24**(4): 279–90.

39. Dawson-Hughes B, Dallal GE, Krall EA, Harris S, Sokoll LJ, Falconer G. Effect of vitamin D supplementation on wintertime and overall bone loss in healthy postmenopausal women. *Ann Intern Med* 1991; **115**: 505–12.

40. Ranstam J, Kanis JA. Influence of age and body mass on the effects of vitamin D on hip fracture risk. *Osteoporosis Int* 1995; **5**: 450–4.

41. Overgaard K, Riis BJ, Christiansen C, Hansen MA. Effect of salcatonin given intranasally on early post-menopausal bone loss. *Br Med J* 1989; **299**: 477–9.

42. Genaht HK, Cann CE, Ettinger B, Gordan GS. Quantitative computed tomography of vertebral spongiosa; a sensitive method for detecting early bone loss after oophorectomy. *Ann Intern Med* 1982; **97**: 699–705.

43. Arjmandi BH, Birnbaum RS, Juma S, Barengolts E, Kukreja SC. The synthetic phytooestrogen, ipriflavone, and oestrogen prevent bone loss by different mechanisms. *Calcif Tissue Int* 2000; **66**(1): 61–5.

6

Postmenopausal hormone replacement therapy and arterial disease

Introduction

Postmenopausal hormone replacement therapy (HRT) with oestrogen was initially developed to relieve climacteric symptoms such as hot flushes and night sweats. The possibility of a reduced incidence of osteoporotic bone fracture (based primarily on biophysical assessment of bone density) soon emerged, but it is the possibility of substantial protection from coronary heart disease (CHD) that has associated HRT with an overwhelmingly positive risk/benefit balance. Even the finding of a two- to three-fold increase in the risk of venous thromboembolism in women using HRT failed to dent the perception of HRT as being of overall benefit in terms of cardiovascular disease

During the 1980s a consensus emerged that oral HRT reduced the risk of diseases such as myocardial infarction (MI) by 50%, more so in women with pre-existing disease or a high cardiovascular risk factor load. Subsequent years saw a switch away from lipids and lipoproteins as the primary mechanism behind this protection towards 'direct' vasoactive properties of oestrogen. As more and more vascular endpoints became established it became harder and harder to predict whether a specific HRT formulation would be better or worse than another. The limitations of surrogate studies had been reached: such data are relatively easy to generate but they cannot give an assessment of net risk.

Formal randomized placebo-controlled trials of different HRT formulations would be needed to resolve these issues. Primarily for reasons of cost, the first study was conducted in CHD patients, a population that could be relied on to generate a high number of clinical events during follow-up. It must be emphasized that at that time the climate of opinion derived from epidemiological, cardiological and animal model studies was that HRT was especially beneficial in damaged arteries and so the use of CHD patients was considered to be an acceptable 'short cut' to understanding the effects in healthy women. A second and potentially vexatious decision was for some investigators to evaluate not just oestrogen but a combination of oestrogen and progestin, the latter steroid needed to prevent oestrogen-induced endometrial disease.

Within the past few years the findings of some of these formal clinical trials have been reported and interim data from others have been presented at scientific meetings. Following over 40 years of perception of postmenopausal oestrogen therapy as an anti-atherosclerotic drug, the failure of these studies to prove that any form of HRT is better than placebo in terms of clinical endpoints such as MI, forces us to regroup and rethink. Indeed a pattern of increased CHD risk, particularly in the early years, has emerged consistently from these studies. Such developments have led to a concern that the surrogate cardiovascular endpoints used for decades may have misled us.

One explanation for these adverse events has quickly emerged: oral oestrogens double or triple plasma levels of C-reactive protein, a marker of inflammation at the level of the endothelium. This major discovery is likely to lead to the identification of the subset of women who respond adversely to oral HRT and also aid the development of novel postmenopausal therapies that do not exert such a pro-inflammatory effect.

Neither the existence of this new cardiovascular problem nor the clinical significance of the increased plasma C-reactive protein levels is universally accepted. Resolution of these issues is unlikely before the planned publication in 2005 of the results from the randomized controlled trial elements of the Women's Health Initiative. Subgroups of this landmark clinical trial include 17 000 healthy women randomized to HRT (alone or in combination with progestin) or placebo and should reveal whether, as has been claimed, the failure of recent studies is related to the progestin component or the health status of the participants (or both). Initial reports from this study argue against these possibilities: a widely leaked letter from the trial organizers to the participants and their doctors refers to a higher incidence of heart attacks, stroke and venous thromboembolic events in the HRT group than in women randomized to placebo. This excess risk of arterial disease is thought to be limited to the early years of therapy, holding out the possibility of protection in the long term.

Heart and Estrogen/progestin Replacement Study (HERS)

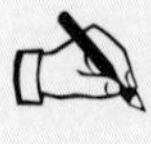

Randomized trial of estrogen plus progestin for secondary prevention of coronary heart disease in postmenopausal women. Heart and Estrogen/progestin Replacement Study (HERS) Research Group.
S Hulley, D Grady, T Bush, *et al. J Am Med Assoc* 1998; **280**: 605–13.

BACKGROUND. Despite widespread acceptance, the belief that HRT reduces a woman's risk of CHD had not been formally tested in a randomized placebo-controlled trial. Some argued that such a trial was unnecessary (even unethical), given the strength of the epidemiological, animal data and risk marker data. In this landmark clinical trial, 2763 CHD patients (mean age 67 years) were randomized to receive either oral HRT [conjugated equine oestrogens (CEE) 0.625 mg/day plus medroxyprogesterone acetate (MPA) 2.5 mg/day] or placebo. The mean follow-up was 4.1 years.

INTERPRETATION. There were no significant differences between the groups in terms of the primary outcome of non-fatal MI or CHD death, nor in secondary cardiovascular outcomes such as angina or stroke. In the first year there was an excess of cardiovascular events in women treated with HRT (Fig. 6.1), despite the expected decreases in plasma levels of low-density lipoprotein cholesterol and increases in high-density lipoproteins.

Comment

The much-awaited findings of this study shattered the hopes of many researchers and clinicians. There was special disappointment as CHD patients had, until then, been thought of as a subset of women whose cardiovascular problems would be remedied quickly by HRT, with some epidemiologists predicting up to a 70% reduction in CHD events in HRT users. The finding of an increased incidence of CHD in the early years of the study was simply astounding. Many commentators subsequently dismissed this trial on the grounds that it was too short a duration, the women were too old and too ill, the HRT formulation was the wrong one and so on. Indeed, some maintain that the study was in fact a success: something went

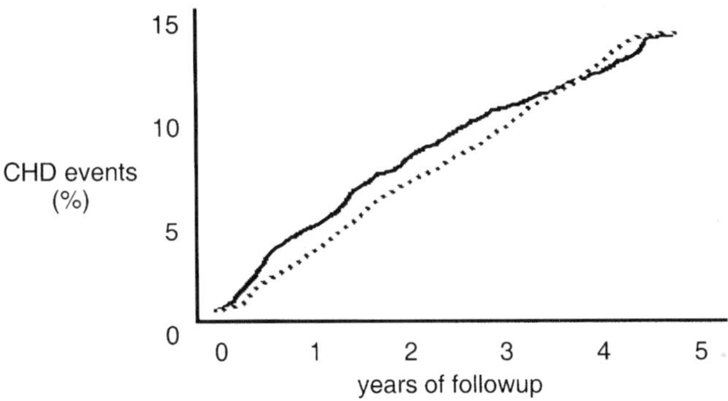

Fig. 6.1 Effect of hormone replacement therapy (HRT; solid line) and placebo (dotted line) on the incidence of coronary heart disease in the Heart and Estrogen/progestin Replacement Study (HERS). Source: Hulley *et al.* (1998).

'wrong' in the placebo group in the early years but towards the end of the study a protective effect can be divined. Others fail to see this benefit.

It is indeed true that this specific study cannot disprove the hypothesis that in the long term (more than 5 years?) HRT does protect women from CHD, but such theories need to be followed up in further formal studies such as the ongoing Women's Health Initiative in the USA. The interested reader is strongly advised to obtain some of the numerous editorials and correspondence generated by this single study, but always to bear in mind that HERS was a well-conducted placebo-controlled trial of 'hard' cardiovascular endpoints, albeit of a specific HRT formulation in a specific patient population.

Oestrogen replacement in atherosclerosis (ERA)

Effects of estrogen replacement on the progression of coronary-artery atherosclerosis.

DM Herrington, DM Reboussin, KB Brosnihan, *et al. New Engl J Med* 2000; **343**: 522–9.

BACKGROUND. The technique of quantitative coronary angiography provides a way to monitor the 'anatomical' response of arteries to drugs such as statins. Studies in fat-fed rabbits and monkeys have been used to explain the low incidence of CHD seen in HRT users as being due to the ability of oestrogen to reduce the size and prevalence of atherosclerotic lesions in coronary arteries. Although the technique can only be justified in women with symptomatic CHD, coronary angiography might be expected to provide a convenient way of comparing the cardiovascular effects of different therapies, such as oestrogen monotherapy versus combined therapy or oral versus transdermal administration. Such studies could be carried out in the setting of relatively small, randomized placebo-controlled trials, at a fraction of the cost of studies using disease endpoints such as MI.

INTERPRETATION. Despite the predicted effect on the plasma lipoprotein profile, neither unopposed oestrogen (CEE 0.625 mg/day) nor continuous combined therapy (CEE 0.625 mg/day plus 2.5 mg/day MPA) affected the progression of angiographically defined atherosclerosis in women with established heart disease (Table 6.1). Analysis of several subgroups and secondary angiographic endpoints ('data torture') failed to show any beneficial effect of either therapy over placebo. The rates of clinical cardiovascular events were the same among the three groups.

Comment

The clear expectation of this study was that HRT would significantly reduce the extent of coronary atherosclerosis, particularly in the group randomized to oestrogen alone. This group, based at Wake Forest University, USA, has been heavily

Table 6.1 The influence of hormone replacement therapy (HRT) on angiographic disease

Minimal coronary artery diameter (mm)	Oestrogen (n = 79)	Oestrogen/ MPA (n = 85)	Placebo (n = 84)	*P* value Oestrogen versus placebo	Oestrogen/ MPA versus placebo
Baseline	1.98 ± 0.03	1.91 ± 0.04	1.98 ± 0.04	0.93	0.17
Adjusted follow-up	1.87 ± 0.02	1.84 ± 0.02	1.87 ± 0.02	0.81	0.23
Adjusted change	–0.09 ± 0.02	–0.12 ± 0.02	–0.09 ± 0.02	0.97	0.38

MPA = medroxyprogesterone acetate.
Source: Herrington *et al.* (2000).

involved in the promotion of standardization procedures for angiographic measurement of disease. If these scientists are unable to demonstrate an improvement in angiographic scores despite a study of such rigour, then it is unlikely that any other group will succeed.

As with HERS, this study was an out-and-out failure. Re-analysis of the data set using stratification and secondary endpoint analysis failed to uncover any subgroup of women who responded well to therapy. The authors concluded that CHD patients should not use oestrogen replacement therapy with the expectation of cardiovascular benefit. At a time when the failure of HERS was being linked to the use of MPA, the finding of no difference between the CEE and CEE/MPA arms is of particular interest: this study suggests that the progestin component of HRT is an irrelevance in terms of cardiovascular outcomes.

The authors attempted to explain their failure by acknowledging that coronary angiography may not necessarily be the best way of following the risk of CHD, citing issues of plaque stability whereby HRT might have a beneficial effect on outcomes even if plaque size (as evidenced by angiography) is unchanged. This is true, but it was axiomatic at the time this study was planned that HRT reduced the number and severity of atherosclerotic lesions. The emerging issue of pro-inflammatory actions of oestrogen on C-reactive protein is also discussed. The authors also postulated that HRT may not be effective in older women with established disease, holding out the prospect of a beneficial effect in primary prevention. This theme has been picked up by others, but it needs to be acknowledged that, up until the publication of the HERS and ERA findings, HRT had been considered to be especially beneficial in the old, the diseased and those loaded with CHD risk markers.

A British case–control cohort study

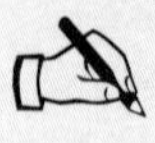

Hormone replacement therapy and incidence of acute myocardial infarction. A population-based nested case-control study.

C Varas-Lorenzo, LA Garcia-Rodriguez, S Perez-Gutthann, A Duque-Oliart. *Circulation* 2000; **101**: 2572–8.

BACKGROUND. **A nested case–control cohort study, unusual in that the data were obtained outside the USA and also that some of the women used transdermal rather than oral HRT.**

INTERPRETATION. A total of 1242 new cases of acute myocardial infarction (AMI) were identified in the UK General Practice Research Database (GPRD). The diagnosis was confirmed in 1013 of these women, and their characteristics compared with a control group of 5000 healthy women from the same cohort. The risk of AMI was reduced by nearly 30% in women who used HRT (relative risk 0.72, 95% CI 0.59–0.89). There was no evidence of any harmful effect in the first year of therapy. Although numbers were small, the authors claim that the protection was less striking in women given combined therapy. Transdermal therapy was associated with protection although this did not reach statistical significance (relative risk 0.75, 95% CI 0.47–1.21). There was no evidence of an oestrogen dose effect.

Comment

A conventional exercise in observational epidemiology, the results of which depended on the ability of the authors to adjust for health status differences between their users and non-users. There was no attempt to adjust for differences in socio-economic status, for example. The novelty of the paper is the data on transdermal therapy, although the authors' claim that this 'might' be protective may be an over-interpretation of the data: many drugs 'might' protect women from CHD.

Review: oestrogen and cardiovascular disease

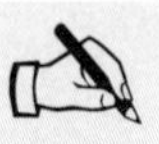

The protective effects of estrogen on the cardiovascular system.

ME Mendelsohn, RH Karas. *New Engl J Med* 1999; **340**: 1801–11.

BACKGROUND. **The rapid pace of investigation into the molecular mechanisms by which oestrogen influences arterial function necessitated an authoritative review. This**

article, part of the classic 'Mechanisms of Disease' series in the *New England Journal of Medicine* is simply superb. The illustrations are outstanding and it is well worth obtaining a colour photocopy of this review.

INTERPRETATION. Starting with an update on the newly described oestrogen beta receptor this review describes the multiple ways in which oestrogen is intimately involved in vascular function, in particular the activation of nitric oxide synthase.

Comment

This is likely to become the classic review in its field. The one problem for the authors is that this impressive pattern of anti-atherogenic properties seen with oestrogen is inconsistent with the failure of HERS. The authors speculate that a small subgroup of women in HERS may have had an adverse reaction to the oestrogen, the progestin or both.

Menopause as a risk marker for MI

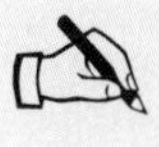

Menopause and risk of non-fatal acute myocardial infarction: an Italian case–control study and a review of the literature.

F Fioretti, A Tavani, S Gallus, S Franceschi, C La Vecchia. *Hum Reprod* 2000; **15**: 599–603.

BACKGROUND. The common belief that HRT reduces the incidence of CHD can be linked to the belief that oestrogen deprivation associated with the climacteric increases the risk of this disease. Data are presented from an Italian case–control study involving 429 women who had suffered an AMI and 863 hospital-based controls.

INTERPRETATION. Postmenopausal women were at higher risk of MI compared with premenopausal women but this excess risk disappeared following adjustment for age and other covariates (Table 6.2). In essence, CHD was common in postmenopausal women, but this was due to the fact that postmenopausal women are older than premenopausal women and CHD risk is strongly influenced by age.

Table 6.2 Distribution of acute myocardial infarction (AMI) cases and controls according to menopausal status

Menopausal status	AMI cases	Controls	Odds ratio (95% confidence interval)
Pre/perimenopausal	141	344	(1)
Postmenopausal	282	517	0.99 (0.64–1.53)

Source: Fioretti *et al.* (2000).

Comment

One of the cornerstones of the belief that HRT reduces CHD risk is the belief that the menopause increases this risk so replacement therapy will reduce the risk. In fact the evidence for a menopausal link has always been weak. The present case–control study suffers from all the inherent flaws of this approach but should not be ignored. The paper contains an excellent review of the literature on menopause and CHD. The issue is not as straightforward as was once thought.

Is it all just a 'healthy user' effect?

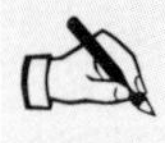

Pre-existing risk factor profiles in users and non-users of hormone replacement therapy: prospective cohort study in Gothenburg, Sweden.

K Rodstrom, C Bengtsson, L Lissner, C Bjorkelund. *Br Med J* 1999; **319**: 890–3.

BACKGROUND. The most impressive evidence that HRT prevents CHD has come from observational epidemiological surveys in which the health of women who take HRT is compared with the health of their neighbours or professional colleagues who do not. Such studies indicate that HRT reduces the risk by 50%. HRT users tend to be healthier than non-users, although the epidemiologists claim to compensate for this bias in their analysis. Such adjustments are often restricted to issues such as educational qualifications, cigarette smoking, body mass index, blood pressure, etc. In this study, 1201 women in Gothenburg, Sweden were followed for up to 24 years. This allowed the authors to look for baseline differences between those women who went on to take HRT and those who chose not to.

INTERPRETATION. Those women who went on to use HRT were clearly in better health than those who did not. A range of statistically significant differences was seen. Those who went on to take HRT started with lower blood pressure, less obesity and, most strikingly, a higher socio-economic status than those who did not. If, at the end of this follow-up, an observational study of these women had been carried out then one would expect HRT users to be protected against CHD, regardless of any drug effect.

Comment

The observational evidence that HRT prevents CHD is impressive but is only as good as the ability of the investigators to adjust for bias and confounding. This study suggests that detailed analysis of CHD risk, especially socio-economic status, would be needed to interpret properly the data from observational studies.

Meta-analysis of CHD from small placebo-controlled trials

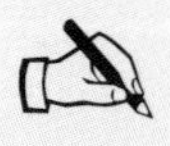

Value of drug-licensing documents in studying the effect of postmenopausal hormone therapy on cardiovascular disease.
E Hemminki, K McPherson. *Lancet* 2000; **355**: 566–9.

BACKGROUND. These authors have previously argued |1| that a prospective randomized placebo-controlled trial of the ability of HRT to prevent cardiovascular disease could be synthesized by pooling data from existing trials in which CHD had not been a primary endpoint. In the current update, new trials submitted by the pharmaceutical industry to regulatory authorities are included. It is of some concern that the authors were forced to go to the Finnish High Court to extract some of this information.

INTERPRETATION. Of the 17 studies analysed, the odds ratio for cardiovascular disease events in HRT users compared with those randomized to placebo was 1.34 (95% CI 0.55–3.30). The number of events (22) was low. The authors maintained that their analysis would have been able to detect a 50% reduction in risk if such protection existed.

Comment

The reaction to the first paper from these authors was quite negative and indeed there is a genuine concern that such a 'patchwork quilt' approach to research may not be wise. However, this update appeared as equally negative results were emerging from formal trials and as the C-reactive protein issue (see below) raised its ugly head. This approach to research will always be unpopular but has now earned the right to be considered as a part of the current debate.

A pro-inflammatory effect of HRT?

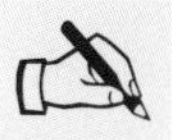

Hormone replacement therapy and increased plasma concentration of C-reactive protein.
PM Ridker, CH Hennekens, N Rifai, JE Buring, JE Manson. *Circulation* 1999; **100**: 713–6.

BACKGROUND. Following the ground-breaking work of the late Russell Ross, atherosclerosis research now firmly focuses on the concept that the disease is due to a deranged inflammatory response to injury. Markers of this response can be detected in plasma and these appear to be more strongly associated with disease than conventional risk factors such as plasma lipoproteins. One small study claimed that postmenopausal oestrogen therapy reduced plasma levels of C-reactive protein, consistent with an anti-inflammatory and anti-atherosclerotic action of this steroid. In this study, plasma C-reactive protein levels were measured in 493 healthy postmenopausal women.

INTERPRETATION. Median plasma C-reactive protein levels were twice as high in HRT users as in controls.

Comment

This finding has now been replicated in formal prospective placebo-controlled trials. There is no doubt that HRT has this unwanted effect on C-reactive protein and it is tempting to use this finding to explain the early increase in arterial disease seen in some women starting HRT. If these women had unstable arterial plaques then the inflammatory response to HRT might be sufficient to start a clinical symptom of the disease, regardless of the other potentially beneficial effects of therapy.

Consensus panel statement

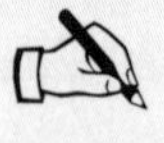

Guide to Preventive Cardiology for Women. AHA/ACC Scientific Statement: Consensus Panel Statement.
L Mosca, SM Grundy, D Judelson, *et al. J Am Coll Cardiol* 1999; **33**: 1751–5.

BACKGROUND. The failure of HERS challenged the preconception that doctors were reducing CHD risk in their patients simply by prescribing HRT. The American Heart Association and the American College of Cardiology convened a meeting to analyse existing data on CHD in women and to make recommendations. This consensus statement was endorsed by the American College of Obstetricians and Gynecologists, among others.

INTERPRETATION. The panel acknowledged that further trials are needed, especially in women free of cardiovascular disease, but considered the evidence strong enough to make the recommendation that women with CHD should not be given HRT. In those women already on HRT it was considered reasonable to continue therapy while awaiting further trial evidence. In healthy women there are insufficient data to make any recommendations concerning HRT and CHD. The role of conventional risk management, especially cessation of smoking and the use of statin drugs, should be at the forefront of CHD risk reduction strategies.

Comment

Some of the previous guidelines from the USA were strongly in favour of a role for HRT in the prevention of CHD. The strength of some of the statements in the current guidelines shows that HERS has clearly made a major impact on the cardiological community in the USA. Note that since this statement was published, further negative studies have been published and that the policy of 'wait and see' recommended for women with CHD taking HRT will need to be revised in the next guidelines. In terms of primary prevention, it should be noted that no drug that has failed in the secondary prevention of CHD has been found to be worthwhile in primary prevention.

Summary

The year 2000 was traumatic for those interested in the cardiovascular effects of HRT. Old ideas about the merits of different progestins in terms of the lipid profile are being discarded and attention is switching to the effect of the oestrogen component on C-reactive protein levels. If an inflammatory action of oestrogen is proven it may be possible to screen out women who will react adversely to HRT. As with most screening procedures, such a strategy requires a vigorous validation before entering clinical practice.

Reference

1. Hemminki E, McPherson K. Impact of postmenopausal hormone therapy on cardiovascular events and cancer: pooled data from clinical trials. *Br Med J* 1997; 315: 149–53.

7

Hormone replacement therapy and breast cancer

Introduction

Endogenous oestrogen is implicated in the aetiology of breast cancer. However, the role of hormone replacement therapy (HRT) remains controversial. In 1997, the Collaborative Group for Hormonal Factors in Breast Cancer (CGHFBC) |1| published their re-analysis of 51 individual observational studies of HRT and breast cancer risk. This constitutes more than 90% of world-wide data and is the most comprehensive review available. The main findings were that per year of use, the risk of breast cancer with HRT exposure was equivalent to that observed with delaying the menopause (2.3 and 2.8%, respectively) and that the lifetime risk of developing breast cancer was significantly increased with current, long-term HRT use [greater than 5 years' use (relative risk 1.35, 95% CI 1.21–1.49)]. This risk, however, falls following cessation of HRT and by 5 years is no greater than that in women without any history of exposure and therefore provides the strongest evidence for HRT acting as a promoter of pre-existing breast cancer rather than initiating malignant transformation in the breast. Paradoxically, the growth-promoting effect of HRT does not appear to have an adverse effect on breast cancer mortality |2|.

Almost exclusively, conclusions about the influence of HRT are based on observational data and as a result, there are many issues about its potential influence on breast cancer that still remain unresolved. Clinical trials published since the re-analysis, for the most part support its findings but have not provided unequivocal evidence about the effect of HRT on breast tumour mortality, the biological behaviour of this disease or whether the growth-promoting effect of HRT is confined to tumours which are considered hormonally responsive [i.e. oestrogen receptor positive (ER +ve)].

The hormone sensitivity of breast cancer

The anti-oestrogenic activity of the selective oestrogen receptor modulator (SERM), tamoxifen, is considered responsible for the efficacy of this drug in the treatment and, potentially, prevention of breast cancer. In conjunction with observational data demonstrating an association of elevated plasma oestrogen levels with an increased risk of developing postmenopausal breast cancer, this has refocused

attention on the link between endogenous oestrogen exposure, breast cancer risk
and progression.

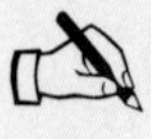

Tamoxifen for early breast cancer: an overview of randomised trials.

Early Breast Cancer Trialists' Collaborative Group. *Lancet* 1998; **351**: 1451–67.

BACKGROUND. Every 5 years since 1984–1985, the Early Breast Cancer Trialists' Collaborative Group (EBCTCG) has undertaken systematic overviews of all randomized trials of any aspect of the treatment of early breast cancer. The most recent overview of adjuvant tamoxifen therapy was based on data collected and finalized in 1995–1996. Information was sought on each of 37 000 women in any randomized trial that began before 1990 of tamoxifen versus no tamoxifen. Overall, data from 55 randomized trials were analysed and this comprised at least 87% of the world-wide evidence. The EBCTCG was able to evaluate the effect of duration of therapy (i.e. 1, 2 or 5 years) on outcome.

INTERPRETATION. Tamoxifen has significant disease-free and overall survival benefits for women with ER +ve, early stage breast cancer ($2P < 0.00001$ for a median of 10 years of follow-up), the degree of benefit progressively increasing with duration of use. Five years of tamoxifen therapy produced a halving of the annual rate of ER +ve contralateral breast cancer incidence, irrespective of menopausal status and the ER status of the primary breast tumours, confirming the findings of a previous EBCTCG overview in 1992.

Comment

Whilst the survival benefit incurred by tamoxifen is greatest in women with ER +ve disease, some women with ER poor disease may also demonstrate a clinical response. It is postulated that this hormonal responsiveness is conferred by the presence of a functional progesterone receptor (PgR). If confirmed by subsequent clinical trials, this could widen the selection criteria for patients treated with endocrine breast cancer therapy.

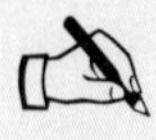

The NSABP P-1 trial. Tamoxifen for prevention of breast cancer: report of the National Surgical Adjuvant Breast and Bowel Project P-1 Study.

B Fisher, JP Constatino, DI Wickerham, *et al.* and other National Surgical Adjuvant Breast and Bowel Project Investigators. *J Natl Cancer Inst* 1998; **90**: 1371–88.

BACKGROUND. The significant reduction in the incidence of contralateral breast cancer reported with tamoxifen exposure led to the initiation of large placebo-controlled randomized tamoxifen chemoprevention trials in women at risk of developing breast cancer in the USA, the UK and Italy (Table 7.1). The largest of these

Table 7.1 Tamoxifen for the prevention of breast cancer: randomized trials

| | Patient characteristics | | | | | Breast cancers/year/1000 women | | |
	Age < 50 years	Primary relative with breast cancer	Breast cancer risk	Sample size	Median follow-up (months)	Placebo	Tamoxifen	*P* Value
NSABP-P1	39%	75%	≥1.66 risk/5 years	13 388	54	6.8	3.6	<0.00001
Italian	38%	18%	Low to normal	5405	46	2.9	2.1	0.6
Royal Marsden Hospital	61%	100%	>3	2471	70	5.0	4.7	0.8

Source: Fisher *et al.* (1998).

trials, the NSABP-P1, recruited 13 388 eligible women between 1992 and 1997 and was stopped prematurely and unblinded in 1997 following the 5-year analysis. At this point, the mean time on the study for the participants was 47.7 months (median 56.6 months).

INTERPRETATION. Tamoxifen exposure was associated with a highly significant reduction in the incidence of both invasive breast cancer (49% reduction, two-sided $P < 0.00001$) and non-invasive ductal or lobular carcinoma in situ (50% reduction, two-sided $P < 0.002$). The decrease in invasive breast cancer was only observed for tumours that were ER +ve (relative risk 0.31, 95% CI 0.22–0.45 comparing tamoxifen with placebo). The duration of follow-up was too short to draw any conclusions about the effect of tamoxifen on cause-specific and all-cause mortality.

Comment

In response to the published findings from the American trial, interim analyses of the UK and Italian chemoprevention trials were undertaken |3, 4|, but neither has demonstrated any risk reduction with the use of tamoxifen. Various explanations have been put forward to account for this discrepancy, including the fact that HRT use was permitted in the European trials but not in the NSABP-P1 trial. Whilst interim analyses do not support HRT antagonizing a preventative effect of tamoxifen, it is important to remember that their combined influence on breast cancer incidence was not a primary hypothesis of either trial. Given the magnitude of the risk reduction reported in the NSABP-P1 trial, it is unlikely that the Royal Marsden trial was under-powered to detect any effect of tamoxifen. Compared with the NSABP-P1 trial, women participating in the Royal Marsden prevention trial were younger and more likely to be selected on the basis of a family history of breast cancer and therefore probably a greater proportion had inherited mutations in the *BRCA1* and *BRCA2* genes. Breast cancers developing in such women tend to be ER –ve and raise the question of whether tamoxifen may be less effective as a preventative agent in this group of women.

Perhaps the most important point about the NSABP-P1 trial is that the short duration of follow-up prevented any meaningful analysis of breast cancer mortality and therefore it is not possible to determine whether the benefit of tamoxifen is due to an absolute reduction in breast cancer incidence, or instead reflects treatment of subclinical disease. Furthermore, it still remains to be determined if the use of tamoxifen in the preventive setting could predispose to the development of endocrine-resistant breast cancer. Despite these caveats, the Food and Drug Administration in the USA has approved tamoxifen for risk reduction in the setting of primary or contralateral breast cancer prevention. However, the European trials are continuing and in the UK tamoxifen is not recommended as a preventative agent outside of the context of a clinical trial.

Confidence in the findings of the NSABP-P1 trial has led to the planning of a further randomized breast cancer chemoprevention trial in the USA, comparing tamoxifen directly with raloxifene [the Study of Tamoxifen and Raloxifene (STAR or NSABP-P2) trial].

The latter has been associated with a significant reduction in the incidence of ER +ve breast cancer (relative risk 0.35, 95% CI 0.21–0.58) at a median follow-up of 40 months in the ongoing randomized Multiple Outcomes of Raloxifene Evaluation (MORE) study, although breast cancer incidence is not a primary study outcome |5|.

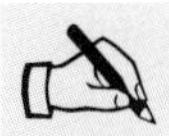

Plasma sex steroid hormone levels and risk of breast cancer in postmenopausal women.

SE Hankinson, WC Willett, JE Manson, *et al. J Natl Cancer Inst* 1998; **90**: 1292–9.

BACKGROUND. This prospective, nested case-controlled study evaluated the relationship between sex steroid hormone levels and the risk of breast cancer development in postmenopausal women enrolled in the Nurses' Health Study. Blood samples were collected between 1989 and 1990 from 11 169 postmenopausal women not using HRT. Two matched controls were selected per case of breast cancer (n = 154) that was diagnosed in this cohort before 1994.

INTERPRETATION. This study provides evidence for a causal relationship between postmenopausal serum oestrogen levels and breast cancer risk. Women who developed breast cancer had significantly elevated serum levels of oestradiol ($P = 0.04$), oestrone ($P = 0.02$) and oestrone sulphate ($P = 0.02$) compared with women who did not progress to develop the disease. Comparison of extreme quartiles of serum oestradiol, oestrone and oestrone sulphate levels demonstrated statistically significant associations with breast cancer risk (oestradiol, multivariate relative risk 1.91, 95% CI 1.06–3.46; oestrone, multivariate relative risk 1.96, 95% CI 1.05–3.65; oestrone sulphate, multivariate relative risk 2.25, 95% CI 1.23–4.17) but these were reduced and not statistically significant when body mass index was controlled for. This is not too surprising given that body mass index is an important determinant of serum oestrogen concentration in postmenopausal women. The positive associations with oestrogen and risk were found to be stronger in women with no previous exposure to HRT, but the calculated 95% confidence intervals were wide and these data should therefore be treated with caution.

Comment

The strengths of this study compared with previous reports are the larger number of incident breast cancer cases (n = 154) upon which the calculated risk estimates were based and the detailed analysis of the different circulating serum oestrogens. The positive association between an elevation in serum oestradiol and breast cancer risk is consistent with earlier studies. Postmenopausal oestradiol replacement, however, is metabolized rapidly to oestrone and oestrone sulphate and associations between increments in the serum levels of these oestrogen metabolites and breast cancer risk have only been explored in this and two other smaller studies and have generated contradictory findings. At present, it would be inappropriate to recommend that serum oestrogen levels could be used as a clinical indicator of breast cancer risk.

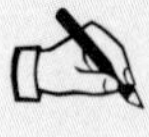

Low biologic aggressiveness in breast cancer in women using hormone replacement therapy.

K Holli, J Isola, J Cuzick. *J Clin Oncol* 1998; **16**: 3115–20.

BACKGROUND. A population-based cohort of 477 Finnish peri- and postmenopausal women presenting with breast cancer at one hospital were interviewed about HRT use and their tumours analysed for sex steroid receptor expression and indicators of biological aggressiveness (i.e. tumour grade and proliferation).

INTERPRETATION. Thirty-six per cent of the women had a history of HRT exposure; of these the majority (64%) had used combined HRT. Current use of HRT was associated with an increase in tumours less than 2 cm in size ($P = 0.0005$), that were better differentiated ($P = 0.04$) and had a lower proliferation rate as assessed by S-phase fraction ($P = 0.009$). These differences predominated in women with ER +ve disease, but no trends were observed for the duration or type of HRT prescribed.

Comment

A significantly greater proportion of women using HRT had their breast cancers diagnosed by screening mammography (42% compared with 32% in non-users, $P = 0.02$). This could account for their tendency to present with tumours with less aggressive tumour characteristics and could contribute to a chance association between ER positivity and decreased proliferation.

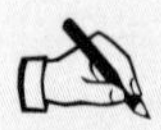

Hormone replacement therapy and high S phase in breast cancer.

MA Cobleigh, FE Norlock, DM Oleske, A Starr. *J Am Med Assoc* 1999; **281**: 1528–30.

BACKGROUND. The prognostic characteristics and sex steroid receptor content of breast cancers arising in a cohort of 331 postmenopausal women presenting consecutively at one teaching hospital in the USA were compared according to prior HRT exposure.

INTERPRETATION. HRT did not influence the expression of tumour sex steroid receptors. However, half the HRT users with ER +ve disease had a high S-phase fraction compared with less than one-fifth of HRT users with ER –ve tumours.

Comment

This study suggests that HRT promotes the proliferation of ER +ve but not ER –ve breast cancer. This is consistent with the findings of the EBCTCG overview and the

NSABP-P1 trial. Stimulation of the growth of a pre-existing breast cancer may lead to its earlier detection and could account for the increase in disease incidence reported in the collaborative re-analysis.

Summary

Current data from clinical trials provide strong evidence that endogenous oestrogen regulates the growth of ER +ve breast cancer, although details of the ER status of tumours diagnosed in women with elevations in endogenous serum oestrogen levels, which would be of further interest, are unavailable. In view of the findings of the collaborative re-analysis, it is biologically plausible that HRT will promote the proliferation of breast cancer cells. However, whether this effect only occurs in ER +ve disease requires verification. One of the main factors hindering interpretation of the latter studies is that it is unclear as to whether HRT was taken up to the day of breast biopsy. The relevance of this is that hormonal therapy has been demonstrated to induce significant changes in breast tumour proliferation indices within a few days of administration |6|. Hence, cessation of HRT, even a few days prior to biopsy, could influence results significantly. It is hypothesized that endogenous serum oestrogen levels may have value as a clinical indicator of breast cancer risk in postmenopausal women. If this is confirmed by further study, is there any relevance to the prescription of HRT, where serum oestrogen levels are far in excess of the normal postmenopausal range and those of endogenous oestrogen reported to be associated with a significant increase in breast cancer risk? If anything, this serves to question our basic understanding of the mechanisms by which oestrogen deprivation or exposure influences breast cancer cell growth.

HRT and the risk of breast cancer development— studies published since the CGHFBC re-analysis

The collaborative re-analysis risk estimates for breast cancer development were based predominantly on the use of unopposed oestrogen replacement therapy. Details of the hormonal constituents of the HRT prescribed to women in the re-analysis were only available for 39% of those taking HRT; of these, 12% had been exposed to progestins. It was concluded that current, long-term use of combined HRT might confer a greater lifetime risk of developing breast cancer than oestrogen alone [relative risk for more than 5 years of use was 1.53 (SE 0.33)], but the number of breast cancer cases upon which this risk estimate was based was considered too small for this finding to be considered definitive.

Recent observational studies of the effect of combined therapy on epithelial proliferation in the breast and breast cancer risk (Table 7.2) have, however, generated significant concern.

Table 7.2 Epidemiological studies of hormone replacement therapy (HRT) and breast cancer risk published since the 1997 Collaborative Group for Hormonal Factors in Breast Cancer (CGHFBC) re-analysis

		Increase in relative risk of developing breast cancer according to duration of use (95% confidence interval) and type of HRT			
Reference	Duration	O [no. of cases]	CHRT [no. of cases]	SHRT [no. of cases]	CCHRT [no. of cases]
CGHFBG	> 5 years of use	1.34 (SE 0.09) [558]	1.53 (SE 0.33) [58]		
Colditz et al.	Per year of use	1.033 (SE 0.84) [not stated]	1.09 (SE 2.5) [not stated]		
Persson et al.	1–6 years	1.0 (0.6–1.4) [23]	1.4 (0.9–2.3) [28]		
	> 6 years	1.1 (0.7–1.7) [35]	1.7 (1.1–2.6) [44]		
Magnusson et al.*	Per year of use	1.03 (0.98–1.08) [137]	1.07 (1.02–1.11) [409]	1.03 (0.94–1.13) [102]	1.19 (1.09–1.31) [135]
	P value for trend	0.44	0.0005	0.27	0.0002
Schairer et al.†	Increase per year of use	0.03 (0.01–0.06) [234]	0.12 (0.02–0.25) [52]		
	P value for trend	0.001	0.01		
	< 4 years of use		1.1 (0.8–1.7) [26]		
	≥ 4 years of use		1.5 (1.0–2.4) [22]		
Ross et al.‡	Per 5 years of use	1.06 (0.97–1.15) [742]	1.24 (1.07–1.45) [425]	1.38 (1.13–2.68) [320]	1.09 (0.88–1.3) [105]
	P value for trend	0.18	0.005	0.0015	0.44

O = unopposed oestrogen; CHRT = combined oestrogen and progestin, type and pattern of progestin prescription not documented; SHRT = sequential combined HRT; CCHRT = continuous combined HRT.
*Values given for women using combined HRT with 19 nor-testosterone progestin derivatives.
†Values given for women with body mass index <24.4 kg/m^2.
‡HRT prescribed predominantly ≤0.625 mg conjugated equine oestrogen ± medroxyprogesterone acetate (i.e. C 21 progesterone derivative).

Hormone replacement therapy with estrogen or estrogen plus medroxyprogesterone acetate is associated with increased epithelial proliferation in the normal postmenopausal breast.

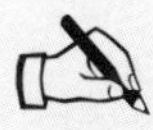

LJ Hofseth, AM Raafat, JR Osuch, DR Pathak, CA Slomski, SZ Haslam.
J Clin Endocrinol Metab 1999; **84**: 4559–65.

BACKGROUND. Steroid receptor status and proliferation indices (i.e. Ki67 and proliferating cell nuclear antigen) were assayed in breast tissue obtained from 86 postmenopausal women who underwent surgical breast biopsy for the diagnosis of a suspicious palpable, or mammographically detected lesion. Fifty-seven women were using HRT and were categorized according to their exposure [i.e. (1) no HRT, defined as not having taken HRT for 1 year before surgery; (2) oestrogen alone, or (3) oestrogen and progestin for at least 3 months up to the day of surgery]. The majority were prescribed conjugated equine oestrogen (CEE) and medroxyprogesterone acetate (MPA) 2.5–5 mg was taken continuously in those requiring combined therapy.

INTERPRETATION. HRT increased breast epithelial proliferation indices and cellular density significantly; combined therapy had the most pronounced effect, especially in the terminal ductal lobular unit of the breast, the site where cancer is believed to develop. A non-significant trend association between duration of HRT exposure and the degree of proliferation and duration was observed. Unopposed oestrogen increased the number of breast lobules per unit area and combined therapy induced morphological changes equivalent to those of the luteal phase of the menstrual cycle. Irrespective of type, HRT had no influence on ER expression.

Comment

This study suggests that combined HRT stimulates proliferation of breast epithelium to a greater extent than oestrogen alone and supports observational studies reporting a greater promoting effect of combined therapy on breast cancer risk. However, the conclusion that the degree of proliferation is directly related to the duration of exposure is tenuous in view of the small patient numbers.

Use of estrogen plus progestin is associated with greater increase in breast cancer risk than estrogen alone.

GA Colditz, B Rosner for the Nurses' Health Study Research Group.
Am J Epidemiol 1998; **147**(S): 64S.

BACKGROUND. This paper reviewed data after 16 years of follow-up (980 000 person-years) of women participating in the Nurses' Health Study. The original cohort consisted of 121 700 registered female nurses in the USA aged between 30 and 55 years who completed a questionnaire every 2 years to determine breast cancer risk and exposure factors which could influence this.

INTERPRETATION. A total of 2035 incident cases of breast cancer were diagnosed in postmenopausal women who provided information about HRT use and did not have a family history of breast cancer. Controlling for all breast cancer risk factors, the annual risk with oestrogen exposure alone per year was 3.3% (SE 0.84%) and for oestrogen plus progestin it was 9.0% (SE 2.5%). Compared with never users of HRT, the long-term use of combined HRT (i.e. up to 10 years) was estimated to incur a greater risk of breast cancer development than oestrogen alone (relative risk of 1.58 compared with 1.11).

Comment

The main problem with the interpretation of this study was the lack of provision of the number of breast cancer cases upon which the analyses were based and for the risk estimate provided with long-term use, the absence of confidence intervals. Whilst figures were given for risk associated with combined HRT, no information was provided about the different regimens prescribed which is relevant for clinical practice.

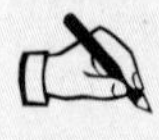

Risks of breast and endometrial cancer after estrogen and estrogen–progestin replacement.

I Persson, E Weiderpass, L Bergqvist, R Bergström, C Schairer.
Cancer Causes Control 1999; **10**: 253–260.

BACKGROUND. This study was based on the long-term findings from prospective follow-up of a cohort of Swedish women established in 1977–1980. In total over 23 000 women who had received a prescription for HRT were enrolled and followed up by mailed questionnaire in 1987–1988. Cancer events were documented through linkage with the National Swedish Cancer Registry for the period from 1987/1988 until 31 December 1993.

INTERPRETATION. A total of 198 incident cases of breast cancer were diagnosed. Short-term use (i.e. 1–6 years) of either unopposed oestrogen or oestrogen combined with a progestin was not associated with a statistically significant increase in risk (relative risk 1.0, 95% CI 0.6–1.7 compared with relative risk 1.4, 95% CI 0.9–2.3, respectively). With longer-term use (> 6 years), however, the risk of breast cancer was increased with exposure to combined HRT (relative risk 1.7, 95% CI 1.1–2.6).

Comment

Although supporting the findings of the collaborative re-analysis, this study was under-powered and positive conclusions were drawn from very small numbers of incident breast cancer cases. As for the Nurses' Health Study data, no information was provided about the type of combined therapy prescribed.

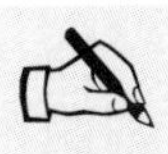

Breast cancer risk following long-term oestrogen and oestrogen–progestin replacement therapy.

C Magnusson, LA Baron, N Correia, R Bergström, HO Adami, I Persson.
Int J Cancer 1999; **81**: 339–44.

BACKGROUND. This population-based case–control study was based on a cohort of 3345 Swedish women aged from 50 to 74 years, who were identified between 1993 and 1995. Subjects completed a postal questionnaire to obtain information about postmenopausal HRT use and risk factors for breast cancer. Incident breast cancer cases were identified through the National Swedish Cancer Registry.

INTERPRETATION. Use of oestrogen with or without the addition of a progestin was associated with an increased risk of breast cancer and this risk increased with increasing duration of use (odds ratio for women treated for at least 10 years 2.43, 95% CI 1.79–3.30 compared with never users). Combined HRT preparations with C21 progesterone-derived progestins were not associated with any increase in breast cancer risk, but this was based on very few breast cancer cases (32 cases and 34 controls). Regimens containing 19 nor-testosterone-derived progestins increased the risk of breast cancer by 8% per year of use (odds ratio 1.08, 95% CI 1.07–1.13). However, this increase in risk only appeared to be associated with continuous combined and not with sequential prescription of these progestins (odds ratio per year of use 1.03, 95% CI 0.94–1.13 compared with 1.19, 95% CI 1.09–1.31, respectively). Subgroup analysis found that risk was significantly increased with HRT if a woman's body mass index was less than 22.0 kg/m^2.

Comment

This was the first study in which differences in combined oestrogen–progestin regimens were evaluated in any detail, suggesting that exposure to testosterone-derived progestins may confer greater risk than progesterone-derived progestins. This supports theoretical arguments, which favour avoidance of the former, as they are relatively androgenic. However, women receiving combined HRT predominantly used continuous 19 nor-testosterone-derived progestins. No increase in risk was observed with the sequential prescription of testosterone-derived or C21 progesterone-derived progestins, but the small number of incident breast cancer cases developing in women so exposed rendered it impossible to make valid risk comparisons between these different preparations.

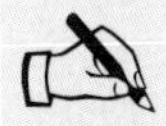

Menopausal estrogen and estrogen–progestin replacement therapy and breast cancer risk.

C Schairer, J Lubin, R Troisi, S Sturgeon, L Brinton, R Hoover. *J Am Med Assoc* 2000; **283**: 485–91.

BACKGROUND. The findings of this study were based on a cohort of 46 000 American women participating in a national screening programme, the Breast Cancer

Detection Demonstration Project. Women were followed up by either telephone or mailed questionnaires.

INTERPRETATION. Based on 2082 cases of incident breast cancer, it was concluded that combined HRT induces a greater increase in breast cancer risk than oestrogen alone and that this is directly related to current or recent use and duration of use. The primary type of oestrogen used was CEE and the primary progestin prescribed was the C21 progesterone derivative, MPA. In women who used combined HRT, the majority used progestins for 15 days or less per month. Oestrogen replacement therapy was found to be associated with an increase in both invasive and in situ breast cancer, whereas combined therapy was only associated with an increase in invasive disease. This relationship was significant only for women with a body mass index less than 24.4 kg/m^2.

Comment

The importance of this study is that it attempted to define risk according to the type of progestin prescribed and the pattern of progestin prescription. Unfortunately, it was insufficiently powered to do so and it is only appropriate to comment about risk associated with sequential MPA and even then the number of breast cancer cases upon which estimated risks have been based were small. The same arguments apply for subgroup analyses respecting extent of disease and tumour histology.

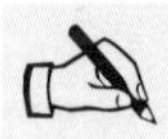

Effect of hormone replacement therapy on breast cancer risk: estrogen versus estrogen plus progestin.

RK Ross, A Paganini-Hill, PC Wan, MC Pike. *J Natl Cancer Inst* 2000; **92**: 328–32.

BACKGROUND. **This population-based case–control study involved American women identified from the Cancer Surveillance Program [which is part of the National Surveillance, Epidemiology and End Results (SEER) Program of the US National Cancer Institute] and the population-based cancer registry of Los Angeles County. Case and control subjects were interviewed in person.**

INTERPRETATION. A total of 1897 incident breast cancer cases were identified over a 4.5-year period, 54% of which had used HRT. The majority of HRT use was unopposed oestrogen. In those using combined HRT, most were prescribed sequential MPA. The data were compatible with a steady increase in risk with increasing duration of use of either unopposed oestrogen (odds ratio per 5 years of use 1.10, 95% CI 1.02–1.18; $P = 0.015$) or combined HRT (odds ratio per 5 years of use 1.24, 95% CI 1.07–1.45; $P = 0.005$). Risk was calculated to be higher in women using sequential rather than continuous combined HRT (odds ratio per 5 years of use of sequential therapy 1.38, 95% CI 1.13–1.68 compared with odds ratio 1.09, 95% CI 0.88–1.35 for continuous therapy).

Comment

The investigators of this study concluded that sequential combined HRT conferred the greatest risk of breast cancer, but again the numbers of incident breast cancer cases in the subgroup analyses were small.

Summary

Whilst the studies evaluating breast cancer risk with combined HRT exposure are limited in the absence of appropriate comparative, randomized control groups, they do provide further evidence that short-term use of HRT for the relief of oestrogen-deficiency symptoms does not appear to be associated with a significant increase in the risk of breast cancer development. They do, however, provide evidence for an increase in breast cancer risk with current, long-term exposure to combined therapy, but as the data from individual studies are expressed in different ways, it is difficult to determine accurately the degree of magnitude of this risk and therefore whether this is equivalent to, or greater than, that conferred by oestrogen alone. The observation that a lower body mass index may be an important predictor of breast cancer development in women exposed to HRT is intriguing and compatible with the collaborative re-analysis, but there is no plausible biological explanation for this at present and no guidance exists to enable the identification of potentially susceptible women in this subgroup.

The study of Hofseth *et al.* (1999) provides biological evidence for a mitogenic effect of combined oestrogen and progestin on the postmenopausal breast which is greater than oestrogen alone, but uncertainty still remains regarding the role of differing classes of progestin (i.e. 19 nor-testosterone and C21 progesterone derivatives) and the pattern of use (i.e. sequential or continuous) on potential modification of this effect. The hypothesis that continuous combined, rather than sequential, HRT will confer protection against the development of breast cancer, as in vitro, the continuous application of progestin with oestrogen induces a sustained, inhibitory effect on cell replication mediated through PgR-driven cellular pathways [7], does not appear to be substantiated by the work of Hofseth *et al.* (1999). Issues surrounding the relative merits, or not, of the 19 nor-testosterone and C21 progesterone derivatives still remain to be resolved in the absence of direct comparisons. Presently, there are insufficient clinical data on which to base clinical recommendations about the use of combined HRT and breast cancer risk.

The effect of HRT on breast cancer mortality and tumour biology

Studies evaluating the influence of HRT on subsequent breast cancer mortality suggest no adverse effect, but potential confounders, such as screening mammography or differences in breast cancer therapy, have often not been controlled or adjusted for in the analysis. The study of Fowble *et al.* (1999) investigated the effect of prior

HRT use on the disease-free and cause-specific mortality of women with breast cancer, but took into account treatment factors that could influence this. The collaborative re-analysis did not explore the question of breast cancer mortality in relation to HRT exposure, but did report that HRT use was associated with a significant increase in the proportion of women presenting with localized rather than advanced stage breast cancer. This has stimulated interest in the question of whether the apparent reduction in breast cancer mortality with HRT is attributable to the promotion of disease with a more favourable prognostic outcome.

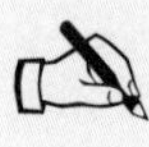

Postmenopausal hormone replacement therapy: effect on diagnosis and outcome in early-stage invasive breast cancer treated with conservative surgery and radiation.

B Fowble, A Hanlon, G Freedman, *et al. J Clin Oncol* 1999; **17**: 1680–8.

BACKGROUND. The pretreatment characteristics and outcome of postmenopausal women with early stage breast carcinoma according to HRT use prior to diagnosis were compared. A total of 485 postmenopausal women were diagnosed between 1979 and 1993 and followed up for a median of 5.9 (range 0.1–15.6) years. Information about HRT use was obtained from questionnaires administered at presentation. One hundred and forty-one women had a history of HRT exposure, but the timing of HRT use in relation to breast cancer diagnosis was unascertainable in a third of these patients.

INTERPRETATION. Women who used HRT were significantly younger ($P = 0.0009$) and had a lower body mass index ($P = 0.004$) than never users. A greater proportion of breast tumours developing in HRT users were ≤ 2 cm in size ($P = 0.02$), but no differences existed with respect to tumour sex steroid expression, lymph node status or grade. The cumulative incidence of ipsilateral breast cancer recurrence was significantly increased in HRT users ($P = 0.02$) despite their being no evidence of any difference in the proportion of women treated with breast conservation surgery, the administration and dosage of radiotherapy, chemotherapy and tamoxifen, or the incidence of positive excision margins. However, prior HRT use was associated with a significant reduction in the cumulative incidence of distant metastases ($P = 0.01$) and a trend, of borderline significance, towards a reduction in cause-specific mortality at 10 years. HRT exposure was not associated with an increase in the incidence of contralateral breast cancer.

Comment

Only tumour size was found to be different in HRT users and this could reflect the fact that, although of only borderline significance, more women with a history of HRT exposure were diagnosed by screening mammography. Whilst this study did take into consideration treatment factors, caution should be exercised in drawing firm conclusions from the calculated cumulative incidences of local and distant recurrence as these were based on a very small number of breast cancer events.

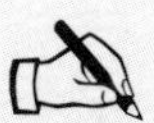

Hormone replacement therapy and risk of breast cancer with a favourable histology.

SM Gapstur, M Morrow, TA Sellers. *J Am Med Assoc* 1999; **281**: 2091–7.

BACKGROUND. Histological classification of breast cancers diagnosed in women taking HRT was analysed from a cohort of 1520 incident breast cancer cases in participants of the Iowa Women's Health Study. Information about breast cancer risk factors and HRT use was obtained from a series of mailed questionnaires.

INTERPRETATION. Thirty-seven per cent of women had used HRT prior to their breast cancer diagnosis; 29% (n = 165) had used HRT for more than 5 years. No evidence was provided for any association between HRT and the risk of developing ductal carcinoma in situ or invasive ductal or lobular carcinoma. However, a positive association was demonstrated with the development of tubular, medullary and papillary carcinoma, irrespective of duration of use (multivariate-adjusted relative risk for current use ≤5 years, relative risk 4.42, 95% CI 2.00–9.75; current use >5 years, relative risk 2.63, 95% CI 1.18–5.89).

Comment

It is difficult to produce a plausible biological explanation for the apparent association of HRT with an increased risk of biologically favourable breast cancer but not invasive ductal or lobular carcinoma. Furthermore, the conclusion of this study, that the lack of an adverse effect of HRT on breast cancer mortality can be explained by its association with the development of breast cancers with a more favourable prognostic outcome, is flawed in that the tumour groupings can be challenged as considerable controversy surrounds the prognosis of women diagnosed with medullary carcinoma.

Summary

Lack of data accrued from randomized comparisons renders it impossible to determine a biological rationale for the observation that HRT does not adversely affect breast cancer mortality and cannot exclude a healthy user effect or selection bias. Lead time bias following more frequent screening mammography or clinical examination could contribute to the apparent improvement in breast cancer mortality with HRT exposure. However, whilst evidence supporting a reduction in breast cancer mortality has yet to be confirmed, mortality does not appear to be increased.

HRT and mammography

HRT increases mammographic breast density and may reduce the effectiveness of mammographic breast cancer screening, increasing the number of women presenting with interval breast cancer. It is important to ascertain the impact of HRT on the prognosis of women presenting with such interval cancers.

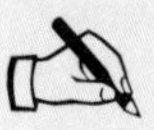

Effects of estrogen and estrogen–progestin on mammographic parenchymal density.

GA Greendale, BA Reboussin, A Sie, *et al.* for the Postmenopausal Estrogen/Progestin Interventions (PEPI) Investigators. *Ann Intern Med* 1999; **130**: 262–9.

BACKGROUND. Subset analysis of 307 women participating in the Postmenopausal Estrogen/Progestin Interventions (PEPI) trial was undertaken to evaluate the effect of HRT on mammographic breast density over a 3-year follow-up period. The randomized treatment comparisons were between placebo, unopposed CEE, sequential combined HRT [CEE plus MPA or CEE plus micronized progesterone (MP)] and continuous combined HRT (CEE plus daily MPA).

INTERPRETATION. Both unopposed oestrogen and combination HRT regimens were associated with an increase in mammographic breast density compared with placebo during the first year of exposure. The proportion of women experiencing an increase in breast density with CEE was 3.5% (95% CI 1.0–12.0%), CEE plus cyclic MPA 23.5% (95% CI 11.9–35.1%), CEE plus cyclic MP 16.4% (95% CI 6.6–26.2%), CEE plus continuous MPA 19.4% (95% CI 9.9–28.9%). Density increases were more pronounced in women taking combined therapy, but no significant difference was found according to the pattern of use of progestin (i.e. cyclical or continuous).

Comment

This was the first randomized placebo-controlled study to evaluate the effect of HRT on mammographic breast density and it supports numerous observational studies reporting an increase with HRT use. The changes induced by HRT were all statistically significant, but the confidence intervals were very wide, particularly for combined therapy. Whilst an increase in mammographic breast density is associated with an increase in the risk of developing breast cancer, it would be premature, based on the results of this study alone, to conclude that changes in breast density with HRT exposure could be used as a surrogate measure of a woman's potential risk of developing cancer of the breast and further controlled investigation of this effect of HRT is required. Rather than elevate actual breast cancer risk, a relative increase in risk could occur due to a delay in breast cancer diagnosis.

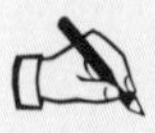

Hormone replacement therapy and accuracy of mammographic screening.

AM Kavanagh, H Mitchell, GG Giles. *Lancet* 2000; **355**: 270–4.

BACKGROUND. Data on the effect of HRT on the specificity and sensitivity of mammographic screening are inconsistent. Here, the accuracy of screening mammography was evaluated in a cohort of 103 770 asymptomatic women attending for their first round of screening during 1994 in Victoria, Australia. Interval cancers

were identified by linkage with the Victoria Cancer Registry. Women completed a questionnaire, which included documentation of current HRT use, at their screening appointment.

INTERPRETATION. Sensitivity was lower in current HRT users (64.8%, 95% CI 57.9–71.8%) compared with non-users (77.5%, 95% CI 73.8–80.9%). In absolute terms, the reduction in sensitivity with HRT use would have accounted for 23 fewer breast cancers being diagnosed by mammography. Among all women screened, the adjusted relative risk of having a small cancer detected was unaffected by HRT exposure. The most plausible explanation for reduced mammographic sensitivity in HRT users is an increase in mammographic breast density. There was no difference in tumour size, grade or axillary lymph node status when comparing screen-detected or interval cancers in HRT users or non-users. Outside the target age group for screening (i.e. 50–69 years), no reduction in sensitivity was found with HRT.

Comment

Although the use of HRT appears to decrease the detection rate of screen-detected breast cancer, prognostic factors were no worse in HRT users presenting with interval cancers that were probably missed in the initial screening round. Regarding the data on the effect of HRT on the sensitivity of mammographic screening in younger women outside the target group for breast cancer screening, the value of mammographic screening has yet to be determined; randomized trials are currently underway.

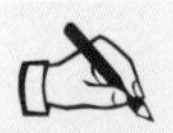

Effect of hormone replacement therapy on the pathological stage of breast cancer: population based, cross-sectional study.

S Stallard, JC Litherland, CM Cordiner, *et al. Br Med J* 2000; **320**: 348–9.

BACKGROUND. **The pathological features of screen-detected and interval cancers in a cohort of 1130 women who underwent mammographic screening between 1988 and 1993 were compared according to HRT use at the time of mammography.**

INTERPRETATION. From the initial cohort, 100 women with screen-detected cancer and 66 with interval cancers were using HRT at diagnosis. A comparison of women according to HRT exposure found no difference in tumour size, grade or histological type of invasive cancer. There was no difference in the proportion of women diagnosed with well-differentiated tumours (tubular, mucoid and invasive ductal grade I cancers) when comparing HRT users with non-users (24 and 22%, respectively, odds ratio 0.98, 95% CI 0.63–1.50). Analysis of screen-detected cancers alone again found no difference between these tumour characteristics according to HRT use.

Comment

Although patient numbers using HRT were small, this study does not support the hypothesis that HRT promotes the development of tumours with more favourable prognostic features. However, as with the findings of Kavanagh *et al.* (2000), HRT exposure was not associated with poorer prognosis disease, particularly in women presenting with interval cancers.

Summary

The findings of an increase in mammographic breast density with HRT exposure, particularly with combined therapy, are not unexpected given the results of the collaborative re-analysis and more recent studies investigating the effect of HRT on normal breast and tumour epithelial proliferation rates. As previously stated, it is premature to assume that changes in mammographic density incurred by HRT confer the same degree of risk associated with natural increases in breast density. The Million Women Study, a survey of HRT use in women attending for mammographic breast cancer screening in the UK, will not provide definitive data on breast cancer risk in the absence of a randomized control group for comparison (Institute of Cancer Research, Epidemiology Unit/National Health Service Breast Screening Programme). Whilst HRT may increase the presentation of interval cancers, this delay in diagnosis does not seem to confer a survival disadvantage, as defined by prognostic indicators. However, long-term follow-up with survival data is necessary to confirm this observation. It has been reported that cessation of HRT for as little as 2 weeks prior to mammography could be sufficient to overcome the problem of reduced sensitivity |8|.

The use of HRT in women at high risk of breast cancer

Considerable controversy surrounds the use of HRT in women with a history of familial breast cancer. Tumours arising in women due to inherited mutations in the *BRCA1* and *BRCA2* genes may have a hormone-resistant phenotype in that they are usually high grade, ER and PgR negative. It has been assumed, therefore, that reproductive factors may not have a significant effect in their development, but the following study challenges this assumption.

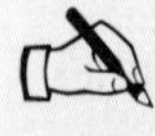

Breast cancer risk after bilateral prophylactic oophorectomy in BRCA1 carriers.

TR Rebbeck, AM Levin, A Eisen, *et al. J Natl Cancer Inst* 1999; **91**: 1475–9.

BACKGROUND. Women with **BRCA1** mutations are at a high risk of developing both cancer of the ovary and cancer of the breast. This study compared the incidence of breast cancer in carriers of **BRCA1** mutations according to whether they had undergone prophylactic oophorectomy for the prevention of ovarian carcinoma. Some women elected to use HRT after their oophorectomy for the amelioration of oestrogen-deficiency symptoms. Therefore, a subgroup analysis was undertaken to determine whether this had any influence on breast cancer incidence.

INTERPRETATION. Forty-three *BRCA1* mutation carriers who had undergone prophylactic oophorectomy were matched with 79 mutation carriers who had not. Breast cancer risk was significantly reduced following oophorectomy (adjusted hazard ratio of 0.53, 95% CI 0.33–0.84). This benefit was limited to women who had oophorectomy at a younger age. Information about HRT was available for 81% of the sample subjects and it did not appear to influence significantly the benefit of oophorectomy in lowering breast cancer risk.

Comment

This study is important as it implies that reproductive factors are important in familial as well as sporadic breast cancer development. HRT would therefore be expected to decrease the benefit conferred by oophorectomy, but this was not the case. As patient numbers were small, it is impossible to conclude whether HRT influences breast cancer risk or not in *BRCA1* mutation carriers. Further study is necessary before making any recommendations about the use of HRT in *BRCA1* mutation carriers undergoing oophorectomy for the prevention of ovarian carcinoma.

Women with benign breast disease are generally considered to be at an increased risk of developing breast cancer and traditionally have been advised to avoid HRT. However, this diagnosis encompasses a spectrum of histological change, not all of which is associated with a significant increase in cancer risk. Studies reviewing the risk of breast cancer in this group as a whole, have not reported HRT to increase risk significantly, but failure to categorize benign breast disease according to histological diagnosis renders accurate counselling of women difficult.

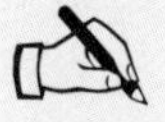

Estrogen replacement therapy in women with a history of proliferative breast disease.

WD Dupont, DL Page, FF Parl, *et al. Cancer* 1999; **85**: 1277–83.

BACKGROUND. This study involved a retrospective analysis of a consecutive series of women who had a biopsy-proven diagnosis of benign breast disease between 1952 and 1978. Follow-up data, which included documentation of oestrogen replacement therapy exposure and the number of incident breast cancer cases, were available for 87.6% (n = 9494) of eligible women. The relative risks of developing breast cancer were calculated with respect to women who took oestrogen replacement but whose benign breast biopsy did not demonstrate any evidence of atypical hyperplasia, complex fibroadenoma or proliferative changes without atypia.

INTERPRETATION. Four hundred and forty-four incident cases of breast cancer were diagnosed during the follow-up period (190 845 person-years). Oestrogen replacement therapy was not found to elevate the risk of breast cancer in women with benign breast

Table 7.3 Breast cancer risk, benign breast disease and the effect of hormone replacement therapy

	Without ERT		With ERT	
Classification of benign disease	**No. of cases**	**RR (95% CI)**	**No. of cases**	**RR (95% CI)**
Proliferative disease with atypical cell changes (atypical ductal or lobular hyperplasia)	5	2.53 (1.0–6.3)	7	2.87 (1.3–6.3)
Proliferative disease without atypia (multiple cysts, duct papillomata, sclerosing adenosis)	21	1.13 (0.69–1.9)	29	1.37 (0.88–2.1)
All proliferative benign disease (duct ectasia, solitary cysts, fibroadenoma)	26	1.27 (0.81–2.0)	36	1.52 (1.0–2.3)
Complex fibroadenoma	4	1.46 (0.53–4.0)	7	1.57 (0.72–3.4)

RR = relative risk; CI = confidence interval; ERT = oestrogen replacement therapy.
Source: Dupont *et al.* (1999).

disease, nor was any association shown for those women who also had a first-degree family history of breast carcinoma (Table 7.3). It was concluded that HRT should not be a contraindicated in women with histologically proven benign breast disease.

Comment

The strength of this study compared with others examining HRT and benign breast disease was that the women were analysed according to their risk of developing breast cancer. This ensured that the calculated risk estimates for HRT were based on women whose benign disease was likely to confer an increased risk of developing breast cancer. Unfortunately, the numbers of incident breast cancer cases upon which the risk estimates were based were small.

Summary

In both women with a family history of breast cancer and benign breast disease, HRT does not appear to increase breast cancer risk, but these studies are not definitive. It is essential that women at high risk are adequately counselled about their personal risk of breast cancer development; for those with a family history, genetic counselling may be appropriate. A patient can only make an informed decision about HRT use when they have a clear idea of their own personal risk and possible preventative interventions.

The incidence of oestrogen-deficiency symptoms in breast cancer survivors

In view of evidence implicating endogenous oestrogen in the aetiology of breast cancer, it would be appropriate to question why HRT should be considered at all in the management of women with a diagnosis of breast cancer. However, the management of problems related to oestrogen deficiency, specifically vasomotor symptoms and vaginal dryness, is an increasing clinical challenge as these symptoms are common side effects of breast cancer therapy that is directed towards suppressing or antagonizing the effect of endogenous oestrogen. As the median age of onset of the climacteric or menopause in women in the UK often coincides with the time of breast cancer diagnosis and treatment, it can be very difficult to determine whether oestrogen-deficiency symptoms are naturally occurring or iatrogenic. A growing number of studies is attempting to define the scope of this problem in more detail.

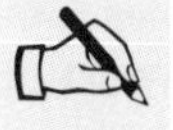

Hot flashes in postmenopausal women treated for breast carcinoma.

JS Carpenter, MA Andykowski, M Cordova, *et al. Cancer* 1998; **82**: 1682–91.

B A C K G R O U N D . **Information on the prevalence and severity of hot flushes in 114 postmenopausal breast cancer patients was elicited by a structured telephone questionnaire.**

INTERPRETATION. The mean time from diagnosis in the study population was 39 (range 4–154) months and an average of 34.4 (range 4–116) months had passed since the completion of breast cancer therapy (i.e. surgery, chemotherapy and radiotherapy). Sixty-five per cent of the study population experienced hot flushes, which were rated as severe in 59%. Symptomatic women were more likely to have received chemotherapy (78%) or adjuvant tamoxifen (72%). Hot flushes were more likely to occur in younger patients and those with a higher body mass index. The incidence of hot flushes in women more than 10 years postmenopause was 54%.

The authors concluded that treatment-induced hot flushes appear to be more bothersome and persist for longer compared with those experienced by healthy postmenopausal women.

Comment

This small cross-sectional study concurs with previous published data suggesting that, at any one time, up to two-thirds of treated breast cancer patients may experience oestrogen-deficiency symptoms. The increase in symptoms in younger patients is probably accounted for by chemotherapy-induced ovarian suppression. The association, however, with increased body mass index is difficult to explain given that this is usually correlated with greater endogenous oestrogen levels and could therefore be a chance finding due to the small patient numbers. With respect to counselling women about the side-effects of their adjuvant therapy, this study is important as it supports anecdotal findings that iatrogenic symptoms may be induced in women who are many years into the postmenopause.

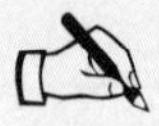

Risk of menopause during the first year after breast cancer diagnosis.

PJ Goodwin, M Ennis, KI Pritchard, M Trudeau, N Hood. *J Clin Oncol* 1999; **17**: 2365–70.

BACKGROUND. A substantial part of the benefit incurred by adjuvant chemotherapy in premenopausal breast cancer patients is mediated through primary ovarian suppression. In some women, chemotherapy induces a premature menopause, the risk of which increases with advancing age. Factors predicting the onset of the menopause in a cohort of premenopausal women with newly diagnosed breast cancer receiving adjuvant polychemotherapy (i.e. cyclophosphamide, methotrexate and fluorouracil or cyclophosphamide, epirubicin and fluorouracil), tamoxifen, both, or no treatment, were examined in this study with the aim of generating a model that could be used to provide clinically useful estimates of the risk of menopause occurring in women receiving adjuvant breast cancer therapy. A cohort of 183 premenopausal women with locoregional breast cancer who had been treated surgically provided information on menopausal status at diagnosis and 1 year later, irrespective of whether they had received adjuvant therapy. Women whose menses stopped during this time and had not returned by the 1-year follow-up were classified as postmenopausal.

INTERPRETATION. Age and systemic chemotherapy were the strongest predictors of the menopause in this cohort. The mean age of women becoming menopausal was greater than that of women who remained premenopausal during the study (45.5 years compared with 42.3 years). The risk of menopause was increased with the addition of tamoxifen. There was no evidence of a difference in risk according to the chemotherapy regimen prescribed. The graphic representation of the multivariate analysis is shown in Fig. 7.1.

Comment

With the more widespread use of adjuvant chemotherapy and tamoxifen in premenopausal women, it is anticipated that the proportion of younger women developing a premature menopause is likely to increase. This is an important study as it provides an aid to clinical decision-making in planning the treatment of premenopausal breast cancer patients. A question that remains to be answered, however, is whether women who regain menses during follow-up are at an increased risk of early menopause at a later stage.

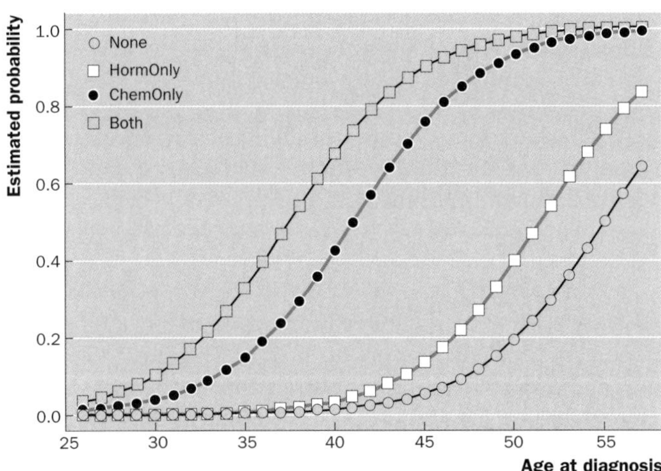

Fig. 7.1 Probability of menopause during the first year after diagnosis. Source: Goodwin *et al.* (1999).

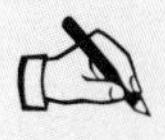

Assessment of quality of life in women undergoing hormonal therapy for breast cancer; validation of an endocrine symptom subscale for the FACT-B.

LJ Fallowfield, SK Leaity, A Howell, S Benson, D Cella. *Breast Cancer Res Treat* 1999; **55**: 89–199.

BACKGROUND. **Information about the frequency of side-effects attributable to endocrine breast cancer therapy in 223 breast cancer patients was accrued in the**

course of this study undertaken to develop and validate an 18-item endocrine subscale to be used in conjunction with a standardized breast cancer quality of life measure [the Functional Assessment of Cancer Therapy (FACT-B)]. Ninety-eight women had advanced breast cancer and 135 had early stage disease. The range of endocrine therapy prescribed included tamoxifen, anastrozole or high-dose megestrol acetate; some women with primary disease used anastrozole and tamoxifen in combination. Forty women with primary disease had developed permanent amenorrhoea following the administration of adjuvant chemotherapy within the previous 6 months. Forty-one patients were not receiving any endocrine therapy.

INTERPRETATION. The most frequently reported symptoms were loss of sexual interest (31%), weight gain (25%) and hot flushes (24%). Loss of interest in sex was most prominent in women with advanced disease treated with tamoxifen or anastrozole and women with early stage disease receiving no current therapy but who had received prior chemotherapy. Weight gain was most common in women taking megestrol acetate. Hot flushes were significantly more common in women who had experienced chemotherapy-induced ovarian ablation (45%) or who had been treated with adjuvant tamoxifen (30.2%). Patients reporting marked vaginal dryness were most likely to be in the adjuvant chemotherapy or megestrol acetate group.

Comment

This confirms that women may experience significant side-effects from endocrine breast cancer therapy and that these are more pronounced in those rendered prematurely menopausal by adjuvant chemotherapy.

Summary

Discussion of treatment side-effects, including the consequences of the long-term sequelae of oestrogen deficiency, is an important aspect of the information required by patients when making decisions about their breast cancer therapy. With the increasing use of adjuvant breast cancer therapy, increasing numbers of women with early stage disease are expected to have a near normal life expectancy and will therefore spend many years in a postmenopausal state. It is essential, therefore, that sensitive, valid methodology to document the incidence and impact of treatment-induced side-effects be developed.

Alternatives to HRT for the management of oestrogen-deficiency symptoms in breast cancer patients

Concern that HRT may increase the risk of developing breast cancer recurrence has led to considerable interest in the use of alternatives for the control of oestrogen-deficiency symptoms. However, few have been evaluated in controlled prospective trials. Recent interest has focused on the use of clonidine, the antidepressant venlafaxine, phyto-oestrogens and low-dose progestins. Whilst tibolone is increasingly being prescribed to breast cancer patients, there is a complete lack of any controlled data of its use in this group of women.

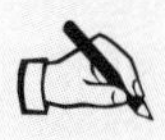

Evaluation of soy phytoestrogens for the treatment of hot flushes in breast cancer survivors: a North Central Cancer Treatment Group trial.

SK Quella, CL Loprinzi, DL Barton, *et al. J Clin Oncol* 2000; **18**: 1068–74.

BACKGROUND. One hundred and eighty-two women with early stage breast cancer who were experiencing hot flushes were randomized to receive three 600 mg soy-containing tablets daily (each tablet contained 50 mg of soy isoflavones: 40–45% genisten, 40–45% diadzein, 10–20% glycitein) or placebo for 4 weeks and then crossed over for a further 4 weeks. A daily questionnaire was completed documenting hot flush frequency, severity and side-effects.

INTERPRETATION. Eighty-four per cent of women completed the follow-up. The soy product tablets had a marginal, non-significant benefit when compared with placebo. At the end of the study, there was no significant patient preference for the use of phyto-oestrogens.

Comment

Soy products are being advocated as a healthy, safe and 'natural' option for the control of menopausal symptoms, but there are few scientific data that support this. Whilst population studies in Asian women with a high dietary soy intake imply that phyto-oestrogens might protect against the development of breast cancer, in vitro data are contradictory as both antiproliferative and proliferative activity has been demonstrated. These plant-derived steroids are weakly oestrogenic and their activity may be influenced by the concentration of circulating serum oestrogen. Significantly more controlled data about the therapeutic and toxic effects of the different phyto-oestrogens are required before any recommendations should be made about their prescription in breast cancer survivors.

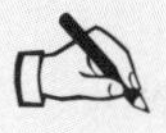

Oral clonidine in postmenopausal patients with breast cancer experiencing tamoxifen-induced hot flushes: a University of Rochester Cancer Centre Community Clinical Oncology Program Study.

KJ Pandya, RF Raubertas, PS Flynn, *et al. Ann Intern Med* 2000; **132**: 788–93.

BACKGROUND. Studies evaluating the effectiveness of the antihypertensive agent clonidine, a centrally acting α-adrenergic agonist, in controlling menopausal hot flushes in breast cancer patients have been inconsistent. Here, 194 symptomatic

women with early stage breast cancer treated with tamoxifen were randomized to receive clonidine (0.1 mg/day orally) or placebo for 8 weeks. The frequency and severity of hot flushes were assessed daily and quality of life was monitored prior to therapy, and at 4-weekly intervals after initiation of therapy.

INTERPRETATION. After 8 weeks, compared with placebo, clonidine reduced hot flush frequency, severity and hot flush score (i.e. mean frequency × mean grade of severity) significantly ($P = 0.006$, 0.08, 0.006, respectively). Global quality of life improved ($P = 0.02$) in clonidine-treated women when assessed using a linear, visual analogue score.

Comment

The withdrawal rate from this study at 8 weeks was high (i.e. 23%), but no information was provided about the women's reasons for doing so. It is left to speculate whether lack of efficacy of clonidine contributed towards this in any way. The fact that clonidine-related side-effects were low in women completing the study does not exclude the possibility that women withdrew due to intolerance of adverse, treatment-induced symptoms. As with other studies of alternative therapies to HRT, the lack of long-term data on the efficacy of clonidine limits its clinical application.

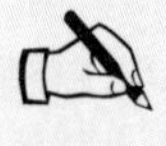

Venlafaxine alleviates hot flashes: a North Central Cancer Treatment Group Trial.

CL Loprinzi, JW Kugler, JA Mailliard, *et al. Proceedings of the (36th) Annual Meeting of the American Society of Clinical Oncology*, Vol. 19, 2000, Abstract 4.

BACKGROUND. **Anecdotal reports that venlafaxine, a serotonin and noradrenaline re-uptake inhibitor used for the treatment of depression, reduces oestrogen-deficiency symptoms prompted the undertaking of a randomized trial comparing venlafaxine with placebo in breast cancer patients. One hundred and eighty women with breast cancer who were experiencing hot flushes were randomized to receive placebo or daily venlafaxine doses of 37.5, 75 or 150 mg for 4 weeks. Women completed a daily hot flush diary for the study duration.**

INTERPRETATION. Venlafaxine was associated with a statistically significant decrease in the hot flush score (i.e. number of hot flushes × mean severity) compared with placebo ($P < 0.0001$). The most efficacious dose was 75 mg, achieving more than a 50% reduction in the hot flush score in 62% of women.

Comment

Venlafaxine appears to be a promising treatment for the alleviation of hot flushes in women with breast cancer. However, controlled data on its longer-term efficacy and side-effect profile are necessary before endorsing it as a valid alternative to

HRT. Whilst the side-effects documented during this study (anorexia, dry mouth and nausea) did not appear to occur very frequently, the use of this antidepressant is associated with disorders of sexual functioning in up to 12% of patients, but this is believed to be considerably under-reported. In the short term, this may not be a problem. However, if vasomotor symptoms are improved, the development of problems relating to sexual functioning could contribute to poor compliance. This is particularly relevant for women with breast cancer as sexual dysfunction is a common side-effect of endocrine breast cancer therapy and a cumulative effect needs to be excluded or confirmed.

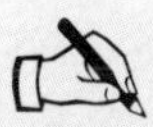

Long term use of megestrol acetate by cancer survivors for the treatment of hot flashes.

SK Quella, CL Loprinzi, JA Sloan, *et al. Cancer* 1998; **82**: 1784–8.

BACKGROUND**. The study population consisted of a cohort of patients who had participated in a previous placebo-controlled randomized trial which demonstrated the superiority of low-dose megestrol acetate (40 mg daily) in the control of hot flushes (symptom reduction of 85% compared with 20% in placebo-treated patients). The maximum duration of the original randomized trial was only 8 weeks, but some patients elected to continue taking megestrol acetate after the study was completed. The perceived benefits and toxicity of long-term megestrol acetate were documented from the responses of 132 of the original study population who completed a semi-structured telephone interview.

INTERPRETATION**. The mean elapsed time since the completion of the randomized trial was 3 years. The randomized trial recruited both men with prostatic cancer, and women with breast cancer who were experiencing hot flushes as a result of their endocrine breast cancer therapy. Fifty-eight of the cohort contacted were female; of these 31% (17/58) were still using megestrol acetate. Whilst 41% (7/17) of these women were still symptomatic, this did not appear to be troublesome. The range of side-effects reported by women who discontinued the progestin was diverse, but the most common complaint was that of abnormal vaginal bleeding, which occurred in one-third of patients. Other symptoms documented included appetite stimulation and weight gain, episodes of chills and depressive mood. Sixty-eight per cent (28/41) of women who stopped taking megestrol acetate experienced hot flushes.

Comment

The uncontrolled follow-up of such a small cohort of breast cancer patients treated with long-term megestrol acetate precludes any firm recommendations from being made about its long-term use. The high incidence of vaginal bleeding may reflect an effect of progestin on a tamoxifen-primed endometrium, but no figures were presented regarding the number of women who were also taking tamoxifen or their menopausal status. This is an issue that warrants further evaluation.

Summary

At present, whilst there appear to be some promising alternatives to HRT for the relief of oestrogen-deficiency symptoms, controlled trials of their long-term efficacy and toxicity must be undertaken before advocating them as safe and effective alternatives. This is particularly relevant in the case of low-dose progestins given that recent epidemiological studies implicate progestin as a mitogen in the postmenopausal breast.

The use of HRT in breast cancer survivors

The contention that a history of breast cancer is an absolute contraindication to HRT is now being challenged, particularly in view of the lack of efficacious alternatives for the alleviation of oestrogen-deficiency symptoms in women with a history of the disease. Consequently, HRT is being prescribed increasingly to symptomatic breast cancer survivors and to date, observational data have not shown a detrimental effect on disease-free or overall survival. However, uncertainty will continue about the safety of HRT in the absence of data from randomized controlled trials.

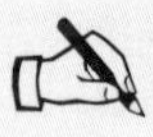

Oestrogen replacement therapy after localised breast cancer: clinical outcome of 319 women followed up prospectively.

R Vassilopoulou-Sellin, L Asmar, GN Hortobagyi, *et al. J Clin Oncol* 1999; **17**: 1428–87.

Background**.** **The effect of HRT was documented on the clinical outcome of a cohort of 319 postmenopausal women with early stage breast cancer followed up for a median of 40 (range 24–99) months. Women included in this study had previously been invited by the investigators to participate in a randomized controlled trial of HRT in breast cancer survivors. Of the original cohort, 62 had consented to take part in the randomized trial, the remaining 257 declined to do so but agreed to be followed up and therefore constituted the control group for this observational study. A total of 39 women took oestrogen replacement therapy (i.e. 0.625 mg CEE).**

Interpretation**.** Baseline comparison of HRT users with non-users failed to demonstrate any differences regarding age at diagnosis or tumour characteristics, although HRT users were more likely to have been premenopausal at diagnosis ($P = 0.014$). One patient who took oestrogen developed a contralateral breast cancer that was positive for both ER and PgR after 27 months of therapy. There were 20 cancer events (i.e. recurrence or contralateral disease) in the control group.

Comment

The number of cancer-related events was considerably greater in the control group, but this cannot be interpreted as evidence that HRT is safe, or reduces the risk of breast cancer recurrence, as this was a small, non-randomized comparison. The selection criteria for the initial randomized trial only included women with early stage disease if their cancer was ER −ve and they had been disease free for 2 or more years, or women with ER +ve disease if they had been disease free for 10 or more years. Such women constitute a very good prognosis group and therefore are at very low risk of developing recurrence. If HRT does have a negative impact on outcome it is unlikely to be detected in such a small sample population as this. However, this study does add to the growing list of published series of patients who have elected to use HRT following a diagnosis of breast cancer and have not reported an obvious adverse effect on prognosis, some of which are reviewed by the authors in their paper. This and earlier studies have been used as justification for the undertaking of randomized controlled trials of HRT in breast cancer survivors.

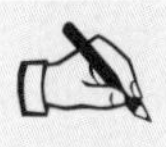

Are randomised trials of hormone replacement therapy in symptomatic breast cancer patients feasible?

J Marsden, NPM Sacks, M Baum, RP A'Hern, MI Whitehead. *Fertil Steril* 2000; **73**: 292–9.

BACKGROUND. The objective of this study was to determine the feasibility of conducting a large randomized trial of HRT in symptomatic women with early stage breast cancer, that is if women were willing to be randomized to receive a therapy which, although providing symptomatic benefit, could equally increase their risk of breast cancer recurrence. This open, randomized study recruited 100 postmenopausal women with early stage breast cancer experiencing vasomotor symptoms and/or vaginal dryness, from out-patient clinics in two London teaching hospitals. Women were stratified according to current tamoxifen use and then randomized to HRT (oestradiol valerate 2 mg daily in hysterectomized women or the same oestrogen plus levonorgestrel 75 µg/day for 12 of 28 days in those with an intact uterus), or no HRT for 6 months. The main outcome measures were acceptance and continuance rates and the reasons eligible women declined study entry.

INTERPRETATION. Oestrogen-deficiency symptoms were associated with a significant, negative impact on patient quality of life. Despite detailed informed consent, which emphasized the uncertainty surrounding HRT and breast cancer recurrence, recruitment was completed in 1 year with an acceptance rate of 38.8% and continuance rates of greater than 80% in each treatment arm. The majority (75%) of patients allocated HRT wished to continue using it after the 6-month study period. Three women developed metastatic disease; two used HRT, one for 2 years and the other for 6 weeks only. Whilst concern about breast cancer recurrence was an important reason for women to decline study entry, prior experience of unexpected and unpleasant side-effects of endocrine breast cancer therapy dissuaded many women from participating in a study of HRT, as this itself was perceived to be associated with unwanted adverse effects. The efficacy of HRT did not appear to be antagonized with concomitant tamoxifen. The results suggested that it is both feasible and justified to conduct a national UK randomized trial of HRT in symptomatic patients and such a trial is to be launched imminently (The Institute of Cancer Research, Sutton, Surrey).

Comment

Whilst the acceptance and continuance rates of this pilot study suggest that a national trial can be implemented, this is only likely to be successful if detailed information about HRT and the oestrogen-deficiency side-effects of breast cancer therapy are provided at the outset and patients have ready access to counselling during the trial.

Summary

Until the results of controlled prospective trials become available, the prescription of HRT in breast cancer patients, which should only be undertaken by the specialist in charge of the patient's care, will necessitate extensive counselling, involving an explanation of the potential positive benefits of HRT being weighed against the clinical uncertainty that it may increase the risk of breast cancer recurrence.

Conclusion

Whilst studies published since the collaborative re-analysis have not resulted in a significant change in clinical practice, they have served to provide a greater basis upon which to advise women about the risk of HRT exposure and breast cancer. In counselling women, it would seem justified to explain that the risk of breast cancer with the use of short-term HRT for the relief of oestrogen-deficiency symptoms, is probably negligible, but there does appear to be a small increased risk of breast cancer with longer-term use (i.e. for more than 10 years), although this falls following the cessation of HRT. At present it is not possible to state with any certainty whether this risk varies with the type of HRT prescribed. Irrespective of the type of HRT, breast cancer mortality, which is the most important endpoint, may not be adversely affected. It is anticipated that results from the ongoing large, randomized trials of HRT in healthy women in the USA (the Women's Health Initiative, which was set up by the National Institutes of Health) and the UK (the MRC WISDOM study; the Women's International Study of Long-duration Oestrogen use after the Menopause) will define risk more reliably. For women at high risk of breast cancer, or breast cancer survivors, whilst there is no evidence suggesting that HRT has an adverse effect on outcome, studies are uncontrolled and therefore inconclusive. In the absence of such data, it is recommended that outside of the context of a clinical trial, the uncertainty about HRT is explained fully to women and the advice of a cancer geneticist or breast cancer specialist be sought as appropriate.

Table 8.1 Low-dose oral hormone replacement therapy preparations in the UK

Preparation	Content
Unopposed	
Climaval®	Oestradiol 1 mg
Elleste-Solo®	Oestradiol 1 mg
Progynova®	Oestradiol 1 mg
Zumenon®	Oestradiol 1 mg
Continuous combined	
Femoston Conti®	Oestradiol 1 mg + dydrogesterone 5 mg
Indivinia®	Oestradiol 1 mg + medroxyprogesterone acetate 2.5 mg
Indivinia®	Oestradiol 1 mg + medroxyprogesterone acetate 5 mg
Kliovance®	Oestradiol 1 mg + norethisterone acetate 0.5 mg
Sequential	
Climagest®	Oestradiol 1 mg + norethisterone acetate 1 mg
Cyclo Progynova®	Oestradiol 1 mg + levonorgestrel 250 μg
Elleste Duet®	Oestradiol 1 mg + norethisterone acetate 1 mg
Femoston®	Oestradiol 1 mg + dydrogesterone 10 mg

response effect). Transdermal oestrogens are available in either patch or gel form. Other non-oral routes include subcutaneous implant, transnasal aerosol and intravaginal pessaries and creams.

Transdermal patch

Estraderm TTS® was the first oestradiol skin patch produced. It contained therapeutic oestradiol in an alcohol reservoir with a membrane-based adhesive layer. The problem with the alcoholic reservoir was that it caused skin reactions. The newer transparent transdermal patch consists of a single transdermal matrix oestradiol dispersal system with an adhesive layer. The dose of oestradiol that is delivered is equivalent to the surface layer of the patch. It causes less skin reactions as the matrix dispersal system does not contain alcohol. It may also be more acceptable in terms of appearance due to its transparency. However, as the matrix patch causes skin occlusion, it may cause more skin reactions in hot and humid climates. The current low-dose HRT patches available in the UK are 25 and 37.5 μg (Table 8.2). Not all oestradiol patches contain progestogen. Women with an intact uterus therefore need additional progestogen when the patch is an oestrogen-only formulation.

Transdermal gel

Transdermal gel has been in use in France for more than 20 years and has recently become more popular elsewhere. Absorption is fast and satisfactory through the skin and effective blood levels are achieved. The gel does not produce the skin reactions which occur with both types of patch and therefore may be more suitable in hot and humid climates. The oestradiol is contained in a hydro-alcoholic gel.

One advantage of the gel is that it allows the possibility of using a low dose. Currently, only two gels are available in the UK (Table 8.3). Both deliver pure oestradiol that can achieve a more physiological oestradiol:oestrone ratio when compared with oral HRT. However, both products can result in variations in the levels of circulating oestradiol, because absorption is dependent on the amount of gel applied by the user and the surface area over which it is applied. As with the patch system, women with an intact uterus need to be given cyclical progestogens to prevent endometrial hyperplasia and neoplastic disease.

Implant

At present, oestradiol implants are manufactured from fused crystalline steroid and are implanted into subcutaneous tissue. They are biodegradable products but the biodegradation rate varies. Insertion of the oestradiol implant requires a minor surgical procedure, except the Riselle 25 mg implant which can be given by injection (not in the UK), and are usually inserted in a hospital clinic setting. The implantation schedule is usually every 6 months, with the conventional dosage being 50 mg. Low-dose pellets containing 25 mg of oestradiol are available in the UK. Testosterone implants (25/100 mg strengths) may also be implanted at the same time in those women who have an incomplete response to the oestradiol implant. Although implants are convenient and ensure treatment compliance for at least 6 months, there are two major disadvantages unique to implants. A minor surgical procedure is required that may run the risk of haemorrhage, bruising and infection. More importantly, the phenomenon of 'tachyphylaxis' can occur with implants. This occurs as a result of repeated implantation based on climacteric symptom recurrence, which may result in supraphysiological serum levels of

Table 8.2 Low-dose oestradiol patches

Preparation	Dose released/24 h, frequency of administration
Dermestril®	Oestradiol 25 µg, every 3–4 days
Dermestril®-septem	Oestradiol 25 µg, every 7 days
Estraderm MX®	Oestradiol 25 µg, twice weekly
Estraderm TTS®	Oestradiol 25 µg, twice weekly
Evorel®	Oestradiol 25 µg, twice weekly
Menorest®	Oestradiol 37.5 µg, twice weekly

Table 8.3 Transdermal oestradiol gels

Preparation	Content and recommended dosage
Oestrogel®	Oestradiol 0.06%, oestradiol 1.5 mg
Sandrena®	Oestradiol 0.1%, oestradiol 0.5/1 mg

oestradiol because of residual oestradiol from previous implants. In a small number of women, climacteric symptoms may be experienced as the serum oestradiol level starts to fall, not when pretreatment values have been reached. Eventually, further re-implantation may not relieve the climacteric symptoms due to oestrogen receptor unresponsiveness.

A lower initiation dose of implant at 25 mg may reduce the risk of supra-physiological levels and tachyphylaxis. It may also lower the risk of endometrial hyperplasia in women with an intact uterus resulting from prolonged endometrial stimulation and at the same time retain the benefits of HRT. The duration and degree of symptom control is similar to the 50 mg dosage.

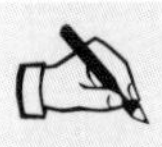

A comparison of 25 mg and 50 mg oestradiol implants in the control of climacteric symptoms following hysterectomy and bilateral salpingo-oophorectomy.

N Panay, E Versi, M Savvas. *Br J Obstet Gynaecol* 2000; **107**: 1012–6.

BACKGROUND. This was a double-blind, randomized, controlled trial to compare the effect of 25 and 50 mg oestradiol implants on serum follicle stimulating hormone (FSH) and oestradiol levels; and to compare effectiveness and duration of climacteric symptom control. A total of 44 women (all under 65 years old) who had total abdominal hysterectomy and bilateral salpingo-oophorectomy for benign causes were recruited and were randomized to receive either a 25 (n = 20) or 50 mg (n = 24) oestradiol implant.

INTERPRETATION. The circulating oestradiol levels remained significantly higher during the last 2 months of the trial in those women who received 50 mg implants, compared with those women who received 25 mg oestradiol implants. The concentration of FSH remained significantly higher in those women who received 25 mg implants compared with 50 mg implants. The control of symptoms was good with both doses. No significant difference in the effectiveness of climacteric symptom control was noted in the two groups. The mean duration of symptom control was similar in the two groups: 5.9 months (SD 2.4) in those receiving 50 mg of oestradiol and 5.6 months (SD 2.3) in those receiving 25 mg.

Comment

The study demonstrated that 25 mg oestradiol implants might be as effective as 50 mg implants in controlling climacteric symptoms. It also demonstrated that the duration of symptom control appeared to be the same in both 50 and 25 mg dosages. This was despite a less significant initial suppression of FSH levels and a more marked decline in the serum levels of oestradiol in the fifth and sixth months after hormone implantation in women who received 25 mg of oestradiol. The study recommended the 25 mg oestradiol implant for those women with normal bone density to control menopausal symptoms as it will maximize the compliance rate.

Intravaginal

There are several intravaginal preparations available for use in the UK in the form of cream, pessary and tablet (Table 8.4). The dose of oestrogen delivered by these preparations is sufficient only to be used for patients suffering from urogenital atrophic problems such as dyspareunia and vaginal dryness. They are usually continued for approximately 3 months.

Intravaginal oestradiol ring

Estring® is an intravaginal HRT ring delivering oestradiol at approximately 7.5 μg in 24 h. The low dose of oestradiol released allows the device to be used without progestogenic opposition. However, due to the small oestradiol dose released, it is only suitable for use in women with postmenopausal urogenital atrophic conditions such as vaginal dryness and dyspareunia. It is not suitable for vasomotor symptom relief or prophylaxis against osteoporosis. It is inserted into the upper third of the vagina and is changed every 3 months. The maximum recommended duration of treatment is 2 years.

Intranasal

The latest addition to the different routes of administration of HRT is intranasal. Aerodiol® is a formulation of oestradiol hemihydrate administered by one spray in each nostril once daily giving a dose of 300 μg oestradiol daily. The efficacy of Aerodiol® 300 μg is similar to oral oestradiol 2 mg [3]. It avoids the first pass metabolic effects of the oral preparation, the skin reactions associated with the transdermal route and the minor surgery associated with implants. Intranasal absorption is made possible by the highly vascularized microvillous nature of the nasal mucosa, resulting in rapid uptake, with maximal plasma levels achieved within 30 min. The plasma concentration returns to 10% of the peak level within 2 h and to the pretreatment level within 12 h. This results in pulse-like oestradiol levels rather than the sustained serum level obtained with the oral and transdermal routes. Studies to date have shown effectiveness in controlling climacteric symptoms and the preparation is well tolerated and accepted by women who choose to use this route [3–5].

Table 8.4 Vaginal oestrogen preparations

Preparation	Content
Ortho-Gynest®	Estriol 0.01% cream
Ortho-Gynest®	Estriol 500 μg pessary
Ovestin®	Estriol 0.01% cream
Vagifem®	Oestradiol 25 μg tablet

Regimens

Sequential and continuous combined therapy regimens

Throughout the world, various schedules of administration of HRT are available. In the UK it has been more common in recent years to administer HRT sequentially. The older combined regimens administered oestrogen in 21-day cycles with the progestogen being given for 7–14 days in the latter half of each treatment cycle. In more modern sequential regimens, the oestrogen is administered in continuous 28-day cycles and the progestogen is added for either 10, 12 or 14 days in the latter half of each cycle. Another sequential regimen is the long cycle sequential HRT. The frequency of withdrawal bleeding is reduced because the progestogen is added only for 14 days every third month whilst the oestrogen is administered continuously. However, at the current time, the product is only available in a high oestrogen dose of 2 mg and therefore cannot be considered as low-dose HRT.

In continuous combined HRT, the oestrogen and progestogen component are combined in a single tablet or patch with the same dosage daily. The aim of continuous combined HRT is to avoid the monthly withdrawal bleed. This is achieved by inducing endometrial atrophy through the antiproliferative effect on the endometrium of the continuously administered low-dose progestogen. The continuous combined schedule should be given only to women who report 12 months of amenorrhoea and are thought to be menopausal or who have received at least 12 months of sequential HRT. If continuous combined HRT is administered to perimenopausal women, erratic vaginal breakthrough bleeding may be experienced due to inconsistent endogenous hormone levels being produced from the ovaries.

Titrating the dose to the requirements of the individual

With clear evidence that side-effects of therapy cause poor compliance and high rates of discontinuation of HRT amongst postmenopausal women, an effective and yet tolerable dosage should be offered at the initiation of therapy. Successful initiation of therapy is crucial, as it will increase the chance of long-term compliance and, hence, maximized benefits. Initiation of HRT in low dosage will reduce the hyperoestrogenic side-effects associated with conventional doses. The issue of avoiding hyperoestrogenic side-effects is particularly important in older women, who may be many years postmenopausal and not able to tolerate conventional doses of HRT following years of oestrogen deficiency.

Initiating HRT at low doses will allow flexibility for dose titration to the requirements of the individual woman's needs. The knowledge that there are options for titrating the dose and, hence, minimizing side-effects and maximizing benefits, may encourage women to continue with the therapy and allow for good compliance [6].

Dose titration according to individual needs is also important because different routes of administration of HRT lead to differing degrees of absorption and metabolism. At low levels, many oestradiol assays are unreliable and also indicate a momentary status as the serum oestradiol levels are subject to numerous changing factors as well as inter- and intra-individual variations |7|. Titration should therefore be based mainly on clinical symptoms and prophylactic therapy requirements with less emphasis on serum oestradiol assays.

Efficacy of low-dose oestrogen

Climacteric symptoms

The most characteristic consequence of the menopause is the experience of climacteric symptoms, which can cause considerable distress to women. Climacteric symptoms can be further divided into subtypes, which include vasomotor instability and urogenital atrophy.

Vasomotor instability symptoms of the menopause are the most common and they include hot flushes, night sweats, insomnia, palpitations, headaches and dizziness. These are often the first symptoms noticed by women and may precede the cessation of menstruation and hence occur during the perimenopausal stage. They usually last for less than 1 year except for 20% of women where they may last longer |8|. Oestrogen replacement therapy is the treatment of choice for postmenopausally related vasomotor instability symptoms. Relatively low doses of oestrogen are sufficient to control the vasomotor instability. Recent studies showed that low-dose oestradiol patches (25 mg) were equally rapid in the significant reduction of the frequency of vasomotor symptoms compared with higher doses |9|. Another study compared two oestradiol implant doses of 25 and 50 mg. The results showed that the higher-dose oestradiol implant at 50 mg did not result in a better control of symptoms compared with lower-dose oestradiol of 25 mg |10|.

Urogenital atrophy occurs in postmenopausal women as a late manifestation of the menopause because the integrity of the female reproductive tract tissue is dependent on collagen, the amount of which reduces with oestrogen deficiency. Oestrogen-deficient vaginal epithelium appears pale due to a decrease in vascularity. The loss of collagen results in the endometrium becoming thin, friable, less elastic, and more prone to infection and bleeding. These atrophic changes result in vaginitis which can lead to vaginal dryness and dyspareunia. Similar changes occur in the urethral tissues and tissues of the lower part of the urinary tract. Inflammation is a common consequence and patients may complain of symptoms of recurrent 'cystitis'. The physiology and function of the urogenital tract are improved by oestrogen, regardless of the route of administration. At low dosages of oestrogen, studies have shown effectiveness in alleviating urogenital atrophy |11|. However, prescribing low-dose oral oestrogen as a prophylaxis against recurrent urinary tract infection in postmenopausal women is inconclusive |12| and at present cannot be advocated.

For women not responding to low-dose oestrogens in either oral, transdermal or implanted forms, intravaginally administered low-dose oestradiol provides a good alternative. It is readily absorbed, providing a direct route to the pelvic venous circulation. Low dosage intravaginal preparations allow administration to be safe and effective if given for a limited period of time, as systemic absorption will be minimal. However, if administration is prolonged, then greater systemic absorption may occur.

Skeletal

Osteoporosis is a disease characterized by abnormalities in the amount and architectural arrangement of bone tissue resulting in impaired skeletal strength and increased susceptibility to bone fracture. It is more common amongst postmenopausal women due to the oestrogen deficiency causing accelerated bone tissue loss. One in three women will suffer an osteoporotic bone fracture in their lifetime and the resulting disability and cost makes osteoporosis an enormous public health problem. The statistics surrounding osteoporotic bone fracture report an alarming picture. Once a patient has suffered a hip fracture, 15% will die within a year, 50% can no longer walk without assistance and 25% are institutionalized in a long-term nursing environment.

With these alarming statistics it is obvious that efforts aimed at prevention are justifiable. Many different prophylactic and therapeutic pharmaceutical products have been suggested, including calcium, vitamin D, bisphosphonates, calcitonin and selective oestrogen receptor modulators, but the cornerstone for osteoporosis is oestrogen. Many studies have now advocated oestrogen, with or without the addition of progesterone/progestogen, in the role of maintaining and even increasing the bone mass in postmenopausal women. It is now a well-recognized and accepted product in both preventing and treating osteoporosis.

For many years, higher doses of oestrogen were thought to be necessary for preventing and treating osteoporosis. This is because the majority of older studies used higher doses of oral oestrogen [6]. High doses of oestrogen are associated with hyperoestrogenic side-effects such as vaginal bleeding and mastalgia. Consequently this leads to treatment non-compliance. If HRT is discontinued, the osteoporotic process will recommence, thereby negating any bone protection effects already achieved.

Although preventing osteoporosis per se is important, the task of reducing rates of discontinuation from HRT is more important, if osteoporosis and its consequences are to be prevented. Correct initiation of HRT will have a great impact on continuation of treatment. One solution to the above problem is to initiate HRT at a lower dose of oestrogen that can reduce the incidence and severity of hyperoestrogenic side-effects.

As mentioned in earlier sections of this chapter, low-dose initiation of HRT is particularly important for older women who may have been postmenopausal for many years. Their circulating oestrogen level may have been insignificant for a very long time and these women will experience quite pronounced side-effects if HRT is commenced at the conventional dose. Initiating HRT at lower doses will also allow titration according to the requirements of the individual woman. This will allow women to gain confidence with the treatment.

Previous prospective studies reported that the minimum oestrogen doses needed for effective prophylaxis against osteoporosis were 625 μg/day oral CEE, 2 mg/day oral oestradiol or 50 μg transdermal oestradiol. However, evidence from recent studies has shown that a lower dosage of oestradiol is effective in preventing osteoporosis. The following study showed that a dosage as low as 0.25 mg/day of micronized 17β-oestradiol was effective in reducing bone turnover when compared with 1 mg/day.

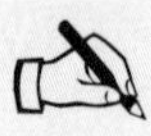

The effect of low dose micronised 17β-estradiol on bone turnover, sex hormone levels and side effects in older women: a randomised, double blind, placebo-controlled study.

KM Prestwood, AM Kenny, C Unson, M Kulldorff. *J Clin Endocrinol Metab* 2000; **85**: 4462–9.

BACKGROUND. This was a randomized, double-blind, placebo-controlled trial examining the effects of three doses (0.25, 0.5 and 1.0 mg/day) of micronized 17β-oestradiol on bone turnover, sex hormone levels and side-effects compared with placebo. The study population was recruited from healthy women over 65 years of age. All women received 1300 mg of elemental calcium with 1000 IU vitamin D/day throughout the study. The primary outcome measures were serum and urinary biochemical markers of bone resorption and formation at baseline, 6 and 12 weeks of treatment and 6 and 12 weeks post-treatment. Markers of bone resorption were N-telopeptides of type 1 collagen, C-telopeptides of type 1 collagen and total deoxypyridinoline cross-links. Bone formation markers were bone alkaline phosphatase, osteocalcin and N-terminal procollagen peptides. Parathyroid hormone, oestradiol, oestrone and sex hormone binding globulin were also measured in serum collected at baseline, 12 weeks of treatment and 12 weeks post-treatment.

INTERPRETATION. Of 107 women randomized into the study, 92 women completed the study. Compliance with the treatment and calcium/vitamin D supplementation was 90 and 84%, respectively. All markers of bone resorption significantly decreased at 12 weeks of treatment compared with placebo and returned towards baseline at 12 weeks post-treatment. Bone alkaline phosphatase and N-terminal procollagen peptides, markers of bone formation, significantly decreased 12 weeks post-treatment. The decrease in osteocalcin varied with time and oestrogen dose. Equivalence testing of doses revealed no significant difference in response of markers of bone turnover with 0.25 mg/day compared with the 1.0 mg/day dosage. Serum oestradiol and oestrone increased significantly compared with baseline in all the treatment groups and also in comparison with placebo in the higher dose groups. Breast tenderness and episodes of bleeding were significantly more frequent in the 1.0 and 0.5 mg groups. Most women who reported bleeding had an increased endometrial thickness of more than 5 mm at week 12 of treatment. Fluid retention was higher in the 0.5 mg/day group.

Comment

The results demonstrated that 0.25 mg/day of micronized oestradiol, when given with adequate calcium and vitamin D supplementation, decreases biochemical markers of bone turnover in older women over a 3-month treatment period compared with placebo. The lowest effective dose of oestrogen for reducing bone resorption and preventing bone loss was a quarter of the dose typically used for the prevention and treatment of osteoporosis and one half the HRT dose used in recent studies. This study did not detect an ineffective dose of oestrogen in their study population and the authors have therefore suggested that it may be possible to use even lower doses of oestrogen to prevent bone loss in older women. The two side-effects that are most commonly cited as reasons for non-compliance, namely mastalgia and vaginal bleeding, were markedly diminished in the 0.25 mg/day oestradiol group and were comparable with the placebo group.

Another study using low-dose CEE of 0.3 mg/day also showed benefits |13|. In this study, all women received calcium supplementation to increase the calcium intake above 1000 mg/day and oral 25-hydroxyvitamin D to maintain serum 25-hydroxy-vitamin D levels of at least 75 nmol/litre. The study demonstrated an increase in bone mineral density in older women who received low-dose oestrogen in the presence of adequate calcium and vitamin D.

In younger postmenopausal women, the use of a lower dose of oestrogen revealed a similar result. A 2-year study from Japan showed that HRT using 0.31 mg of CEE and 2.5 mg of medroxyprogesterone acetate (MPA) on younger women (mean age 55 years) was effective in increasing lumbar bone mineral density in either naturally menopausal or oophorectomized women. The problems inherent in previous studies lie in the type of diagnostic equipment available for the detection of bone loss. This study from Japan addressed this issue by using a more accurate instrument, dual-energy X-ray absorptiometry, for measuring bone mineral density.

Prevention of postmenopausal bone loss with minimal uterine bleeding using low dose continuous estrogen/progestin therapy: a 2-year prospective study.

H Mizunuma, H Okano, M Soda, *et al. Maturitas* 1997; **27**: 69–76.

BACKGROUND. This 2-year prospective, open-label, randomized study examined the minimal effective dose of conjugated oestrogen–progestogen HRT on postmenopausal bone loss and uterine bleeding. The study subjects comprised 52 postmenopausal women with at least 1 year continuous administration of CEE 0.625 mg/day; CEE 0.625 mg plus MPA 2.5 mg/day; CEE 0.31 mg plus MPA 2.5 mg/day; or control.

INTERPRETATION. Forty-nine patients completed 1 year of therapy and 36 patients completed 2 years. The percentage changes in lumbar bone mineral density at 2 years of CEE alone, CEE 0.625 mg plus MPA and CEE 0.31 mg plus MPA were 8.52% (95% CI

4.6–12.4), 7.40% (95% CI 0.60–14.2) and 3.20% (95% CI 0.61–5.84), respectively, and were significantly higher than pretreatment values. The control group showed a significant decrease in lumbar bone mineral density over the 2 years ($P < 0.05$). The serum calcium, phosphate, alkaline phosphatase and intact osteocalcin levels showed a significant decrease in the CEE-treated group, suggesting that CEE at a dose of 0.31 mg is effective in suppressing bone resorption. No significant differences were seen in the lipid profile in the groups taking CEE 0.31 mg plus MPA and controls. The incidence of bleeding was significantly lower in women taking CEE 0.31 mg plus MPA.

Comment

The study demonstrated that the effect of CEE on postmenopausal bone loss is dose dependent. A daily dose of 0.31 mg of CEE is effective in increasing lumbar bone mineral density in postmenopausal women for at least 2 years. The rate of vaginal bleeding was reduced in patients taking 0.31 mg of CEE. Patients who previously had vaginal bleeding and defaulted from the CEE dose of 0.625 mg plus MPA regimen were retreated and thereafter showed no episodes of vaginal bleeding, suggesting that CEE 0.31 mg plus MPA is superior to conventional HRT. Therefore a daily dose of 0.31 mg of CEE may be an appropriate option for women with a normal lipid profile requiring HRT who wish to avoid unscheduled bleeding.

With recent evidence that low-dose HRT is effective in both the prevention and treatment of osteoporosis, women should be informed of this and fears regarding hyperoestrogenic side-effects should be allayed. This may result in greater confidence in the use of HRT for osteoporosis prevention.

Cardiovascular

Studies on the cardioprotective effects of HRT have been based mainly on conventional doses. Large studies have been conducted which showed beneficial effects on lipid changes by reducing low-density lipoprotein (LDL) cholesterol and increasing high-density lipoprotein (HDL) cholesterol. These lipid changes are thought to be beneficial due to an associated reduction in cardiovascular risk. Evidence from the Nurses' Health Study in the USA showed similar changes [14]. However, combined oestrogen and progestogen therapy in postmenopausal women with coronary heart disease revealed a surprising result in the Heart and Estrogen/Progestin Replacement Study (HERS). At the end of the first year, improved lipid levels were found in the hormonally treated group, but more coronary heart disease events occurred. It has been suggested that the study was stopped prematurely before the benefit of longer-term therapy became apparent.

Studies using low-dose HRT on cardioprotective effects are limited. The most recent study by Utian *et al.* [9] reported improvements in the lipid profile of patients in all treatment groups. The lowest oestrogen dose used in the trial was a 25 μg oestradiol transdermal patch. Triglyceride levels decreased in the study with reduction occurring in both the 25 and 50 μg oestradiol transdermal groups. With these improvements in lipid profile, it suggests potential clinical benefits for lower-dose oestradiol in relation to risk factors for cardiovascular disease.

Central nervous system/Alzheimer's disease

Alzheimer's disease is a disease of the central nervous system characterized by severe progressive cognitive deterioration and is a leading cause of dementia. Its prevalence doubles every 4.5 years after the age of 65 years and is more common in women than men |8|. Oestrogen deficiency after the menopause is thought to increase a woman's risk of dementia. There is an increasing number of studies looking at oestrogen as prevention and treatment for Alzheimer's disease, but all use conventional dose HRT. There are no studies yet reported using low-dose HRT, but one may expect some benefit in view of the fact that higher-dose oestrogen therapy appears to be associated with a 30% reduction in reporting of Alzheimer's dementia.

Safety and side-effects

Endometrium and vaginal bleeding

One of the problems of oestrogen replacement therapy is an increased risk of endometrial cancer. This results from the proliferative effect of unopposed oestrogens causing cystic hyperplasia, atypical complex hyperplasia and subsequent development of cancer in some individuals. Evidence has shown that the addition of progestogen to oestrogen replacement therapy would prevent hyperplasia and virtually remove the risk of cancer. It has been reported from various studies that the addition of progestogen in either a sequential or continuous regimen lowers the risk below that conferred by unopposed oestrogen but does not completely eliminate the risk of oestrogen administration |15|.

The number of oestrogen receptors in the endometrium decreases with age; therefore withdrawal bleeding can also cease during cyclic oestrogen therapy. Therapy with low-dose sequential HRT may lead to early cessation of bleeding due to low proliferative stimulus |7|. This is an important fact if compliance is to be maintained, as bleeding problems are one of the major issues in non-compliance.

Breast

Mastalgia is a common side-effect that has been frequently quoted by patients as a reason for stopping HRT. As demonstrated already, the use of low-dose HRT can reduce this common side-effect to the extent that patients do not consider it serious enough to discontinue treatment.

The relationship between HRT in conventional dose and breast cancer has been studied widely. Epidemiological studies have found an increased risk of breast cancer after long-term HRT whilst other data suggest a higher risk with combined oestrogen–progestogen therapy than with oestrogen alone. Although one might postulate a dose–response effect, there are no data regarding the use of low-dose HRT and breast cancer risk. The following study by Lundstrom *et al.* showed that mammographic density was less in those women using low-dose oral oestrogen compared with conventional dose continuous combined HRT. Mammographic breast parenchymal density was suggested to reflect the increased proliferation of epithelium and stroma and has been identified as a strong independent risk factor for breast cancer.

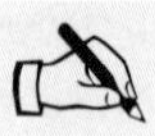

Mammographic breast density during hormone replacement therapy: effects of continuous combination, unopposed transdermal and low-potency oestrogen regimens.

E Lundstrom, B Wilczek, Z von Palffy, G Soderqvist, B von Schoultz.
Climacteric 2001; **4**: 42–8.

BACKGROUND. This study evaluated the impact of different HRT regimens on mammographic breast density. Mammographic breast density is an independent risk factor for breast cancer. At the first mammogram, all the participants were non-users of HRT. Thereafter, they used the same HRT regimen throughout the study. The study population comprised 158 women. Fifty-two women used continuous combined HRT (CEE 0.625 mg plus MPA 5 mg), 51 women used low-dose oestrogen alone (oestriol 2 mg daily) and 55 women used unopposed transdermal oestrogen given as a patch (oestradiol 50 μg/24 h). The films were coded and analysed by an independent radiologist specializing in mammography who was blind to the treatments.

INTERPRETATION. There was no significant difference between the groups with respect to findings prior to therapy. The type of HRT regimen had a significant impact on mammographic breast parenchymal density at the first visit following initiation of therapy. An increase in mammographic breast density was much more common among women taking continuous combined HRT (40%) than those using oral low-dose oestrogen (6%) and transdermal (2%) therapy. The mammographic breast density recorded at the first visit after the start of the HRT remained stable at subsequent examinations in most women using oestrogen alone.

Comment

The study demonstrated that different HRT regimens have differing effects on the normal breast. The authors stated that efforts should be made to define HRT regimens that minimize breast epithelial proliferation but retain their advantages. The effects of different doses, routes of administration and types of oestrogen and progestogen requires further exploration. The study also found a marked difference in breast density response among women using the same hormonal therapy. Factors regulating differences in individual sensitivity are presently unknown. Further studies are needed to ascertain the nature and the significance of mammographic breast density changes during the treatment and, in particular, its relation to symptoms and risk of breast cancer.

Venous thromboembolic disease

The risk of thromboembolic disease appears to be increased two- to three-fold in postmenopausal women who are on HRT. There is a theoretical possibility of venous thromboembolic disease and HRT being dose related, but there are currently no data regarding this possibility.

Progestogenic side-effects

Progestogen is given in various schedules to women with an intact uterus who are taking oestrogen replacement therapy to prevent endometrial hyperplasia and endometrial cancer. However, with the addition of progestogen, women may experience monthly or breakthrough bleeding which may be unpleasant, heavy and painful. They may also experience premenstrual syndrome-type side-effects. Symptoms of fluid retention are produced by the sodium-retaining effect on the renin–aldosterone system. The testosterone-derived progestogens such as norethisterone can produce side-effects on the skin, lipids and vasculature. The skin effects include acne, greasy skin and darkening of facial hair. The C19 progestogens such as norethisterone and levonorgestrel can oppose the beneficial increase in HDL produced by oral oestrogen.

Use of low-dose oestrogen replacement therapy gives a greater potential for manipulation of the dosage and duration of progestogen in order to reduce the unpleasant symptoms and improve compliance |16|. For example, in 1 mg continuous combined preparations, the daily dosage of progestogen can be halved compared with the dosage used in other preparations. Use of local progestogenic opposition from the levonorgestrel-releasing intrauterine system, vaginal progesterone gel and vaginal progesterone pessaries can also minimize progestogenic side-effects.

Tibolone

Tibolone (Livial®) is a steroid hormone that has oestrogenic, progestogenic and androgenic properties. The unique properties of tibolone stem from its metabolites and the parent compound binding to varying degrees to steroid receptors. One of its metabolites, the δ-4 isomer, confers progestogenic and androgenic properties. Different hormonal effects occur in various tissues affecting climacteric symptoms and bone, while progestogenic effects predominate in the endometrium and androgenic effects benefit libido |17|.

Tibolone is mainly indicated for women who are more than 1 year after their last menstrual period. It is particularly suitable for older women (over 65 years) who have not received HRT, as it does not produce withdrawal bleeding or spotting and has minimal stimulation of breast tissue. A review of clinical studies up to 1998 by Moore |17| revealed clear beneficial effects on menopausal symptoms, mood, libido, vaginal atrophy and bone density. However, two areas of uncertainty regarding tibolone are its effects on cardiovascular disease, due to a lack of studies measuring clinical events such as myocardial infarction, and atherosclerosis. Further studies with clinical endpoints are required to allow a balanced comparison with the known problems encountered with conventional HRT.

Conclusion

Current research data have shown that low-dose HRT is effective in providing the beneficial effects of conventional dose HRT. Low-dose therapy also has the advantage of reducing the unwanted side-effects of high oestrogen levels. The potential for lowering progestogenic side-effects is also immense. As the commonest reason for non-compliance with HRT is problematic side-effects, clinicians should therefore consider commencing women on lower initiation dosages of HRT and then titrate the dose according to the response. This is particularly important when prescribing HRT for the first time in older women whose tolerance to the conventional dosage may be lower.

Phyto-oestrogens

Phyto-oestrogens are plant-derived substances with oestrogen-like activity. The oestrogenic activity is found in diphenolic compounds such as isoflavones, lignans and coumestans that are converted into oestrogenic substances in the gastrointestinal tract. These diphenolic compounds have a steric structure similar to steroidal oestrogens which allow them to occupy the oestrogen receptor (Fig. 8.1). The slight differences in their structure result in a lower affinity in the activation of the oestrogen receptors. However, interest in phyto-oestrogens' potential for exerting oestrogenic activity stems from a high level of these substances present in the blood through its consumption in the diet of certain cultures. Most studies have been conducted using isoflavone due to its higher oestrogenic potency and because higher levels are found in the diet. Isoflavones are common in legumes such as soy. Soy products are relied upon in greater capacity as dietary protein in communities in the Far East compared with communities in the West.

The prevalence of menopausal symptoms such as hot flushes and sweating is reported to be lower in women in the Far East compared with women in Western countries [18]. This lower prevalence has been partially attributed to the traditional Far Eastern diet being rich in phyto-oestrogens. The incidence of diseases attributed to oestrogen changes, such as cardiovascular disease, breast cancer and osteoporosis, is also lower in populations with a high phyto-oestrogen-containing diet. Phyto-oestrogens have been thought to produce these advantageous hormonal effects with an altered urinary oestrogen metabolite ratio found following their consumption.

Despite the lower prevalence of menopausal symptoms, such as hot flushes, in Far Eastern women, studies of the effect of phyto-oestrogens on hot flushes are

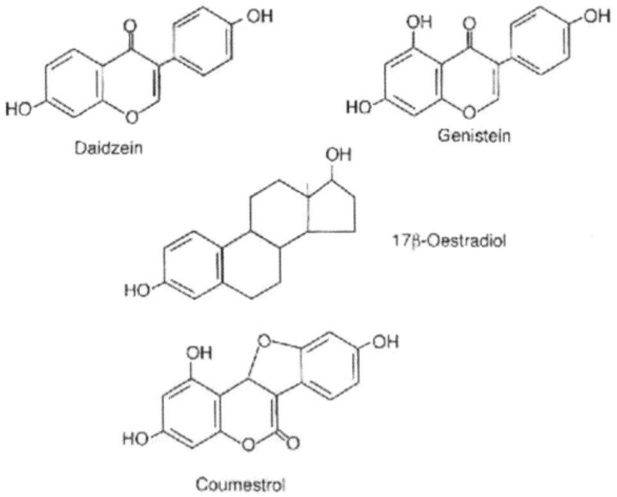

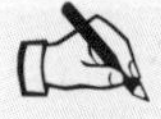

Fig. 8.1 Structural similarities between oestradiol and phyto-oestrogens.

inconclusive. Recent small, double-blind, placebo-controlled trials, such as the one presented below, have not shown a significant difference in the incidence of hot flushes. Previous uncontrolled trials with isoflavones on menopausal symptoms may have been confounded by a large placebo response.

The effect of Promensil™, an isoflavone extract, on menopausal symptoms.

DC Knight, JB Howes, JA Eden. *Climateric* 1999; **2**: 79–84.

BACKGROUND. The ability of Promensil™ to alleviate menopausal symptoms was evaluated in this randomized, double-blind, placebo-controlled prospective trial. A total of 37 menopausal women were recruited from St George Hospital (Sydney) using strict inclusion and exclusion criteria. There were three arms: placebo (12 subjects), 40 mg (12 subjects) and 160 mg (13 subjects) of isoflavone. Assessment of symptoms was carried out using subjective frequency of hot flushes, menopause symptom score (Greene Menopause Scale) and biological measurements of oestrogenic activity. The pretrial assessment phase lasted 1 week, while the trial lasted 12 weeks.

INTERPRETATION. This study provides evidence that Promensil™ does not affect menopausal symptoms or objective measurements of oestrogenic activity over the short period of this study. Flushing frequency was reduced in the groups taking isoflavone (–29% with 40 mg and –34% with 160 mg). However, it was also reduced in the placebo arm (–35%). Ultimately there was no difference between symptoms of flushing between the three arms. There was, however, an increase in urinary isoflavone excretion in the control group. All biological parameters were unchanged in all groups, including FSH levels, sex hormone binding globulin levels and vaginal pH values. However, serum non-fasting HDL levels were the exception, as there was an 18% increase in the 40 mg group ($P = 0.038$). Interestingly, HDL levels in the 160 mg arm did not show any difference compared with placebo subjects.

Comment

Epidemiological data have suggested that phyto-oestrogens may play a role in the modification of menopausal symptoms. A decrease in flushing in the treatment groups was matched by a fall in the control group. The rise in urinary isoflavones in the placebo group may well represent an increase in dietary phyto-oestrogens during the course of the trial. At present, no positive relationship has been found between isoflavones and blood parameters (FSH and sex hormone binding globulin) and vaginal parameters (pH and epithelium). This has been mirrored in other studies. The effect on HDL is interesting and needs further evaluation. The authors suggested the need for further larger studies.

An important cardioprotective effect of phyto-oestrogens on systemic arterial compliance has been shown, where a significant dose-dependent improvement occurred in menopausal women taking isoflavone supplements derived from red clover. It is reported that diminished arterial compliance leads to systolic hypertension and may increase left ventricular work. This finding may indicate a potential for a new treatment for improving cardiovascular function after the menopause.

Isoflavones from red clover improve systemic arterial compliance but not plasma lipids in menopausal women.

PJ Nestel, S Pomeroy, S Kay, *et al. J Clin Endocrinol Metab* 1999; **84**: 895–8.

BACKGROUND. This prospective double-blind study considered the relationship between oral isoflavone administration and the risk of ischaemic heart disease. The parameters evaluated included arterial compliance, mean arterial pressure and plasma lipid levels. Arterial compliance was measured by ultrasound as a volume and pressure relationship. Women were invited to participate through newspaper advertisements. A total of 26 women were enrolled using strict criteria including, a body mass index less than 32, absence of cardiovascular disease as well as no concurrent HRT or evening primrose oil usage. Some women dropped out of the study leaving three placebo controls, 13 women who completed all four phases while one subject only completed three phases. The phases were divided into an initial 3-week run-in period, a 5-week placebo period, and a period of 5 weeks of 40 mg of isoflavone followed by 5 weeks of 80 mg of isoflavone. The phyto-oestrogen used was Promensil (Novogen) whose four

isoflavone constituents were genistein 4 mg, daidzein 3.5 mg, biochanin 24.5 mg and formononetin 8 mg.

INTERPRETATION. This study provides evidence for the possible cardioprotective role of the group of phyto-oestrogens, the isoflavones. The placebo group served to show that there were minimal changes over time with respect to arterial compliance and baseline urinary isoflavone excretion. These three subjects were not used in the statistical analysis. Therefore, the subjects in the treatment arms acted as their own controls. Arterial blood pressures did not show any changes in any of the groups. There was approximately a 10% reduction in the LDL/HDL cholesterol levels between the placebo and treatment arms. However, this was not statistically significant. During the placebo, 40 mg isoflavone and 80 mg isoflavone phases the arterial compliances were found to be 19.7 ± 5.7, 23.7 ± 5.3 and 24.4 ± 4.9, respectively. Using paired t-test, the increase in compliance between placebo and 40 mg was statistically significant ($P = 0.039$). Placebo compared with 80 mg was also significant ($P = 0.018$). There was no difference between 40 and 80 mg dosages.

Comment

This study, although having a small number of subjects, produced some interesting results. It is known that postmenopausal women have an increased risk of cardio-vascular disease resulting from a number of factors, including a rise in LDL choles-terol, endothelial dysfunction and changes in carotid arterial pulsatility. Previous studies have shown that oestrogen replacement therapy improves arterial com-pliance. This study appears to mirror those findings. The authors postulated that isoflavones may well act through endothelium-related arterial relaxation mechanisms. These drugs, therefore, have the future potential of preventing post-menopausal cardiovascular disease, especially in those where oestrogen is contra-indicated.

Phyto-oestrogen is also thought to have an anticarcinogenic biological property and could have a role in the prevention of breast cancer. The case–control study by Ingram *et al.* has shown that increased excretion of some phyto-oestrogens is asso-ciated with a substantial reduction in breast cancer risk. Cell culture studies also indicate that phyto-oestrogens can exert an antiproliferative effect on breast cancer cell lines.

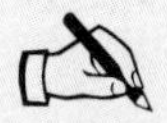

Case controlled study of phyto-oestrogens and breast cancer.

I Ingram, K Sanders, K Marlene, D Lopez, DJ Hunter. *Lancet* 1997; **350**: 990–4.

BACKGROUND. **This case-controlled study evaluated the relationship between dietary phyto-oestrogens and the risk of breast cancer development in both pre- and**

postmenopausal women (cases were aged between 30 and 84 years). A total of 341 women with newly diagnosed breast cancer were recruited from an unnamed private clinic and Sir Charles Gairdner Hospital (Perth) between December 1992 and November 1994. A total of 144 were eligible for the study. Each case had an age and demographically matched control; these were obtained from the 1993 Perth electoral role. Data were obtained in the form of one 72-hour urine collection, blood tests and a food frequency questionnaire. The urine samples were assayed for nitrogen compounds, the isoflavonic phyto-oestrogens daidzein, genistein and equol, and the lignans enterodiol, enterolactone and matairesinol. Genistein proved difficult to analyse, as there were technical difficulties. Nitrogen measurement was used as an assessment of calorific intake.

INTERPRETATION. The results of this study provide evidence for a relationship between high dietary phyto-oestrogens and a reduction in breast cancer risk. Women with proven breast cancer were found to have lower excreted levels of phyto-oestrogens. This had been adjusted for confounders including age at menarche, parity, length of lactation, alcohol intake and fat consumption. All types of phyto-oestrogens assessed revealed a reduction in breast cancer risk. However, two were statistically significant in terms of quartile trends. Equol odds ratios were 1.00, 0.45 (95% CI 0.20–1.02), 0.52 (95% CI 0.23–1.17) and 0.27 (95% CI 0.10–0.69). The test for trend had a value of $P = 0.009$. This therefore represents a four-fold reduction in risk. Enterolactone was the other phyto-oestrogen that revealed a significant trend ($P = 0.013$). The odds ratios were 1.00, 0.91 (95% CI 0.41–1.99), 0.65 (95% CI 0.29–1.44), 0.36 (95% CI 0.15–0.86). This represents a three-fold reduction in risk. It was reported that there were no differences in the trends between pre- and postmenopausal cancers.

Comment

Previous observational studies have reported higher levels of excreted phyto-oestrogens in populations with a low frequency of breast cancer. Apart from one case-controlled study looking at soya consumption and breast cancer, this was the first of its kind. The strengths of this study included using matched case and control pairs. Additionally, a quantitative measurement of urinary phyto-oestrogens as a reflection of dietary intake is more accurate than dietary diaries. Lastly it involved a large number of breast cancer cases (n = 144). The postulated antiproliferative mechanisms of phyto-oestrogens include its nuclear anti-oestrogen effects, stimulation of sex hormone binding globulin production as well as inhibition of aromatase. At present there are no dietary recommendations with respect to phyto-oestrogens, but it is clear that they have a potential role in the prevention of breast cancer. Long-term prospective studies are required to evaluate this.

Conclusion

The use of phyto-oestrogens as an alternative for the therapy of postmenopausal women is still controversial. These plant-derived products have been implicated because of epidemiological studies based in South-East Asian countries. This interest has sparked off a multitude of trials evaluating their role in hormone replacement. Furthermore, an antiproliferative role has been implicated for breast and gynaecological cancers. The result is a surge of these natural products in health shops promoting the above benefits in the absence of concrete evidence. Pharmaceutical studies using naturally occurring products tend to be problematic. It is impossible to control or cease dietary intake during a trial. Newspaper and magazine reporting of these beneficial effects has probably caused an increased intake in women who are health conscious. Additionally, research is hampered by a lack of availability of pure phyto-oestrogen products; those obtainable tend to be of mixed components. Hence, an active component may well be masked by an inactive competitor.

The evidence regarding the control of subjective symptoms appears to be conflicting. It is likely that some women do obtain benefit. However, as of yet there are no pharmacological explanations available. From the point of view of cardioprotection, the most positive finding appears to lie in the improvement in arterial compliance. The effect on HDL/LDL profiles may well be beneficial, but this needs further investigation.

Further vigorous research on dietary phyto-oestrogens is essential. The potential advantageous effects studied so far suggest that they could be a very useful substance in the prevention and treatment of menopausal complications, especially in those where oestrogens are contraindicated. Until data from large controlled prospective trials are available, firm conclusions should not yet be drawn. Despite these inconclusive findings, it is reasonable to advise postmenopausal women to have a diet rich in legumes, cereals and fruits.

References

1. Ryan P, Harrison R, Blake G, Fogelman I. Compliance with hormone replacement therapy after screening for postmenopausal osteoporosis. *Br J Obstet Gynaecol* 1992; **99**: 325–8.

2. Schneider H, Gallagher J. Moderation of the daily dose of HRT: benefits for patients. *Maturitas* 1999; **33**: S25–9.

3. Panay N, Toth K, Pelissier C, Studd J. Dose-ranging studies of a novel intranasal estrogen replacement therapy. *Maturitas* 2001; **38**(S1): S15–22.

4. Studd J, Pornel B, Marton I, *et al.* for the Aerodiol Study Group. Efficacy and acceptability of intranasal 17β-oestradiol for menopausal symptoms: randomised dose–response study. *Lancet* 1999; **353**: 1574–8.

5. Gompel A, Bergeron C, Jondet M, *et al.* Endometrial safety and tolerability of AERO-DIOL® (intranasal estradiol) for 1 year. *Maturitas* 2000; **34**: 209–15.

6. Gallagher J. Moderation of the daily dose of HRT: prevention of osteoporosis. *Maturitas* 1999; **33**: S57–63.

7. Huber J, Campagnoli C, Druckmann R, *et al.* Recommendations for estrogen and progestin replacement in the climacteric and postmenopause. *Maturitas* 1999; **33**: 197–209.

8. Fraser I, Jansen R, Lobo R, Whitehead M. *Estrogens and Progestogens in Clinical Practice.* Churchill Livingstone, Edinburgh, 1998.

9. Utian W, Burry K, Archer D, *et al.* Efficacy and safety of low, standard and high dosages of an estradiol transdermal system (Esclim) compared with placebo on vasomotor symptoms in highly symptomatic menopausal patients. *Am J Obstet Gynecol* 1999; **181**: 71–9.

10. Panay N, Versi E, Savvas M. A comparison of 25 mg and 50 mg oestradiol implants in the control of climacteric symptoms following hysterectomy and bilateral salpingo-oophorectomy. *Br J Obstet Gynaecol* 2000; **107**: 1012–6.

11. Botsis D, Kassanos D, Kalogirou D, Antoniou G, Vitoratos N, Karakitsos P. Vaginal ultrasound of the endometrium in postmenopausal women with symptoms of uro-genital atrophy on low-dose estrogen or tibolone treatment: a comparison. *Maturitas* 1997; **26**: 57–62.

12. Cardozo L, Benness C, Abbott D. Low dose oestrogen prophylaxis for recurrent urinary tract infections in elderly women. *Br J Obstet Gynaecol* 1998; **105**: 403–7.

13. Recker R, Michael Davies K, Dowd R, Heaney R. The effect of low-dose continuous estrogen and progesterone therapy with calcium and vitamin D on bone in elderly women. *Ann Intern Med* 1999; **130**: 897–904.

14. Grodstein F, Stampfer M, Manson J, *et al.* Postmenopausal estrogen and progestin use and the risk of cardiovascular disease. *New Engl J Med* 1996; **335**: 453–6.

15. Shoupe D. HRT dosing regimens: continuous versus cyclic—pros and cons. *Int J Fertil* 2001; **46**: 7–15.

16. Panay N, Studd J. Progestogen intolerance and compliance with hormone replacement therapy in menopausal women. *Hum Reprod Update* 1997; **3**: 159–71.

17. Moore RA. Livial: a review of clinical studies. *Br J Obstet Gynaecol* 1999; **106**: 1–21.

18. Eden J. Phytoestrogens and the menopause. *Baillier's Clin Endocrinol Metab* 1998; **12**: 581–7.

9

Hormone replacement therapy in older women

Introduction

Although some of the most important indications for hormone replacement therapy (HRT) relate to the prevention of age-related health problems, the majority of women who take HRT are around the age of the menopause. Few women in the age of greatest incidence of osteoporotic fracture, myocardial infarction, stroke and dementia are taking HRT. Likewise the use of HRT for symptom relief has tended to focus on the symptoms of the climacteric, such as hot flushes and mood changes, much more than on those of the postmenopausal years, such as urogenital atrophy symptoms, falling and cognitive decline. One could speculate on the reasons for this. Prescription of HRT still tends to be patient led, with some of those most in need of symptom relief or protection not presenting for discussion of HRT. This could be because of a lack of knowledge, fear, prejudice, or simple stoicism on the part of the woman, but it remains the doctor's responsibility to explore the patient's needs and fears, and to offer HRT as a possible solution if appropriate. The older woman is probably less likely to arrive asking about HRT specifically and, ironically, as the older woman probably has the most to gain from preventative medicine, there is a tendency not to discuss prevention with her, particularly if she already has health problems. The symptoms she may be experiencing may be intimate and difficult to discuss, and perhaps easier for both patient and doctor to ignore. There is more of a worry on the part of the doctor about side-effects and interactions with other medication, and possibly a lack of understanding about what the real risks and benefits of HRT may be.

The anxieties about the use of HRT in the older woman are very real, and have perhaps limited research as well as prescription. Some issues are very clear, and yet are still not universally heeded, such as the fact that there are HRT regimens which do not cause vaginal bleeding, while others are much less clear and perhaps need further research. Into this category perhaps would go stroke and cardiovascular disease, as well as cognitive function and falls.

This chapter cannot provide a comprehensive review of the use of HRT in the elderly, and care has been taken not to duplicate information in the other chapters. Issues about safety in terms of breast and cardiovascular disease and about appropriate preparations will be found elsewhere in this book.

Recent papers have been reviewed in four sections:

- Issues about the use of HRT in the older age group, attitudes of women and doctors, reasons for use or non-use of HRT;
- Cognitive decline, the risk of Alzheimer's disease (AD) and the possible use of HRT in the treatment of dementia;
- Osteoporotic fracture and falls;
- Urogenital symptoms and the use of HRT.

Issues around the use and non-use of HRT

These papers do not seem to suggest anything new about women's views on HRT, but deserve repeating. The message about the importance of the prescriber's views must be heeded if the use of HRT is to be targeted more effectively.

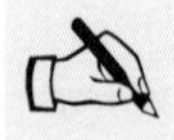

Older women and hormone replacement therapy: factors influencing late life initiation.
SG Leveille, AZ LaCroix, KM Newton, NL Keenan. *J Am Geriatr Soc* 1997; **45**: 1496–1500.

BACKGROUND. **Starting from the premise that HRT can be beneficial in terms of prevention of osteoporotic fracture and cardiovascular disease, it is important to question whether it needs to be initiated at the menopause, or whether later initiation may be as good, or better. This study aimed to explore the differences between those women who began taking HRT after the age of 60 years and those who did not.**

INTERPRETATION. This work was part of a large study performed in 1995, looking at a group of women aged 50–80 years, and their use of preventative health services. Participants were a random sample of female enrolees to the Group Health Cooperative of Pugent Sound, a large health maintenance organization. Of the original 1520 women, 1395 were invited to participate in a telephone interview about HRT use, after those for whom telephone contact was not practical had been excluded. A total of 1119 responded, of whom 671 women were older than 65 years, of which 521 (77.6%) were interviewed. One hundred and eight were current HRT users, having begun before the age of 60 years, which when excluded, left 413 women who could have started HRT after the age of 60 years. Fifty-one women had done so and 123 had not.

The interview addressed socio-demographics, health status and history, reproductive and hormone use history, as well as beliefs about HRT and information received from health care providers.

There were differences between the groups in that those who began HRT were less likely to describe their health as fair or poor, less likely to smoke and more likely to exercise, less likely to have had a myocardial infarction or breast cancer, and more likely to have hypertension, or to have had a fracture since the age of 50 years. The differences in these respects were slight, and not all were statistically significant. Significantly, however, the results also showed that HRT initiation was increased four-fold with the occurrence of hysterectomy after the age of 60 years. HRT starters were also more likely to have received more information from their providers about both the benefits and risks of HRT, and to believe that HRT was beneficial in terms of osteo- and cardioprotection. They were more likely to have had contact with a gynaecologist. Reasons for starting HRT were that it was prescribed by the doctor (41%), osteoprotection (33%), cardioprotection (22%) and symptoms (18%). Reasons for stopping included side-effects, doctors' advice, fear of cancer and dislike of taking pills, with no single reason predominating.

Comment

By the nature of the sample population the participants in this study tended to be white, educated and with concern for their health. The effect of socio-economic status, which has been seen in other studies, was thus selected out. Access to health care was also similar across the sample. Although the results show, as is well recognized, a tendency for women selecting HRT to have healthier lifestyles than those not, this study also suggests that the attitude of the health care provider has a large effect on a woman's choice. The effect of having a late hysterectomy on the choice to take up HRT is interesting, and may simply be a factor of increased contact with a gynaecologist, whom, the study assumes, will tend to counsel towards HRT. This study does suggest that increased discussion of HRT with older women may encourage its use.

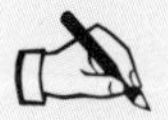

Effect of age on reasons for initiation and discontinuation of hormone replacement therapy.

B Ettinger, A Pressmens, P Silver. *Menopause* 1999; **6**: 282–9.

BACKGROUND. This study involved telephone interviews with random samples of two populations registered with the Kaiser Health Foundation in Northern California, the first being women who began or restarted HRT at the age of 65 years and the second being women who began or restarted HRT at the age of 50–55 years. It followed on from an earlier study by the same team which had looked at women aged 45–65 years. The aim was to understand the reasons for initiating and discontinuing HRT in older women, and how they compared with a younger group. This work was prompted by a recognition of the potential benefits of HRT in older women, and that despite this, uptake and continuation of HRT use is very poor in this age group.

INTERPRETATION. Women were selected by searching for prescriptions showing simultaneous dispensing of oestrogen and medroxyprogesterone acetate during 1996 to women who had not received such a prescription for at least 1 year. It was assumed that a prescription for 2.5 mg medroxyprogesterone acetate indicated a continuous combined regimen, and that higher doses indicated a sequential regimen. Those who were aged 65 years at the time of the first prescription made up the first population and those aged

50–55 years made up the second. From each population a random sample of 1200 women was selected for interview. Although the studies were performed 1 year apart, care was taken to use the same interviewers, and to select women from the same 550 prescribers.

The interview consisted of an open question about the main reason for starting HRT, followed by 14 specific closed questions asking about secondary reasons. A similar set of questions was asked about stopping treatment, if appropriate. Each woman was also asked whether she believed that she had osteoporosis. Information about continuation or discontinuation of HRT was also sought from the prescription records.

The older women had more difficulty remembering details of HRT use than the younger women, and were less willing to be interviewed. The interviewers still managed to interview 604 older women and 866 younger women. The results showed that older women were four times as likely to be using very low-dose preparations, i.e. 0.3 mg conjugated equine oestrogen (CEE) as younger women, and that whereas about half of the younger group were prescribed a continuous combined regimen, this predominated in the older group. Thirty-five per cent of older women started HRT primarily for osteoprotection or treatment of osteoporosis (14% of younger women), but the percentages starting primarily to prevent cardiovascular disease or stroke were much the same. Only 7% of older women (34% of younger women) started primarily because of flushes. Older women were more likely to quote vaginal dryness and urinary symptoms than younger women as a primary reason for HRT, but in fact equal numbers quoted these as a main or secondary reason (24.5%). Older women were less likely to be aiming to improve mood, energy or sexual function, but were more likely to want to improve memory.

The interview was conducted at an average of 11.5 months after the first prescription in the older women and 20.3 months after the first prescription in the younger age group. By the interview 31.7% of the older group and 21% of the younger group had stopped using the HRT. Vaginal bleeding was quoted as the reason in most cases (60% of the older women who stopped and 40% of the younger women who stopped). This did not seem to be affected by whether they were using a continuous combined or sequential regimen. Mastalgia was also a common reason for discontinuing, more so in the older group. The younger group was more likely to have mixed reasons for stopping, and more likely to be worried about breast cancer. The relative risk of stopping in older versus younger women was 1.4 (95% CI 1.2–1.6). Of the older group, 24.4% believed that they had osteoporosis, but these women were just as likely to discontinue as those without osteoporosis. Among the factors which did not appear to be associated with a significantly increased or decreased continuance rate was the type of regimen.

Comment

These results do provide some useful information about older women's attitudes to HRT. This was not a representative population, and there may have been recall bias and also bias introduced by the fact that more of the older women refused to be interviewed, and those that did refuse were more likely to have discontinued therapy. However, it shows that one of the commonest reasons for older women to take HRT is osteoprotection, but the fact that a woman knows she has osteoporosis does not seem to make her any more likely to continue with treatment. Urogenital atrophy symptoms are also important reasons for starting HRT. Vaginal bleeding is still a major reason for stopping; taking a continuous combined regimen did not seem to improve this. It is possible that the women were not sufficiently counselled about the likelihood of bleeding despite this type of regimen, and that more support and encouragement may be needed in this respect. Breast tenderness was also important.

Despite its limitations this is a useful paper, the messages of which need to be taken seriously by health care providers. Better information and support appear to be needed, but also perhaps more use of alternatives such as tibilone and raloxifene which may be less likely to cause bleeding than continuous combined therapy. From a British viewpoint it would be interesting to know whether the 0.3 mg dose of CEE has advantages in terms of continuance over the higher doses, as this is not yet available to us.

Cognitive functioning and dementia

Over the years a great deal has been written about the effect of oestrogen on the brain. Evidence from experimental studies suggests that there is a scientific basis for hypotheses that oestrogen deficiency after the menopause may impair cognitive function and thus that replacement might improve it, and that oestrogen treatment might reduce the risk of Alzheimer's disease (AD) or delay its onset, at least in some women. There is also some fascinating evidence [1] that cognitive function scores in childhood may be related to the age of the natural menopause, with higher cognitive function at 8 years being related to a later natural menopause. These authors plan to repeat cognitive function tests on their large cohort of women when they reach the age of 53 years. This may shed light on whether women who reach menopause early are at risk of clinically significant cognitive decline, and if so, whether this was predestined or as a result of early ovarian failure.

We appear to know [2]:

- That there are oestrogen receptors in the brain, especially in the areas known to be important for memory and cognitive functioning;
- That neuronal plasticity and structural neuronal loss may be affected by oestrogen levels, via a sex steroid effect on the growth proteins that control neuronal growth and repair;
- That oestrogen deficiency increases noradrenergic tone and cholinergic neurones may be preserved by oestrogen replacement;
- That oestrogen may have an effect on the vascular system of the cerebrum and cerebellum, in the order of about 30%, as it does elsewhere in the body, and thus improve brain perfusion;
- That oestrogen has a positive effect on cerebral glucose utilization;

- That vasomotor symptoms are mediated via the hypothalamus, with hot flushes and sweats being due to a temporary derangement of the thermoregulatory centre;

- That surgical or spontaneous menopause is associated with a fall in circulating beta endorphin, which may be involved in changes in mood and behaviour;

- That oestrogen affects the metabolism of monoamines and serotonin, the neurotransmitters involved in mood and arousal. Both mood and arousal can affect performance on memory tests;

- That oestrogen positively affects the synthesis of acetyl choline which is a vital transmitter in terms of learning and memory, and disturbance of which is important in the pathogenesis of AD;

- That oestrogen promotes the breakdown of amyloid precursor protein.

Evidence from epidemiological studies is conflicting, but tends to suggest that there is a positive effect of oestrogen, and probably combined HRT, on mood and well-being. Some studies, particularly those looking at younger women who have undergone surgical menopause, have suggested an improvement in memory and cognitive function with HRT, some have disputed this, and there is controversy over whether any effect on cognitive function is primary or secondary to improved mood. It may be that both are true.

The literature is conflicting at present, both in terms of the effect of oestrogen on cognitive function in healthy postmenopausal women, and in terms of a possible role for oestrogen in the prevention of cognitive impairment, dementia or AD. Several large, long-term studies are in progress at present, which should inform the debate further. These include the following.

The Wisdom COG section of the Wisdom trial will recruit until 2002 and is due to report in 2010. It aims to test the hypothesis that HRT reduces incident dementia and cognitive decline in postmenopausal women. The study includes 22 000 women and will look at long-term HRT use, with longer follow-up than has been achieved previously [3].

The Women's Health Initiative Memory Study [4] is also in progress at present, with recruitment between 1993 and 1998 and a planned average of 9 years of follow-up per subject. This study aims to assess the incidence of all causes of dementia in women over the age of 65 years in a cohort of women taking part in the HRT trial of the Women's Health Initiative. The work will try to assess the effect of HRT on the incidence of dementia, taking into account any difference between oestrogen alone and combined oestrogen and progestogen regimens, and will allow for any effect conferred by differences in age, ethnicity and geographical site. It will also try to comment on any effect of HRT on the progression of dementia symptoms in the cohort.

The studies presented here attempt to answer some of the questions about oestrogen and cognitive function.

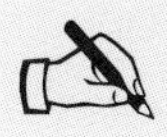

The effect of hormone replacement therapy on cognitive function in elderly women.

E Hogervorst, M Boshuisen, W Riedel, C Willeken, J Jolles.
Psychoneuroendocrinology 1999; **24**: 43–68.

BACKGROUND. This paper describes two studies performed in an attempt to answer three salient questions about the relationship between oestrogen replacement and cognitive function.

- **Is there a short- or long-term protective effect of oestrogen on cognitive function?**

- **If there is an effect, is it specific to any aspect of cognitive functioning or is it a global effect, for example on well-being?**

- **Is any effect of oestrogen replacement compromised by the addition of progestogen to the regimen?**

INTERPRETATION. The first study reported was small, part of a larger study into the effect of HRT on the vessel wall. Women were recruited through an information-giving meeting and 11 who chose to take HRT were compared with a group who chose not to, matched for age, postmenopausal symptom level and social class. All were aged over 45 years and were at least 1 year postmenopause. Any woman more than 10% from the population weight norm or who had any known factor which might affect cognitive function was excluded.

The HRT group took 17 beta oestradiol 2 mg with 12 days of 2.5 or 5 mg of progestogen (presumably medroxyprogesterone). All subjects received cognitive testing at baseline, 6 months and 12 months, and also at 2 weeks, 1 month and 3 months, so that the effect of learning of the tests could be accounted for. All testing was carried out in the progestogenic phase of the HRT regimen, so that the effect of progestogen was studied. The tests comprised a visual learning test with distraction, a questionnaire to assess subjective energy and tension levels, and a neurovegetative complaints list, which assessed emotional vulnerability, psychosomatic or tension-related complaints, cognitive complaints (such as slowness of working and concentration), flushes and quality of sleep. The results were analysed with respect to time from baseline and at each test moment HRT users were compared with controls.

Immediate recall showed only a learning effect in both groups, but the HRT group did show an improvement from baseline in long-term recall, which was not seen in the control group. HRT users also reported feeling more vigorous and activated than controls after 6 and 12 months, and less stressed than controls after 6 but not 12 months. The neurovegetative scale showed the groups to be similar at baseline, but HRT users had a lower score on emotional vulnerability at 12 months than controls, and less cognitive complaints than controls, which showed a trend at 6 months and became significant at 12 months. Not surprisingly, flushes were reduced over time in the HRT group, compared with controls; sleep quality similarly improved.

The authors criticized the small numbers (11 in each group) and the number of drop-outs (two HRT and one control) and recognized that this might explain the absence of significant differences between the groups. This is important as it has been previously suggested that larger differences between women using oestrogen than between controls can make inter-group differences difficult to detect. They also recognized that a cross-over design allowing a subject to be her own comparison, is more sensitive to slight changes with time than the case–control design used here. They commented that the addition of progestogen to the regimen did not cause a decrease in subjectively reported activation and stress.

Because the improvement in subjectively assessed factors could have been explained by an expectancy of benefit from HRT on the behalf of the women, a second study was performed using a group of HRT users who were unaware of the purpose of the study. In this study, women born between 1929 and 1949 were selected from the Maastricht Aging Study database and exclusions made on the basis of conditions which could affect cognitive function, whether these were previously reported, or detected during a semi-structured interview at the beginning of the study. This yielded a group of 342 women, 23 of whom were taking HRT of various regimens. Three cognitive performance tests were performed, the main dependant variables being memory, sensorimotor speed and cognitive flexibility. Subjective information was also collected by means of questionnaires about memory complaints and perceived health. Statistical analysis comprised direct comparison of the two groups and linear multiple regression analyses to compare the effects of age, years of education, health risk factors, and perceived health with the weight of the HRT effect on cognitive function.

The results showed that age and years of education had the strongest effect on cognitive function, with HRT users having more years of education. HRT was positively associated only with sensorimotor processing speed, independent of age and education. Interestingly, the HRT group tended to complain more of anxiety and depression, and forgetfulness than the control group. The authors' tentative explanation for this, apart from the fact that these women were unaware of the researchers' expectations, was that doctors in The Netherlands are more reluctant to prescribe HRT to postmenopausal women without a strong medical indication. This might mean that the HRT group would include women with a pattern of subjective complaints that may or may not be independent of the climacteric syndrome.

Comment

These small studies seem to suggest a general activating effect of HRT use, rather than any specific effect on memory or cognitive function. The numbers were too small for this to answer the questions posed, but this work does show how carefully studies have to be designed to overcome the 'healthy user' effect of HRT. As the authors concluded, larger, longer-term studies of older women are needed to investigate whether or not HRT confers any protection against long-term cognitive decline.

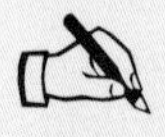

Cognitive decline in women in relation to non-protein-bound oestradiol concentrations.

K Yaffe, LY Lui, D Grady, J Cauley, J Kramer, SR Cummings. *Lancet* 2000; **356**: 708–12.

BACKGROUND. Previous studies, including one from some of these authors [5], have not demonstrated an association between levels of endogenous serum oestradiol and

cognitive function. The hypothesis behind this paper is that because most of the circulating oestradiol is protein bound, and thus not able to pass the blood–brain barrier, the total oestradiol level is not the relevant measurement. Instead, levels of non-protein-bound and loosely protein-bound oestradiol should be measured. Testosterone levels were also measured in this study, but were not found to relate to cognitive function.

INTERPRETATION. The Study of Osteoporotic Fractures was a large prospective study involving 9704 community-dwelling women aged 65 years or above. The study population was largely white, as this is the racial group thought to be most at risk of osteoporotic fracture, and also excluded some women who were unable to walk without assistance. A subsection of this study looked at hormonal risk factors for breast cancer. A group of women who went on to develop breast cancer, and a group of controls, had their baseline blood samples tested retrospectively for non-protein-bound and bioavailable (non-protein-bound and loosely bound) oestradiol, and total and free testosterone levels. This group consisted of 425 women, 116 of whom went on to develop breast cancer. Each woman underwent cognitive testing by a trained examiner at the baseline visit and then as many as possible were retested 6 years later. The test used was a modified Mini Mental State Examination (mMMSE). The MMSE is a test routinely used in the diagnosis of dementia and tests long- and short-term recall, cognition and judgement. The standard MMSE has questions about orientation which produce consistently high scores in women who do not have dementia. These questions were omitted in the mMMSE in an attempt to improve discrimination in non-demented women. Each patient also performed a shortened geriatric depression scale soon after baseline testing. Details of HRT use before and during the study were requested and checked by examining medicine package labels.

Thirty-nine patients died before the 6-year retest and 94 survivors were not retested. This left a group of 292 who were retested. The hormone levels were not rechecked, as there is evidence from other work that postmenopausal sex steroid levels are consistent for any given woman, at least for 3 years. Baseline characteristics of groups corresponding to tertiles of sex hormone concentrations were compared by analysis of variance (ANOVA) and χ^2-test as appropriate. Linear regression analyses were used to compare baseline cognitive scores between the groups and the 6-year change score between the groups. Adjustments were made for age, years of education, body mass index, exogenous oestrogen use, and history of surgical menopause. Analyses were also repeated excluding those with exogenous oestrogen use, to see if there was a difference in the relationship of cognitive function and hormone levels between users and non-users of HRT.

The results showed that women in the low tertile for non-protein-bound oestradiol were older, had a lower body mass index, were less likely to be taking oral oestrogen and less likely to develop breast cancer than women in the other two tertiles. Women in the low tertile for bioavailable oestradiol were also more likely to have had a surgical menopause than women in the other two tertiles. Mean depression scores were similar across the tertiles. Baseline cognitive scores were similar across the tertiles, but it was noted that the group who were not able to be retested at 6 years were older, less educated, did less exercise, had higher depression scores and lower baseline cognitive scores than those who were retested. Their sex hormone concentrations, however, were not significantly different from the retested group.

The mMMSE scores tended to decline over the 6 years, but women in the high tertile for non-protein-bound oestradiol showed on average stable scores, as opposed to significant decreases in those in the mid and low tertiles. The effect was similar for bioavailable oestrogen. There was no difference related to the different tertiles of testosterone concentration. Cognitive impairment (defined as a decrease of three or more points on the mMMSE) occurred in 16% of women in the low tertiles for non-protein-bound oestradiol and 5% of those in the high tertile. This means that women in the high tertile had a 70% lower risk of cognitive impairment than those in the low tertile. The results were similar for bioavailable oestradiol, and those in the mid tertiles did not show a significantly lower risk of cognitive impairment than those in the low tertile.

Using hormone concentrations as continuous variables showed a 50% lower risk of cognitive impairment per standard deviation increase in non-protein-bound oestradiol. The results were similar when women taking exogenous oestrogen were excluded from the analysis.

The authors concluded that there was an association between bioavailable oestradiol concentrations and cognitive decline in this study group. They recognized that this was not a representative population, in that women with reduced cognitive function at baseline were likely to be excluded from the study by the fact that they were volunteers and had a rigorous and lengthy introductory interview. They felt that this may explain the similar mMMSE scores across the group at baseline despite the difference in hormone levels at that point. The group was also unusual in the high proportion of women with breast cancer included.

Comment

These findings tend to support the hypothesis that there is a relationship between oestradiol levels and cognitive decline. The suggestion is that there may be a critical level of bioavailable oestradiol needed to preserve cognitive function, and thus that low-dose replacement may be sufficient to increase the levels above that threshold, and only necessary in the group of women whose bioavailable oestradiol levels are low. This would be very exciting in practical terms in that it could allow targeted use of HRT in older women. This was not a representative population, however, due to the fact that the study was part of another larger work with different end-points. It must also be remembered that a causal relationship was not necessarily proven. Although educational attainment was taken into account, there could be other confounding factors that have not yet been recognized.

This study is helpful in that it looks at the problem of the relationship between postmenopausal oestrogen levels and cognitive function from a different angle, and adds biological plausibility to the suggestion that HRT may be helpful. It also raises the possibility that protection of cognitive function may be possible with very low-dose regimens.

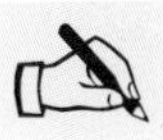

Estrogen use, APOE and cognitive decline. Evidence of gene–environment interaction.

K Yaffe, M Haan, A Byers, C Tangen, L Kuller. *Neurology* 2000; **54**: 1949–53.

BACKGROUND. In order to understand further why studies have produced conflicting results in terms of oestrogen and cognitive decline, this paper explored whether there could be a genetic basis involved. The apolipoprotein E (APOE) gene appears to be associated with later life onset of AD, with the APOEε4 allele being strongly implicated. Some studies have suggested that APOEε4-related AD is significantly more prevalent in women than men. There is also evidence from animal studies of an interaction between oestrogen and APOE mRNA expression.

This was an observational study in which changes in score on a mMMSE were analysed as a function of oestrogen use, APOE genotype and internal carotid artery wall thickening. The latter was an attempt to find a biological explanation for any changes in cognitive decline that might be detected. Recruits came from the Cardiovascular Health Study and were all aged over 65 years.

INTERPRETATION. A total of 3393 women were recruited into the Cardiovascular Health Study. In order that any oestrogen effect was not modified by progestogen, 154 women who were taking progestogen, either alone or with oestrogen, were excluded from the study. A total of 2716 women had cognitive testing performed at baseline of this study and at least once subsequently, and of these 2586 had APOE genotyping performed. At baseline a detailed questionnaire provided background medical data, current and past oestrogen and progestogen use was documented, and a depression score was administered. Common and internal carotid artery wall thickness was also measured ultrasonographically. The mMMSE was then administered annually for between five and seven yearly follow-up visits.

Subject characteristics at baseline were analysed by oestrogen use, defined as never, current and past use. Repeated cognitive scores were analysed in association with oestrogen use, APOE genotype and carotid artery wall thickness, and the effect of oestrogen on the association between APOEε4 and cognitive decline was assessed. Relevant factors such as age, education, race and stroke history were also incorporated into the analysis.

The results showed that at baseline 11% were taking oestrogen and these women tended to be white, younger, better educated, drink slightly more alcohol and have a lower body mass index. They tended to have a younger age at menopause and they had less common and internal artery wall thickness. The past users were more similar to the never users in baseline characteristics. Baseline cognitive testing showed the current users to have higher scores than past users who in turn were higher than never users, although that difference was less marked. Similar numbers from each group died or dropped out. As in other studies those who did not continue with yearly testing were older, scoring less well and more depressed. They did not appear to differ in oestrogen use or genotype.

Average mMMSE scores declined with time, and initially it appears that current users declined significantly less than past or never users. When the models were adjusted for age, education, race and stroke, however, the difference was no longer significant.

On genetic testing, 26% of the women had one or more APOEε4 alleles, and there was no difference between racial groups or oestrogen use groups in this respect. APOEε4-negative women declined on average by 1.7 ± 0.4 points over the average 6 years of follow-up, ε4 heterozygotes declined by 4.6 ± 0.8 points, and APOEε4 homozygotes declined by 11.9 ± 2.6 points (all 95% CI). Adjustment for age, education and stroke left a difference of 3.6 ± 0.7 between the heterozygous women and the negative women, and of 7.8 ± 2.4 between the heterozygous and homozygous groups. For APOEε4-positive women there was no effect from oestrogen use, but for APOEε4-negative women current users had a 1.5 ± 1.0 point smaller decline than past and never users. Adjustment did not remove this difference but reduced the statistical significance to $P = 0.06$.

Ten per cent of the women had cognitive impairment as defined by the mMMSE at baseline and 13% developed impairment during the course of the study. Among APOEε4-negative women, cognitive impairment occurred in 8% of current users and 15% of never users. Among APOEε4-positive women, 18% in each group became impaired. When adjustments were made, APOEε4-positive women had an adjusted hazard risk of 1.47 (95% CI 1.13–1.90) compared with APOEε4-negative women, and among APOEε4-negative women, current use of oestrogen produced an adjusted hazard risk of 0.59 (95% CI 0.36–0.99) compared with never users. Past use was not significantly different from never use, with a hazard risk of 0.72 (95% CI 0.48–1.08). Among APOEε4-positive women, oestrogen use had no effect on the risk of cognitive decline.

Carotid artery wall thickness showed a similar pattern of oestrogen use affecting thickness in APOEε4-negative women. The wall was thicker in APOEε4-positive women and this was not affected by oestrogen use.

Comment

This fascinating study may help to explain why results of other studies have been conflicting, as the genetic make up of other study populations has not been explored. Clearly APOE status has a major effect on the risk of dementia, and the effect of oestrogen appears to be relevant only in APOEε4-negative genotypes. It must be noted, however, that the inclusion of educational level into the multivariate analysis does reduce the statistical significance, so education is again a major player in the risk of dementia.

The effect on carotid artery wall thickness introduces a possible biological explanation for the effect of oestrogen. Carotid artery atherosclerosis is known to increase the risk of AD, vascular dementia, and mild cognitive decline. APOE is a carrier protein involved in the distribution of lipids generally in the body, and the APOEε4 genotype is associated with central nervous system atherosclerosis. This suggests various mechanisms by which oestrogen may protect against cognitive decline, by protecting against central nervous system atherosclerosis, inducing vasodilatation, as well as effects on smooth muscle, platelets and lipids. It can be seen that there could come a point in the extent of the damage that oestrogen can make no further difference which would explain the findings of other studies that oestrogen may delay the onset of dementia, but not help once it is established.

More work needs to be done before this type of work translates into practice. This study did not include women using progestogen and, of course, most women who need HRT have not had a hysterectomy. It does suggest that if oestrogen is to be useful, it needs to be continued long term, as past use did not appear to be as helpful. The benefit really does need to be understood more, therefore, if we are to look at women needing HRT, albeit probably low dose, into their ninth decade, so that it can be targeted correctly.

Prevention and treatment of AD

Although there is clearly not a consensus of opinion about whether HRT use improves cognitive functioning in healthy women, there may be more clarity about the effect of HRT on the risk of developing the commonest cause of dementia, AD. AD pathology consists of neuronal loss and deposition of beta amyloid in brain tissue. Metabolism of acetyl choline is impaired, which has effects on learning and memory. The characteristic postmortem finding, along with shrinkage of the brain tissue, is of intracellular neurofibrillary tangles, and extracellular senile plaques which are the result of the cell damage and deposition of debris. The hippocampus, basal forebrain, and the cholinergic mechanism appear to be particularly affected by the disease. Symptoms include progressive loss of short-term memory, confusion when dealing with complex tasks, personality and mood changes, and loss of inhibition. The greatest risk factor is increasing age, with 0.1% incidence at ages below 65 years, rising to 4–5% above 65 years and 20% at 80 years. Other estimates show an incidence of 47% by the age of 85 years and over. The disease is more common in women than men with a ratio of 3:1. Women also tend to have more severe cognitive impairment than men. There is a recognized genetic component with amyloid precursor protein (APP), presenilin-1 and presenilin-2, being responsible for early onset disease, and weaker links with ApoE4, and ApoE3. ApoE2 genotype appears to be protective.

Animal and epidemiological studies throughout the 1990s have explored the association between AD and HRT use. Animal studies suggest that oestrogen affects several aspects of brain function that impact on memory and cognition, that oestrogen deficiency reduces synaptic connections to the hippocampus, and that oestrogen replacement reverses this effect. There is also evidence that oestrogen may prevent the accumulation of beta amyloid in brain tissue. Results of epidemiological studies have been conflicting, with studies being made difficult by issues such as the usual tendency for HRT-taking women to be healthier, of higher socioeconomic class, and having had more years of education. In particular, higher educational attainment appears to be negatively associated with the development of AD. Retrospective studies are thwarted by poor recall of details of HRT use by both subjects and their carers.

Tang *et al.* [6] reported a significant delay in the onset of AD in women who had taken oestrogen, and a reduced relative risk of developing the disease in oestrogen users as opposed to non-users. This paper also suggested a dose effect in that longer duration of use appeared to confer a greater protective effect.

Since then several papers have continued to look at this association. As previously mentioned, several large studies with longer-term follow-up are awaited.

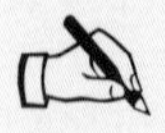

Postmenopausal oestrogen replacement therapy and risk of AD. A population based study.

SC Waring, WA Rocca, RC Petersen, PC O'Brien, EG Tangalos, E Kokmen. *Neurology* 1999; **52**: 965.

BACKGROUND. **This study aimed to improve on previous studies by avoiding the problems of recall bias experienced by other workers. The records linkage system used allowed complete medical records to be available for review retrospectively after a diagnosis of AD was made.**

INTERPRETATION. A total of 222 patients were identified as having a probable diagnosis of AD made between 1980 and 1984. These were selected by taking all the possible cases and allowing a neurologist access to the records, so that a diagnosis could be made from the information recorded using accepted diagnostic criteria. AD is difficult to diagnose and standard criteria could not be used because of the difference in information available for each patient. Autopsy reports were used when available as the only definite way of making a diagnosis of AD. A total of 222 matched controls were selected by age and length of time within the health care system (as assessed by the clinic registration number). A patient could only act as a control if there was sufficient information in the medical records for the neurologist to exclude dementia at entry to the study.

A trained nurse abstractor reviewed all the notes without being aware which were cases and which were controls. This was not a true blinding as she did have access to the records containing diagnostic information. She collected information about HRT use from the menopause to the time of the AD diagnosis in the case. Various other related information was extracted so as to assess potential selection bias. HRT use was recorded as never, less than 6 months and more than 6 months; total cumulative dose was also recorded.

The results showed that cases and controls were similar in terms of age at menarche, age at menopause, number of live births and number of years in education. The median age at onset of AD was 82 years. For those exposed to HRT for more than 6 months, the onset appeared to be delayed to a median of 84 years. The frequency of postmenopausal HRT use was higher in the control group than the cases (10 versus 5%). Thus, control patients were more likely to have used more than 6 months of oestrogen than AD patients with an odds ratio of 0.42 (95% CI 0.18–0.96). The odds ratio was not significantly changed by controlling for the effects of education, age at menopause or parity. The results were not changed by excluding women who had undergone surgical menopause or by only including those who had taken oestrogen for 12 months or more. Investigation of the dose–response relationship showed a trend of decreasing risk of AD with greater duration of HRT. No statistically significant effect of cumulative dose was seen.

Comment

The major problem with this study was the difficulty in making an accurate diagnosis of AD retrospectively, but it was useful to have objectively recorded information on dose and duration of oestrogen therapy in as much detail as possible, given that note keeping varies in completeness and accuracy. Selection bias was reduced by taking all the known AD cases in the time scale and area, and this appears to have been successful in that cases and controls were similar in terms of educational experience. Using incidence instead of prevalence excluded any possible effect of greater longevity in HRT users.

However, it is not possible to determine if the timing of HRT use has any effect on the risk of AD, as it was not clear from the paper how many of the patients were taking HRT at the time of the diagnosis, and whether this had any effect. This may be important in practical terms if it is considered that women could be advised to take HRT to reduce the risk of development of AD as more information about the timing of use and the dose required would be needed.

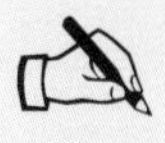

A prospective study of estrogen replacement therapy and the risk of developing Alzheimer's disease: the Baltimore Longitudinal Study of Aging.

C Kawas, S Resnick, A Morrison, *et al. Neurology* 1997; **48**: 1517–21.

BACKGROUND. This, being a prospective study, had few problems with recall bias and allowed tighter diagnostic criteria to be used in the diagnosis of dementia. There does not appear to have been a problem with HRT users being better educated than non-users because this unrepresentative population tended to have high educational levels across the sample.

INTERPRETATION. The Baltimore Longitudinal Study of Aging is a longitudinal study of normal ageing and has been recruiting women since 1978. Data on HRT use have been collected from the outset. The study population is known not to represent the general population, and the sample used in this study was predominantly (92%) white, and had generally high levels of educational attainment, with 62% having college or graduate degrees. The study group comprised 514 women who were peri- or postmenopausal at recruitment. The mean age was 61.5 years and the mean age of menopause was 46.4 years. Twenty-nine per cent had undergone hysterectomy. The women had already been followed for up to 16 years by the time of recruitment into the present study.

The women attended for interview and examination every 2 years, including sufficient neuropsychological tests and investigations to allow diagnosis of dementia. Dementia and probable AD were diagnosed by standard criteria. HRT use was recorded at each visit, which aimed to reduce recall bias and allowed detailed recording of HRT regimens. The aim of the statistical analysis of the results was to calculate a relative risk of developing AD in association with oestrogen use. A model was used which allowed each case of AD that occurred to be compared with all women of the same age who had not developed the disease. This analysis divided women into HRT users or non-users and used a measure of education as greater or less than 16 years of education. A second analysis explored the duration of HRT use into categories (never, 0–5 years, 5–10 years and more than 10 years).

Of the 514 women, 472 had complete data on HRT use. Those with missing data were excluded, but as a group did not have different educational levels or incidence of AD during the study period. Of the remaining study group, 34 developed AD, nine of whom had used HRT. This gives a relative risk of 0.457 (95% CI 0.209–0.997) of developing AD when comparing HRT use with non-use. There was not a significant increase in protective effect with duration of use of HRT and when HRT use was divided into duration of use categories the relative risk for each category was less than one but not statistically significant. Adjusting for years of education did not significantly affect the result, and HRT users and non-users were similar in terms of years of education.

Interestingly, this study also looked at non-steroidal anti-inflammatory drug use and found a relative risk of 0.49 of developing AD for women who took non-steroidal anti-inflammatory drugs. This appeared to be independent of HRT use.

Comment

There are problems with this study, but it does contribute usefully to the debate. The long-term use of HRT seen in the study could have provided useful information about optimum duration of HRT use, and possibly optimum timing. Unfortunately, once the HRT users were divided into groups by duration of use, the confidence intervals for relative risk crossed 1, suggesting that larger numbers would be needed to provide the information sought. Because the relative risk calculated actually came from a never versus ever use divide, we need to know more about how much use was needed to be categorized as an ever user. Because the numbers developing AD were small, this type of information could affect the final conclusion of the study.

As ever the conclusion is that larger studies are needed.

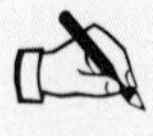

Estrogen for Alzheimer's disease in women: randomised, double-blind, placebo-controlled trial.

VW Henderson, A Paganini-Hill, BL Miller, *et al. Neurology* 2000; **54**: 295.

BACKGROUND. Given accumulating evidence of benefit from oestrogen in terms of cognitive function and prevention of AD, the authors hypothesized that oestrogen might improve cognitive function and daily life of women with AD. This study was small and had to be short term, because of the decision to use unopposed oestrogen, even in those women who had an intact uterus. It was, however, randomized, double blind and placebo controlled. The authors noted that prior to this work, several studies had suggested a benefit from oestrogen use in women with AD, but these studies were small and not randomized. Several also looked at women who were on HRT at

baseline, so it was not clear whether the oestrogen effect was short or long term. The four randomized trials preceding this had shown conflicting results. All were shorter duration and used smaller numbers than this study. The studies that suggested benefit appeared to involve less careful neuropsychological testing than that used here.

INTERPRETATION. This study was designed to have an 80% chance of detecting a clinically significant change in cognitive ability with a 0.1% significance level. The subjects were all postmenopausal (natural or surgical) and met strict criteria for the diagnosis of AD. They had been assessed as having mild to moderate dementia. It was decided to use unopposed oestrogen (CEE 1.25) because of concerns that the addition of progestogen might compromise any beneficial effect of the oestrogen. Thus, the trial was limited to 16 weeks, but despite this some women experienced vaginal spotting and mastalgia, which could have led their carers to suspect that they were in the active treatment group.

The tests used covered a wide range of cognitive tasks, a depression score, Clinical Global Impression of Change (CGIC) and a caregiver's assessment of daily functioning. Specific memory tests were used to try to assess if short-term oestrogen therapy had specific effects on some skills. Testing was at baseline, 4 weeks and 16 weeks. Compliance based on pill counting was found to be good in both groups. By 16 weeks, three women had dropped out from each group, with no evidence of this being because of oestrogen-related problems.

The results did not show any significant difference between the groups on cognitive testing, with a non-significant tendency for the treatment group to decline more than the placebo group. For those who did improve, there was slightly more improvement in the placebo group. Specific cognitive tasks did not show a pattern favouring either group consistently. CGIC, caregivers' assessments and mood scores were not different between the groups.

Comment

This study was carefully randomized and blinded, and testing appears to have been rigorous. The other important feature of this study design is that it placed importance on a woman's actual ability to function on a day to day basis, as well as to score on tests. The study would appear to have had quite high expectations of finding improvement with oestrogen, in that the level of change on cognitive testing that was considered to be clinically relevant was equal to the deterioration one would expect over the space of a year. However, any biases involved would probably favour the treatment arm, and there were no trends towards improvement with oestrogen even if one looks at non-significant results. It is possible that a larger study would yield more informative results, perhaps if subgroups of AD differ. It is also necessary to look at longer-term oestrogen therapy, bearing in mind the short-term deterioration that one sees with HRT, for example, in cardiovascular function.

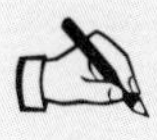

Estrogen replacement therapy for treatment of mild to moderate Alzheimer disease. A randomised controlled trial.

RA Mulnard, CW Cotman, C Kawas, *et al. J Am Med Assoc* 2000; **283**: 1007–15.

BACKGROUND. This was again a randomized, double-blind, placebo-controlled trial. Again, the study was well performed, with careful randomization and blinding; the numbers were larger and the follow-up longer than the previous study. The results, however, are much the same. To allow for oestrogen-only use, and longer-term use, women who had undergone hysterectomy were recruited from 32 sites of the Alzheimer's Disease Cooperative Study, which is supported by the National Institute on Ageing. All women had a diagnosis of probable AD and were categorized as mild to moderate by MMSE scores. They were older than 60 years and not suffering from major depression. Criteria were included to ensure that they were suitable for treatment with oestrogen. Patients taking donezepil (a reversible inhibitor of acetylcholinesterase used in the treatment of mild to moderate dementia) were initially excluded, but this rule was changed during the study to allow women who had been taking it for 4 weeks or more to be recruited.

This set out to be a definitive trial, aiming to assess whether oestrogen has a beneficial effect on cognition in AD, independent of any mood-enhancing effect. It also aimed to establish by what mechanism memory is improved by oestrogen, and whether or not oestrogen has any other clinically relevant benefits in AD.

INTERPRETATION. The 120 women recruited were randomly assigned to one of three groups: placebo, CEE 0.625 mg and CEE 1.25 mg, each for 12 months. Each group then had a single blind placebo washout period for 3 months.

Testing was performed at baseline, and 2, 6, 12 and 15 months, with the primary measure being a version of the CGIC scale. The MMSE and the Clinical Dementia Rating (CDR) scale were used and two measures of depression were used to separate out mood and direct cognition effects of oestrogen therapy. Several tests specific to memory were administered to try to investigate how any effect of memory might be mediated. Safety monitoring for HRT was incorporated into the visits, and any adverse events were reviewed by the independent safety monitoring committee. Ninety-seven of the 120 recruits completed the trial.

The results were analysed twice, first comparing both treatment groups as one to the placebo group, and second comparing all three groups to each other. The two-group comparison did not show any lessening in cognitive decline in those treated with oestrogen, and the two specific differences found were both in favour of the placebo group. The three-group comparison again did not show any benefit from oestrogen therapy. The CDR showed a benefit from low-dose oestrogen, but this did not persist with continuing treatment. No benefit was seen at any point in terms of mood or memory.

Separate analyses revealed that in the low-dose treatment group only, women with prior exposure to oestrogen had better CGIC scores at 12 months. This group contained significantly more women who had used oestrogen in the past than the placebo or high-dose treatment group. Analysis between donezepil users and non-users showed no significant difference.

years), with a median time postmenopause of 3 years. All the women had been referred because of vasomotor symptoms. Thus, any positive findings from the study are only referable to this population, and cannot necessarily be extrapolated to an older, vasomotor symptom free population. However, the findings are interesting, and the study methods could presumably be extended to other population groups.

INTERPRETATION. Loss of balance may be the endpoint of a fault in any part of the complex balance system. Balance depends on an intact vestibular system to recognize the position of the head and its dynamic changes, usually an intact visual system that can input into the vestibular system, and intact proprioception to recognize small tension changes within the muscles and tendons. Information from these systems is processed in the cerebellum and brainstem, and information sent to the motor system to allow correction. There is also an element of conscious perception and memory, involving the cerebral cortex. A tool called dynamic posturography has been developed which can objectively evaluate the three components of the balance system and their integration. This consists of a platform and a visual surround, both of which move to challenge the woman's balance. The platform can measure vertical forces between feet and ground and also horizontal forces. The tests involve multiple combinations of moving platform and surround, with the subject's eyes either open or closed, so that different components of the balance system are tested. Because the tests are usually used to assess patients with vertigo or balance problems, they had to be made more challenging for this research, from which women with known balance problems were excluded.

Nineteen women completed the study. They had routine gynaecological and otoneurological examinations prior to the study and blood samples for follicle stimulating hormone and serum oestradiol. In the two pretreatment weeks, a Kupperman index was used to assess climacteric symptoms and a diary of hot flushes was kept. The treatment phase consisted of 12 weeks of transdermal oestrogen 50 µg, followed by 2 weeks of oestrogen with 5 mg/day of medroxyprogesterone acetate. All subjects were tested with dynamic posturography before treatment and at 4, 12 and 14 weeks.

The results showed that symptoms and flushes improved in all women during the treatment phase. All women had balance results in the normal range at the beginning of the test, and showed significant improvement during the treatment phase, which continued through the progestogenic phase.

The authors concluded that these tests show an improvement in the balance system with oestrogen treatment in women with climacteric symptoms. They postulated that this might be because of an increase in cerebellar blood flow, as previous studies have demonstrated differential increases in the brain and cerebellum with oestrogen therapy. They recognized that the effect could be due to a general improvement in well-being with the HRT, in particular improved sleep patterns due to a reduction in hot flush frequency. Previous studies have shown that there is not a learning effect with dynamic posturography, and in fact it is used for assessing improvement or deterioration in balance-related conditions. It was, therefore, valid to use the subjects as their own controls. They suggested that a prospective double-blind placebo-controlled study using oestrogen in postmenopausal women without climacteric symptoms would be the next step. They also recognized that a demonstration of benefit in women with normal balance at the outset does not necessarily extrapolate to benefit in women with balance impairment.

Comment

Although this study only represents a first step in the assessment of balance problems in postmenopausal women, and their possible improvement with oestrogen, it is valuable. Studies like this, which attempt to assess issues which are relevant to the day to day risk of falling, and also take into account the effect of progestogen, which is an essential part of HRT for most women, are very relevant to the aim of reducing the real fracture risk in the older population.

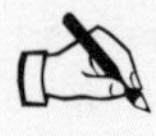

Hormone replacement therapy increases isometric muscle strength of adductor pollicis in post menopausal women.

DA Skelton, SK Phillips, SA Bruce, CH Naylor, RC Woledge. *Clin Sci* 1999; **96**: 357–64.

BACKGROUND. This study looked at the effect of HRT on age-related decline in the strength of the adductor pollicis muscle of the thumb. This muscle has been extensively studied over the years, because simple, reliable tests have been developed. The ratio of the maximum voluntary force (MVF) to its cross-sectional area (CSA) is more reliable than in the larger muscles of the leg, which may seem more directly relevant to the problem of falls. Falls aside, this muscle is essential for daily activities that involve grip, such as holding door handles, opening jars and doing up buttons. The authors have reported previously a cross-sectional study demonstrating a rapid decline in the MVF/CSA ratio, which corresponded with the age of the menopause, and was not seen in men, or in women taking HRT. Another study by different authors showed similar results, looking at the muscles of the knee. Both these studies may have suffered from selection bias, because women who choose to take HRT are generally fitter and stronger than those who do not. They also could not assess if the apparent effect of the HRT would be seen if it was started after the menopause-related decline in strength, or if it would be protective only if started before this decline occurred. Studies have also shown strength changes corresponding to the menstrual cycle in the hand and in the quadriceps, which provides further evidence of some degree of hormonal influence.

This study was a prospective randomized placebo-controlled study of CEE 0.625 mg for 12 months in women 5–15 years postmenopause, aiming to assess if the loss of strength could be reversed. It was not blinded as it was felt that blinding of the subjects would not be possible because of the bleeding to be expected with HRT, and that blinding of the observers was unnecessary because of the objective nature of the tests.

INTERPRETATION. Well-validated tests of MVF and CSA of the adductor pollicis muscle were performed on 102 women, 52 of whom were randomized to the placebo group and 50 to the HRT treatment group. Women were not included if they had any condition causing pain or stiffness of the thumb, relevant medication, or evidence of wasting or generalized neuromuscular disease. Other exclusion criteria included hysterectomy, use of HRT in the previous year or oestrogen implants in the previous

3 years, or conditions that could contraindicate HRT usage. The treatment group was given 13 cycles of CEE 0.625 mg. The tests were performed at baseline, and 2, 4, 6, 13, 26, 39 and 52 weeks. Oestradiol and oestrone levels were measured in all patients at baseline and in the HRT group at weeks 4 and 13.

There were four drop-outs in the control group and 13 in the HRT group, these latter being due to side-effects of treatment, mainly bleeding and weight gain. Forty-four of the treatment group remained at 6 months and these were included in the analysis. The HRT group showed an increase of at least 50% in oestradiol and oestrone levels, and an increase in bone mineral density, suggestive of successful absorption.

The results of the strength testing were presented as each measure of strength divided by the overall average strength for the individual subject. This was so that increases could be compared, and because it was expected that any increase would be in proportion to the strength of the individual. This showed a significant increase in MVF at and after 13 weeks in the HRT group and a significant decrease in the control group at and after 26 weeks. The CSA did not change significantly in any subject, so the change seen in MVF was not due to an increase in the size of the muscle. Looking at the change for each individual showed an increase in strength in 20 subjects in the control group and a decrease in 29. The HRT group showed an increase in 36 patients and a decrease in three (only those who completed 39 weeks of the study were included in this analysis).

Factors such as age, years past menopause, initial hormone levels, change in hormone levels, body weight, and initial MVF were examined to see if they had any predictive value for changes in MVF. Only initial oestrone level and initial MVF showed significant correlations, and a multiple regression model using these two variables showed that they only accounted for 34% of the variance between individuals in the increase in MVF over the year of treatment. It was interesting that the weaker the initial MVF, the more benefit was obtained by the treatment. The amount of bone mineral density increase did not relate to the increase in strength.

The authors commented that these finding are generally consistent with other studies, although the isometric contractions measured here seem to show an improvement with HRT, whereas isokinetic contractions which depend on the speed of muscle contraction as well as strength, do not seem to show the same effect. They suggested that the most likely mechanism for an oestrogen effect on muscle strength is at the level of the cross bridges, and is in terms of force per cross bridge rather than number.

Comment

Again, this appears to be the early stages of work looking at HRT use and muscle strength. There was no selection bias in this study, as the two groups were similar in every characteristic at the outset. This is important because HRT users are usually fitter and more active than non-users. Because any women with pre-existing muscle stiffness or wasting were excluded, however, the results may not be relevant to women with, for example, arthritis of the hands who may be looking for help in this direction. This would have to be studied separately. There may be bias introduced by the high drop-out rate in the HRT group in favour of an increase in muscle strength with HRT if there was a tendency for the drop-outs to be not improving with treatment. There was no suggestion of this in the paper and the results were highly significant, so it is unlikely that this effect would make a difference to the conclusions of the study.

The difference between the different types of muscle activity may be relevant when one looks at clinical endpoints such as falls. Ideally, we therefore need studies with clinical endpoints to follow on from this useful work, but as there are so many factors involved in, for example, the risk of falling, this would involve very large and complex studies.

Urogenital atrophy and incontinence

Although vaginal dryness is frequently mentioned as a symptom of the menopause, it is a subject for which women may find it difficult to seek help, as are the related symptoms of urinary frequency and dyspareunia. Perhaps for this reason, many women suffer these problems in silence, and the area has not been well researched over the years. The first study reviewed here looked at the problem of urogenital ageing and possible cultural influences on help seeking. The second paper looked at a subject that can be even more difficult to discuss, faecal incontinence.

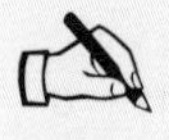

A study of European women's experience of the problems of urogenital ageing and its management.
DH Barlow, G Samsoioe, JM van Geelen. *Maturitas* 1997; **27**: 239–47.

BACKGROUND. **This study was performed to assess to what extent there may be international differences in women's experience and presentation of postmenopausal urogenital problems. This was felt to be important because the sensitivity of the subject could make it difficult for women to seek help, and because working in a multicultural society demands knowledge of how a woman's cultural background may affect her presentation.**

INTERPRETATION. This study took the form of a survey of a stratified random sample of the populations of Denmark, France, Germany, Italy, The Netherlands and the UK. A total of 3062 women were interviewed face to face by female interviewers, asking about dysuria, incontinence of urine, urinary frequency, recurrent urinary tract infection, vaginal itching or burning and dyspareunia. Because of the potential embarrassment of the interview, patients were able to answer using show cards. Questions about severity of symptoms had a choice of answers ranging from 'a minor problem with no effect on everyday life' to 'a very irritating problem strongly affecting everyday life over a long time'. Care was taken to ensure that questions were understandable in all the languages, but also retained a consistent meaning.

The results showed that the population surveyed was fairly evenly spread in age from 55 to 74 years and 58.7% were either married or living with a partner, but this percentage reduced with increasing age. The median age at menopause was 50 years in all countries apart from the UK, where it was 49 years. In total, 20.6% had undergone hysterectomy, which was performed premenopausally in 75.8% of cases. In 48.8% of hysterectomies both ovaries were removed, a unilateral oophorectomy was performed in 13.1% and in 33.8% both ovaries were conserved; 4.3% of the women did not know if their ovaries had been removed or not. Dutch women were most likely to have undergone hysterectomy (24.3%) and Italian women the least (14.9%).

A total of 29.3% of the women said that they had experienced at least one of the urogenital atrophy symptoms in question. This broke down into more than 35% of Italian and British women and less than 25% of Danish and Dutch women. Fifty-two per cent considered the problem to be moderate or severe. Urinary frequency was reported by 12.7% (13.5% severe, 39.1% moderate). Vaginal itching or burning was reported by 10.6% (16.5% severe, 40.7% moderate). Dysuria was reported by 8.3% (17% severe, 45.6% moderate). Urinary incontinence was reported by 7.4% (22.1% severe, 41.7% moderate). Recurrent urinary tract infection was reported by 7.4% (20.7% severe, 45.5% moderate). Dyspareunia was reported by 6.7% (12.7% severe, 48.0% moderate). A total of 49.1% of the women had been sexually active in the previous year. The symptoms rarely occurred in isolation, with urinary frequency and vaginal itching frequently accompanying other symptoms.

In terms of the action taken by the women, 58% had consulted a doctor and 10.9% had visited a pharmacist. Thirty-three per cent of the women felt that their problem was embarrassing (ranging from 'maybe embarrassing' to 'absolutely embarrassing') and 13.1% said they would be embarrassed to discuss the problem with a doctor.

Of the women who consulted a doctor or a pharmacist, 43.6% received no treatment. Of those who did receive treatment, most were given HRT. Of these prescriptions, 27.7% were for oral HRT and 31.2% were vaginal creams or pessaries. Twelve per cent of women used transdermal patches or gels. The efficacy as reported by the women was high in all cases, with the best relief being from local vaginal preparations. Tablets and transdermal gel were not significantly less effective, and patches slightly less so. Of the whole population, 11.2% had used HRT at some time and by the time of the interview, 48% of those who had ever taken HRT were still using it. When asked about symptoms experienced in the last month before their interview, 8.4% of the group had experienced urinary frequency or vaginal itching/burning and 2.2% had experienced dyspareunia or urinary tract infection.

Comment

The actual purpose of this paper was to compare women's experiences across Europe, and it contains some fascinating details of cross-cultural differences which are not reported here. The paper contains some interesting lessons about urogenital atrophy in general. It shows that although the incidence of atrophy symptoms is lower than one might have expected, a huge number of people across Europe are significantly affected by it. The symptoms seemed to occur in clusters, which means that if a woman presents with one of these recognized urogenital atrophy symptoms, the others should be actively asked about, and a specific treatment may not be as effective as oestrogen therapy. Vaginal treatment in this study appeared to be as effective as systemic HRT, and it is possible that the better side-effect profile that one can see with local oestrogen might have been responsible for the relatively high use of HRT and the relatively good continuance seen in this study.

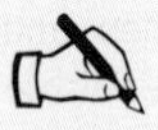

The influence of oestrogen replacement on faecal incontinence in postmenopausal women.

V Donnelly, PR O'Connell, C O'Herlihy. *Br J Obstet Gynaecol* 1997; **104**: 311–5.

BACKGROUND. Faecal incontinence is another problem which is distressing, and often causes such embarrassment that seeking help is difficult. Most affected women are parous and postmenopausal, and it occurs eight times as frequently in women as men. It is likely that the initial insult relates to childbirth, but that the integrity of the pelvic floor connective tissue compensates until oestrogen deficiency occurs. There is evidence that there may be a hormone-dependent factor in the muscles and ligaments of the pelvic floor, and of oestrogen receptors in the tissue of the external anal sphincter. This would suggest that oestrogen replacement might be helpful in faecal incontinence as it has been shown to be in some women with postmenopausal urinary incontinence.

INTERPRETATION. Twenty women were recruited from gynaecological, menopause and coloproctology clinics at two hospitals in Dublin. Their average age was 61 years, they were all postmenopausal and oestrogen deficient with an oestradiol level of less than 50 pg/ml. They had all been incontinent of faeces for some years (average 6.1 years). Women with other relevant disorders were not included.

Before the treatment phase all the women completed a questionnaire detailing bowel function and a continence grading score. This records the frequency with which a woman experiences solid or liquid faeces or flatus, or soils, or has her lifestyle been affected by incontinence. The effect of the incontinence on each woman's daily life was assessed by means of a visual analogue score. Anorectal physiology, consisting of anal manometry, anal endosonography, measurement of rectal sensation, anal electrosensitivity and pudendal nerve terminal motor latency was performed at baseline and after 6 months of treatment. The treatment consisted of a 50 μg transdermal patch twice weekly for those women who had undergone hysterectomy, and the same patch regimen with 1 mg of norethisterone acetate orally for 12 days of each cycle, for those who had not.

All women completed an obstetric history questionnaire. This showed them to be parous (range three to eight deliveries). One related the onset of incontinence to childbirth, but only five of the women had memories of difficulty in labour or delivery. Two women felt the incontinence had begun after hysterectomy, and 12 felt that it had become worse at the menopause. Eighteen per cent recorded an improvement in their symptoms after 6 months of HRT, and 25% reported themselves as symptom free by the end of the treatment period. This was reflected in improved continence scores and improvements in daily life.

The anorectal physiology tests showed significant increases in the mean resting and maximum resting anal canal pressure and mean maximum voluntary squeeze. There was an increase in the maximum tolerated rectal volume, but the other sensory indicators were unaffected by the oestrogen treatment. The anal ultrasonography revealed that 30%

of the women had an anal sphincter defect that had not been recognized previously. This group still showed improvement with the treatment.

The symptoms that showed most improvement were those that would generally be considered minor: defaecatory urgency, faecal staining and lack of flatus control. These do, however, cause a great deal of distress. They are unlikely to be presented directly as a symptom, but a survey at the menopause clinic at the National Maternity Hospital in Dublin showed that 4% of women attending had some degree of faecal incontinence, and most felt that the symptoms had become worse since the menopause. There is a debate about whether benefit from HRT is direct on the strength of the pelvic floor, or whether it is due to an indirect effect of the improved well-being that is recognized with this treatment. The physiological test results presented here tend to suggest that at least part of the effect is direct, probably due to an increase in the collagen and elastic content of the pelvic floor.

Comment

This study needs to be followed up by larger, randomized studies to explore these issues further. At present it serves to heighten awareness of the frequency of faecal incontinence postmenopause, as it does appear to be a symptom that will only be presented after direct questioning, and is perhaps more common than most clinicians would have expected. It is clearly worth arranging anal endosonography to exclude sphincter damage and referral to a centre that can investigate the complaint carefully.

Summary

Reviewing the literature on the subject of HRT and the older woman seems to produce more questions than answers, but the fact that the questions are being asked is a positive step. As the female population ages, any strategies that might reduce the morbidity of ageing have to be taken seriously.

It is evident from the attitude studies that there is more reluctance on the part of prescribers to recommend HRT to older women than to younger women. More knowledge of the balance of benefit versus risk is vitally important if we are to prescribe correctly and with the confidence that is clearly needed to encourage continuance.

More work is needed on assessing the true risks, but our understanding of some of these is increasing. It is vitally important, however, that benefit is proven before prescribing for indications such as cognitive decline and falls becomes commonplace. It is very encouraging to see more studies using clinical endpoints, and also recognizing that the effect of the progestogen component has to be assessed as this is essential for the majority of women. There needs to be much more communication between specialists if we are to understand the real issues about ageing in order to improve our care of our older patients.

To make HRT more acceptable to those who may benefit from it, the issue of vaginal bleeding needs to be taken very seriously. Low-dose continuous combined regimens should improve acceptability, but this appears not always to be the case, and it may be that our explanations to women considering HRT need to be more comprehensive.

Newer preparations such as tibilone and the selective oestrogen receptor modulators may prove very useful here, but it must be remembered that the effects of these drugs for each indication will need to be explored and not assumed.

References

1. Richards M, Kuh D, Hardy R, Wadsworth M. Lifetime cognitive function and timing of the natural menopause. *Neurology* 1999; **53**: 308.

2. Genazzi AR, Spinetti A, Gallo R, Bernardi F. Menopause and the central nervous system: intervention options. *Maturitas* 1999; **31**: 103–10.

3. National Research Register, Cochrane Library.

4. Shumaker S, Reboussin B, Espeland MA, *et al.* The Women's Health Initiative Memory Study (WHIMS): a trial of the effect of estrogen therapy in preventing and slowing the progression of dementia. *Control Clin Trials* 1998; **19**: 604–21.

5. Yaffe K, Grady D, Pressman A, Cummings S. Serum oestrogen levels, cognitive performance and risk of cognitive decline in older community women. *J Am Geriatr Soc* 1998; **46**: 816–21.

6. Tang MX, Jacobs D, Stern Y, *et al.* Effect of oestrogen during menopause on risk and age at onset of Alzheimer's disease. *Lancet* 1996; **348**: 429–32.

7. Recker RR, Davies KM, Dowd RM, Heaney RP. The effect of low-dose continuous estrogen and progesterone therapy with calcium and vitamin D on bone in elderly women. *Ann Intern Med* 1999; **130**: 897–904.

8. Hayashi T, Ito I, Kano H, Endo H, Iguchi A. Estriol (E3) replacement improves endothelial function and bone mineral density in very elderly women. *J Gerontol Biol Sci* 2000; **55A**: B183–90.

9. Hunt K, Vessey M, McPherson K. Mortality in a cohort of long-term users of hormone replacement therapy: an updated analysis. *Br J Obstet Gynaecol* 1990; **97**: 1080–6.

Part III

Other gynaecology

10

Gynaecological malignancies

Introduction

Genital tract cancers represent a major disease burden in women in the UK and world-wide. Ovarian cancer is the most common gynaecological cancer in England and Wales, causing approximately 4000 deaths per year, and is the fourth leading cause of cancer-related death in women aged 55–74 years in the USA, with approximately 13 000 deaths per year. Mortality from cervical cancer in the UK has decreased to approximately 1000 deaths per year, but cervical cancer remains the most common form of cancer in women in developing countries, and the second most common form of cancer in women in the world as a whole. It is estimated that there are 450 000 new cases of invasive cervix cancer per year in developing countries.

This chapter will focus on new developments in ovarian cancer treatment and screening and two new developments in the treatment of cervical cancer.

Ovarian cancer

Only 30% of women with ovarian cancer survive 5 years or more after diagnosis, compared with 70% of patients with breast cancer. The reason for this is two-fold. First, over 75% of women with ovarian cancer present with stage III or IV disease. Second, despite the recent successes seen with the use of newer cytotoxic agents such as taxoids and topoisomerase 1 inhibitors (camptothecins), the median survival for stage III disease is 20–30 months, whereas the survival for disease confined to one ovary (stage IA) is over 90%.

Thus, the challenges in ovarian cancer are to increase the proportion of women presenting with early stage disease, which is most likely to be done by an organized screening programme, and to improve the survival of women who still present with late stage disease. This chapter will consider the recent work in screening for ovarian cancer, and then analyse the current work on surgical therapy for stage III disease.

Ovarian cancer screening

There are major problems with the detection of epithelial ovarian cancer. The ovaries are intra-abdominal organs making them relatively inaccessible to direct examination. Unlike cervical cancer, no premalignant stage has yet been identified and the natural history of ovarian cancer is unclear. It is unlikely that benign ovarian cysts progress to become malignant, and indeed the literature supports the fact that removing persistent cysts does not result in a reduction in the incidence of epithelial ovarian cancer. It is even less clear whether borderline cancers lie along a continuum from normal to frank invasion. Knowledge of the molecular events in the progression of ovarian cancer is lacking, so it is difficult to target biological markers which may facilitate early detection.

A suitable screening test must fulfil various criteria. These include the likelihood of a test being positive in patients with the disease (specificity) and the likelihood of a test being negative in patients who do not have the disease (sensitivity). As the specificity of a test is increased, the sensitivity is decreased and vice versa. In ovarian screening, women who test positive will require abdominal surgery, so the specificity needs to be such that the number of unnecessary procedures and consequent operative morbidity are kept to a minimum.

The current candidates for screening for epithelial ovarian cancer are ultrasound scanning (transvaginal ± abdominal) and measurement of the serum biochemical tumour marker CA125, a glycoprotein of unknown function. For ultrasound scanning, abnormal morphology constitutes any cystic ovarian mass with solid or papillary projections. The addition of colour Doppler has been used in an attempt to improve the specificity. CA125 measurements were initially used with a specific cut-off level to define abnormal and normal, but have now been shown to be more sensitive if used serially to include rises in levels occurring below the absolute cut-off level.

Three studies are reviewed here; two involve ultrasound scanning of women, the third differs in its approach as it is based on screening with CA125 initially, with the addition of ultrasound in cases of CA125 elevation.

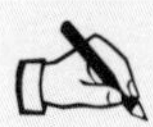

The efficacy of transvaginal sonographic screening in asymptomatic women at risk for ovarian cancer. University of Kentucky Ovarian Cancer Screening Project.

JR van Nagell, PD DePriest, MB Reedy, *et al. Gynaecol Oncol* 2000; **77**: 350–6.

BACKGROUND. The annual prevalence of ovarian cancer is low, with a lifetime risk of 1.4% for a low-risk population. This means that a large number of women need to be included in a trial to detect a single case. Women with a family history of ovarian cancer are at a higher risk. The purpose of this study was to examine the effectiveness and justification of screening for ovarian cancer in a group of asymptomatic high-risk women using transvaginal ultrasound scanning.

INTERPRETATION. A total of 57 214 scans were performed in 14 469 women who were either above 50 years of age or were aged above 25 years and had a family history of ovarian cancer.

Seventeen cancers were detected: 11 stage I, three stage II and three stage III tumours. Eleven of these were epithelial ovarian cancers, three were borderline cancers and three were granulosa cell tumours.

Transvaginal ultrasound screening in this group of high-risk women was associated with a sensitivity of 81%, a specificity of 98.9%, a positive predictive value of 9.4% and a negative predictive value of 99.97%. The overall survival of the patients who were screened annually was $95.0 \pm 4.9\%$ at 2 years and $88.2 \pm 8.0\%$ at 5 years. When only epithelial ovarian cancers were included, the survival decreased to $92.9 \pm 6.9\%$ at 2 years and $83.6 \pm 10.8\%$ at 5 years. This compares with a 5-year survival of 50% in unscreened women ($P = 0.001$).

Comment

Seventy-two per cent of patients were detected at stage I or II, fulfilling one of the criteria for screening (detecting early stage disease). All these patients were alive without evidence of recurrence after a median time of follow-up of 4.5 years after diagnosis.

However, four patients developed stage II or III disease within 12 months of a normal scan. What is not clear is the length of time between the ovaries appearing recognisably abnormal on ultrasound and transabdominal spread of the cancer (stage III). Methods to improve this aspect would be to increase the frequency of scans to every 6 months, or to add a serum marker such as CA125 and incorporate this into a clinical algorithm. However, the authors point out that 78% of the patients with stage I/II disease did not have an elevated CA125 level.

The positive predictive value in this study was low at 9.4%, and was partly due to a high rate of benign ovarian tumours (mainly simple cysts in postmenopausal women) surgically removed. One case of cancer was detected for every 10 operations.

Overall, this study shows that transvaginal scanning can improve the detection of early stage disease, with a likely improvement in survival. Measures need to be taken, however, to improve the sensitivity.

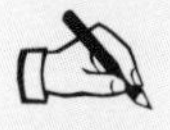

Usefulness of mass screening for ovarian carcinoma using transvaginal ultrasonography.

S Sato, Y Yokoyama, T Sakamoto, M Futagami, Y Saito. *Cancer* 2000; **89**: 582–8.

BACKGROUND. The efficacy of transvaginal ultrasound may be increased by the addition of serum tumour markers. This study evaluated the effectiveness of a secondary screen, after an initial abnormal ultrasound, comprising a repeat scan with measurement of the serum markers CA125, CA19-9, carcinoembryonic antigen, alpha-fetoprotein and lactate dehydrogenase.

INTERPRETATION. A total of 51 550 women presenting for cervical screening underwent ovarian screening with ultrasound. The criteria for an abnormal scan differ to the previous study and constituted an increase in the long axis of the ovary >30 mm rather than ovarian volume. Of the 51 550 women, 5309 (10.3%) had an abnormal scan, and had secondary screening with tumour marker estimation. Of these, 2554 women had persistently abnormal scans and proceeded to diagnostic imaging in the form of computed tomography or magnetic resonance imaging. A total of 324 women underwent laparotomy where 22 primary cancers were diagnosed along with two metastatic cancers. Of the 22 primary tumours, 17 (77.3%) were stage I, a similar rate to the 72% detection of stage I/II tumours in the previous study. Again, 70.6% of these women did not have an elevated tumour marker (cf. 78% in the previous study).

A positive predictive value of 4.9% was obtained using transvaginal scanning and serum markers. A total of 24 tumours were detected in 51 550 women, giving a detection rate of 0.047%. No follow-up data were available, so no comment could be made on survival.

Comment

This study shows that stage I tumours can be detected with ultrasound screening, although 20 operations were performed for each case of cancer (10 per case of cancer in the previous study), which could be attributed to the alternative criteria for an abnormal scan. Tumour markers were elevated in 50% of women. Most of these had late stage disease, so it is unclear therefore what the benefit of additional tumour markers is in this group of women. Criticisms of this study include the lack of a control group and the fact that the women being screened were undergoing cervical screening at the time of the first scan. These women were therefore highly motivated and health conscious, which must introduce great bias in the overall outcome. However, it does show that screening can be beneficial in a low-risk population.

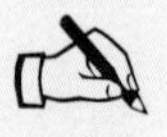

Screening for ovarian cancer: a pilot randomised controlled trial.

IJ Jacobs, SJ Skates, N MacDonald, *et al. Lancet* 1999; **353**: 1207–10.

B A C K G R O U N D . Jacobs *et al.* have previously shown that if elevated CA125 is combined with an abnormal scan finding, these women have an increased risk of ovarian cancer of 327-fold compared with that of the general population. This randomized controlled trial evaluated the feasibility of using a combination of CA125 and ultrasound scanning in screening for ovarian cancer in postmenopausal women. Postmenopausal women were selected as this group has the peak incidence for this disease, and avoids some of the conditions that also elevate CA125, such as endometriosis, fibroids and menstruation.

I N T E R P R E T A T I O N . This prospective study included 22 000 postmenopausal women aged over 45 years who were randomized either to screening (10 997 women) or to follow-up with no screening (10 958 women). The primary screen in this study consisted of serum CA125 measurement rather than an ultrasound scan, unlike the two previous

Five-year survival rates for cervical tumours confined to the cervix are in excess of 90%. However, once the tumour has spread to only one pelvic lymph node group, this figure drops to 60%. The more nodal groups affected, the more the 5-year survival decreases. Radiation is the mainstay of treatment for cervical tumours that have spread outside the cervix. Recent studies have shown that concurrent chemotherapy can increase the efficacy of radiotherapy.

Radical trachelectomy and laparoscopic node dissection

For early invasive cancer of the cervix (IA2–IB1), the standard treatment has been radical hysterectomy and pelvic lymph node dissection in young women and radical pelvic radiotherapy in older women. For young women who are nulliparous, and who present with a small tumour, the need for removal of the uterine corpus has been questioned. A new technique, radical trachelectomy and laparoscopic pelvic node dissection, has been described for small volume, early stage tumours found in younger women who wish to retain their fertility. The cervix is radically excised ensuring surgical clearance, and pelvic lymphadenectomy is performed via a laparoscopic approach. Thus, the uterus and fertility are preserved.

Dargent was the first to use this approach in 1987. Although no large, randomized controlled trials have been undertaken, small, mainly retrospective studies have reported on survival and pregnancy rates.

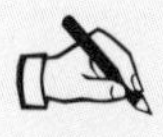

Radical trachelectomy: a way to preserve fertility in the treatment of early cervical cancer.

JH Shepherd, RA Crawford, DH Oram. *Br J Obstet Gynaecol* 1998; **105**(8): 912–6.

BACKGROUND. The extent of radical surgery in the treatment of early stage cervical cancer is being questioned. The treatment of FIGO stage IA (superficially invasive cervical cancer) in the form of a cone biopsy is common practice, and maintains fertility. For stage IIA and IB tumours, radical hysterectomy has been the standard surgical treatment. The radical trachelectomy is a stage between cone biopsy and the radical hysterectomy, and represents conservative surgery, which is nevertheless locally radical, excising the tumour and draining lymph nodes. The procedure of pelvic lymphadenectomy and vaginal radical trachelectomy is a specialized procedure performed in tertiary referral centres. In this paper, the authors describe a modification of the initial procedure performed on women who had been referred for a second opinion in view of their wish to maintain their fertility.

INTERPRETATION. Of the 10 women in this pilot study who underwent a pelvic lymphadenectomy and a vaginal radical trachelectomy, no recurrence was reported, although follow-up was very short (1–35 months). Three women went on to have further treatment as residual tumour was discovered at the resection margins. The inclusion of cervical cerclage resulted in three live births and no late miscarriages in this series of patients.

Comment

This report describes the technique of radical trachelectomy in detail; it differs slightly from the operation as described by Dargent in that the pouch of Douglas is not entered. A permanent cerclage suture was placed at the uterine isthmus (the lowest remaining part of the uterus) to prevent incompetence of the uterine canal. No information on operative time or complications related to surgery was given.

The importance of pelvic lymphadenectomy is demonstrated as three patients were found to have pelvic node involvement, one went on to have adjuvant pelvic radiotherapy and all three were free of recurrent disease at the time of the report. A clear margin of between 5 and 8 mm in the trachelectomy specimen is normally considered adequate; two patients in this series had disease at 1.5 and 5 mm from the resection margins and underwent completion radical hysterectomy.

It is imperative that patients are thoroughly counselled. They must understand that high cure rates are obtained from the standard surgical treatment of radical hysterectomy, and that the cure rates from this new technique are not proven. They must also understand the possible need for further treatment if pelvic lymph node involvement is discovered or if residual disease is seen at the excision margins of the cervical specimen.

This study demonstrates that this procedure, when performed by skilled surgeons in a tertiary referral centre, can result in adequate control of disease whilst enabling women to retain their fertility potential.

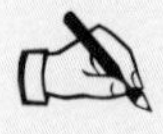

Pregnancies after radical vaginal trachelectomy for early-stage cervical cancer.

M Roy, M Plante. *Am J Obstet Gynecol* 1998; **179**: 1491–6.

BACKGROUND. As the procedure of radical trachelectomy combined with pelvic lymphadenectomy is a comparatively new technique with only few patients, specific criteria have not yet been established to define which patients are eligible. This study evaluated this treatment primarily in terms of fertility potential but also with regard to cure rate.

INTERPRETATION. This study reviewed the authors' experience with their first 30 radical trachelectomy procedures. All women included had no indications of subfertility. All six women who attempted pregnancy succeeded. Four women had healthy live deliveries by caesarean section at 39, 38, 34 and 25 weeks. Two patients at the time of submission of the paper were 8 and 33 weeks pregnant. The recurrence rate was 3.7% (one patient out of 30). She developed a parametrial recurrence 18 months after surgery, but despite pelvic radiation therapy rapidly developed metastatic disease, and died soon after.

Comment

Dargent first described the technique in 1986, and since then only a few centres have taken up this approach because considerable skill is required and it is only appropriate that gynaecological oncologists with expertise in laparoscopic procedures and vaginal surgery should be performing radical trachelectomies. Two such operators are Roy and Plante, and in this paper they described their experience over a 7-year period (1991–1998). Women with early stage invasive cervical cancer who wished to preserve their fertility were offered this procedure. Although the majority of cancers were stage I, two stage IIA cancers were included, with tumours measuring more than 2 cm, and four cases had vascular space invasion. This latter finding is often considered a poor prognostic indicator, and should be treated more aggressively, in some cases with adjuvant radiation therapy.

The one patient who developed recurrence in this series had a stage IIA, 3 cm poorly differentiated squamous cell lesion. Recurrence was diagnosed in the parametrium, with disease initially confined to the pelvis. Despite pelvic radiation therapy, distant metastases in the lung soon developed, and after stopping radiotherapy the disease rapidly progressed and she died. Parametrial recurrences have occurred in other studies, and underlines the importance of wide surgical excision of the tumour. These authors ensured wide excision by only regarding the procedure successful if the upper endocervical margin on the specimen was clear of cancer by at least 8–10 mm. Parametrial recurrence could be considered a trachelectomy failure, but other factors such as size of initial tumour, grade of the lesion and the presence of vascular invasion could pay a role in determining outcome. In retrospect, these authors considered that they should probably not have offered conservative treatment to a patient with such a large tumour. Although definite criteria have not yet been established, it could be suggested that the following are appropriate for a radical trachelectomy:

(i)   desire to retain fertility;

(ii)   stage IA and IB lesions, no larger than 2 cm in size;

(iii) no vascular space involvement.

All six patients who attempted to become pregnant were successful without medical intervention. Patients were advised to wait 6 months before trying to conceive, as this is the time when cervical re-epithelialization has taken place. All patients were delivered by caesarean section because of the cerclage suture; two at term and two after premature labour, at 34 and 25 weeks. In the latter case, it is unclear whether cervical dilatation occurred due to premature labour, or that labour started because of cervical incompetence. The authors recommended more frequent antenatal visits precisely because of the risk of this occurring, with a repeat of the cerclage if the original suture is found to be inadequate.

The median operating time was 285 min. However, this is a new technique, and as expertise improves, so the length of surgery will decrease. More important is the rate of complications, which in this study was not unduly high. Here, four patients (13%) had intra-operative complications, two as a consequence of the laparoscopy and two from the trachelectomy procedure with three of the four requiring a laparotomy. The uterus was preserved in all cases. The median blood loss was 200 ml, with no patients requiring a blood transfusion, and the median hospital stay was 4 days. Interestingly, one patient developed continuous vaginal spotting post-operatively and this was found to be due to persistent granulation tissue caused by the non-absorbable cervical suture.

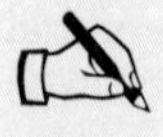

Laparoscopic vaginal radical trachelectomy. A treatment to preserve the fertility of cervical carcinoma patients.
D Dargent, X Martin, A Sacchetoni, P Mathevet. *Cancer* 2000; **88**: 1877–82.

BACKGROUND. Conservative treatment in the form of laparoscopic pelvic lymphadenectomy followed by vaginal radical trachelectomy for early stage carcinoma of the cervix may conceivably carry with it the risk of a higher incidence of recurrence compared with the more aggressive surgical approach. Second, preserving the uterus without the cervix may not enable it to preserve its function of fertility and subsequent full-term live births. This study, representing the experience of the authors over a 10-year period, set out to address these two questions.

INTERPRETATION. Forty-seven patients with stage IA1–IIB were entered into the study. The patients first underwent a laparoscopic lymphadenectomy and if the lymph nodes proved to be free of disease on frozen section, a vaginal radical trachelectomy was then performed. The specimen was also sent for frozen section to confirm that the endocervical margin was clear, otherwise more endocervix would be removed or a total hysterectomy performed. If the embedded specimen later showed poor prognostic features, such as vascular space involvement, then the patients were advised to proceed to a total radical hysterectomy.

The mean duration of the laparoscopic procedure was 62 min and for the vaginal radical trachelectomy was 67 min. After a median follow-up period of 52 months (7–123 months), two patients (4%) developed recurrence. One patient died from disease progression. Despite a 25% rate of late miscarriage, 13 pregnancies resulted in live births.

Comment

Operating times were not prolonged as this centre has much expertise in these surgical techniques. Only one intra-operative (cystotomy) and seven minor postoperative (pelvic collections) complications occurred.

The recurrence rate of 4% (two cases) is comparable with that after open radical hysterectomy. These two patients had large primary tumours (2 cm adenocarcinoma and 2.5 cm squamous carcinoma) with negative pelvic lymph nodes but with vascular space involvement in the specimen. It is well recognized that the frequency of parametrial involvement and distance spread increases with larger tumour size. These recurrences occurred at sites not contiguous with the primary tumours, emphasizing the importance of careful patient selection and wide parametrial resection in each case.

Sixteen patients in this series conceived and 13 were successful in delivering a live child by caesarean section. No cerclage procedure was performed at surgery. In the early part of the series, there was a high late miscarriage rate. This prompted the authors to perform the Saling procedure, first described by Saling in 1981 to prevent miscarriage. This method involves complete obliteration of the cervix at 12–14 weeks of gestation. Consequently, the miscarriage rate in this study decreased to less than 20% compared with 33%, and 11 term deliveries occurred after the Saling procedure was instituted, compared with only two when no form of cervical cerclage was performed. The overall results from this study in terms of survival and term pregnancy rate are very encouraging, and show that this technique is acceptable in a carefully selected, well-informed patient population.

The authors made three stipulations for a successful outcome: first, a stringent pre-operative work-up; second, adequately trained surgeons, competent in both laparoscopic and vaginal oncological surgery; and third, that pathologists give clear information regarding presence or absence of disease near the margins of excision.

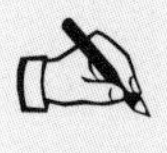

Is radical trachelectomy a safe alternative to radical hysterectomy for patients with stage IA-B carcinoma of the cervix?

A Covens, P Shaw, J Murphy, *et al. Cancer* 1999; **86**: 2273–9.

BACKGROUND. Ideally, the legitimacy of radical trachelectomy for early stage cervical cancer should be tested by a randomized controlled trial. This would be difficult from an ethical viewpoint. Furthermore, as the recurrence rate is small in this group of women (approximately 5%), 300 women would need to be recruited to detect a difference in recurrence rate between the two forms of treatment. As the number of women fulfilling the criteria for trachelectomy is small, it is extremely unlikely that this number of women could be recruited. Evidence of survival has so far been based on small case series. This study aimed to improve the standard of the evidence by a case–controlled trial technique.

INTERPRETATION. This was a prospective study, over 5 years, of the outcome of pelvic lymphadenectomy and radical vaginal trachelectomy. Controls were obtained from the computerized database accrued since 1984 of all radical hysterectomies performed at the University of Toronto. The control groups consisted of patients who underwent radical hysterectomy for stage IA-B cervical carcinoma, with tumours measuring ≤ 2 cm and negative pelvic lymph nodes, the first group having adjuvant radiotherapy and the second group having no adjuvant treatment. The cases were matched for age, tumour size, histology, depth of invasion, capillary lymphatic space involvement and lymph node metastases.

Thirty-two patients who had radical trachelectomy were compared with one group of matched and another group of unmatched controls. The recurrence rates were 5, 0 and 3% at 2 years, respectively. The actuarial conception rate at 12 months was 37%.

Comment

The tumour-free resection margin was 5 mm in this report, compared with 8–10 mm in the Roy and Plante report. Even though this study restricted radical trachelectomy to just stage IA-B lesions, one patient developed recurrence (a rate of 5%, in line with other studies). She had an adenocarcinoma with capillary lymphatic space involvement and developed parametrial recurrence 13 months after diagnosis, which did not respond to pelvic radiotherapy. The authors doubted that she would have had a more favourable outcome with a radical hysterectomy, as similar amounts of parametrial tissue are removed in the two procedures. As almost half of their patients with cervical cancer were found to have capillary lymphatic space involvement, the authors felt that this factor, in the absence of other poor prognostic indicators, should not in itself exclude patients from this procedure. Making the criteria too stringent may deny the technique to women who have small and highly curable cancers. It is encouraging that in all series no recurrence has been found in either the cervical stump or the uterus. So essentially Covens *et al.* were very much in favour of this technique for women determined to retain fertility who may have one risk factor for recurrence, where the alternative treatments would not allow child bearing.

Operative time was longer for the trachelectomy group, but conversely blood loss and incidence of blood transfusions were much less. The complication rate was relatively high at 25%. This was accounted for mainly by six cystotomies which were easily repaired with no long-term sequelae. Again this demonstrates the higher than normal complication rate with a new technique.

The 12-month fertility rate was 37%. This is lower than in the Roy and Plante study because women with known subfertility were included. Three patients had anovulation which corrected with medical treatment and pregnancies were achieved. Even though women may not have evidence of infertility, Covens *et al.* point to various factors associated with the radical trachelectomy procedure itself which may compromise fertility. These include subclinical salpingitis as a consequence of sexually transmitted diseases, which may be higher in women with cervical cancer compared with the general population, postoperative adhesions, cervical stenosis, damage to uterine arteries compromising uterine blood flow and the uncertain role of cervical mucus.

In summary, this study confirms findings from other series showing that radical trachelectomy is an acceptable procedure for early stage cervical cancer for women who wish to preserve fertility.

Table 10.1 summarizes the results of the studies on radical trachelectomy.

Summary

The approach to treatment of early stage cervical cancer is changing. A more conservative surgical approach is being considered. Combined laparoscopic lymphadenectomy and a radical vaginal trachelectomy is a feasible approach to treat early stage cervical carcinoma with a view to cure. Operative morbidity and recovery

Table 10.1 Summary of studies on radical trachelectomy

Study	No. of women	Stage	Recurrence rate (%)	Operative time (minutes)	Operative complications (%)	No. of live births
Dargent *et al.*	47	IA–IIB	4	129	11	13
Shepherd *et al.*	10	N/A	0	N/A	N/A	3
Roy and Plante	30	IA–IIA	3	285	13	4
Covens *et al.*	32	IA–B	5	180	25	5

Source: Covens *et al.* (1999).

time are low, and women who wish to preserve their fertility have a reasonable chance of delivering a live child. Importantly, conservative treatment must not compromise long-term survival. These studies have demonstrated that recurrence rates are not increased. Recurrence rates were approximately 4%, comparable with those with radical hysterectomy. It is imperative that surgeons are skilled in laparoscopic and vaginal surgery.

Concurrent chemoradiation for later stage cervical cancer

The mainstay of treatment for stages IB2 to IVA has been intracavity and external beam radiotherapy, giving an overall 5-year survival of approximately 65%; 70% for stage IB2–IIB, 50% for stage IIIA, 30% for stage IIIB and 15% for stage IVA. If recurrence occurs, disease is found in the pelvis in between 35 and 90% of cases. Therefore, locoregional control is important. The dose of radiotherapy that can be given to the pelvis is, however, limited by the toxicity to normal tissue and severe late complications of high-dose radiation. Therefore, strategies have been sought to improve outcome by the addition of adjuvant treatments.

The most effective strategy has been to combine radiotherapy with chemotherapy. It has been suggested that these two modalities act in a synergistic manner by (a) inhibiting the repair of lethal damage caused by radiation, (b) inducing proliferation in cells which are not proliferating, (c) synchronizing cells into a radiation-sensitive phase of the cell cycle and (d) reducing the number of hypoxic cells which are resistant to radiation.

Furthermore, concurrent treatment ensures that the overall treatment time is kept as short as possible thereby minimizing repopulation of tumour cells. Retrospective studies have clearly shown that local control of tumour and long-term survival are diminished with increased length of treatment time. An acceptable duration of therapy would be less than 55 days in general.

The overall effect is for chemotherapy to act as a radiosensitizer and to destroy distant micrometastases. This would have the added advantage of reducing the distant spread of disease in women with pelvic or para-aortic lymph node involvement.

Chemotherapeutic agents investigated include hydroxyurea, mitomycin, fluorouracil and cisplatin. Whilst the aim of combining different treatment modalities is to improve survival, patients will experience adverse effects from each type of therapy. The challenge is therefore to devise a regimen giving an increased survival advantage without causing substantial toxicity.

Three prospective randomized controlled trials are reviewed here: two by GOG, GOG 120 and GOG 123, and one by the Radiation Therapy Oncology Group, RTOG 9001.

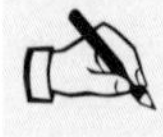

Concurrent cisplatin-based radiotherapy and chemotherapy for locally advanced cervical cancer. Gynecologic Oncology Group 120 trial.

PG Rose, BN Bundy, EB Watkins, *et al. New Engl J Med* 1999; **340**: 1144–53.

BACKGROUND. The ability of radiotherapy to cure locally advanced cervical cancer is limited by the size of the tumour, because the doses required to treat large tumours exceed the limit of toxicity in normal tissue. Severe complications occur in approximately 5–10% of women after radical pelvic radiotherapy, mostly to the small bowel, rectum and bladder. This damage can substantially reduce quality of life. The addition of chemotherapy can theoretically increase the efficacy of treatment without increasing the overall dose of radiotherapy. Hydroxyurea has been shown to increase the rate of complete response, progression-free survival and overall survival. Myelosuppression is a limiting toxic effect of treatment with hydroxyurea. Thus, cisplatin, which is less myelotoxic and can be given weekly during the radiotherapy with acceptable levels of toxicity, was included in the trial.

INTERPRETATION. In this study, 526 women with stage IIB, III or IVA cervical cancer without para-aortic lymph node involvement were randomized. Almost 50% of the patients in this study had either pelvic wall involvement (stage IIIB) or involvement of the bladder (stage IVA).

There were three treatment arms; single agent cisplatin (40 mg/m^2 weekly for 6 weeks); a three-drug combination of cisplatin (50 mg/m^2 on days 1 and 29) followed by fluorouracil (4 g/m^2 over 96 h on days 1 and 29) and oral hydroxyurea (2 g/m^2 twice weekly for 6 weeks); oral hydroxyurea (3 g/m^2 twice weekly for 6 weeks). The latter group was used as the control arm in line with GOG practice.

The dose of radiation was 80.8–81 Gy to point A, with a median duration of treatment of 63 days.

Toxicity in terms of grade 3 (moderate) and grade 4 (severe) adverse haematological effects was twice as high in the three-drug combination (group 2) as compared with the other two groups ($P < 0.001$). However, there was no mention of late complications due to the radiation therapy, which are often severe, permanent and disabling.

The addition of chemotherapy in the form of single agent cisplatin (group 1) or the combination of cisplatin, fluorouracil and hydroxyurea (group 2) to radiation treatment increased the progression-free survival rates at 24 months significantly (67 and 64%, respectively) as compared with group 3 which received hydroxyurea and radiotherapy (47%)($P < 0.001$ for both comparisons). The relative risks of disease progression or death were 0.57 for group 1 and 0.55 for group 2, as compared with group 3. Patients in groups 1 and 2 had a lower incidence of local progression (19 and 20%, respectively) than group 3 (30%), and a lower frequency of lung metastases (3% in group 1, 4% in group 2 and 10% in group 3). Toxicity was least with single agent cisplatin.

Comment

Chemoradiation with either cisplatin alone or a combination containing this agent is clearly effective in increasing survival in this poor prognostic group. Hydroxyurea was shown to give a worse outcome in terms of survival, progression of pelvic disease and incidence of distant metastases. Early randomized studies investigating the effectiveness of hydroxyurea in combination with radiotherapy found an increased response rate, longer median progression-free interval and survival. The GOG 56 trial randomized patients to receive either radiotherapy and hydroxyurea or radiotherapy with misonidazole, a hypoxic cell sensitizer. Survival between the two groups was not statistically different. A subsequent trial (RTOG 80-05) compared radiation therapy alone with the combination of radiotherapy and misonidazole. The latter group had a similar or slightly worse outcome than the radiotherapy-only group. This led to the concern that the observed benefit of hydroxyurea in the GOG 56 trial was due to the comparison with the misonidazole group, as there was no control group receiving only conventional radiotherapy. The added fact that survival with hydroxyurea is worse, makes the use of this drug in the treatment of cervical cancer questionable, if not obsolete.

Criticisms of this study include the absence of a control arm consisting of patients treated with radiotherapy only, and that the length of time of radiation treatment was prolonged (median 63 days). Retrospective studies have shown that increased treatment duration can result in decreased efficacy of local tumour control and survival. What was clearly shown, was that the combination of radiotherapy and single agent cisplatin was superior in the treatment of late stage cervical cancer and also had a lower incidence of acute toxicity than the multiple agent chemotherapy regimen and hydroxyurea.

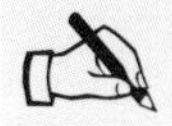

Cisplatin, radiation and adjuvant hysterectomy compared with radiation and adjuvant hysterectomy for bulky stage IB cervical carcinoma. Gynecologic Oncology Group 123 trial.

HM Keys, BN Bundy, FB Stehman, *et al. New Engl J Med* 1999; **340**: 1154–61.

BACKGROUND. **Although early stage cervical cancer has a good outcome, bulky stage IB tumours have a worse prognosis. The objective of this study was to determine whether concurrent radiotherapy and cisplatin, as weekly infusions, improved the progression-free survival and overall survival over radiotherapy alone. As the GOG 120 trial showed, cisplatin is effective when used with radiotherapy in improving survival in**

women with advanced stage (IIB–IVA) cervical cancer. This study examined the benefit of this treatment regimen in women with less advanced disease (stage IB) who nevertheless may develop local recurrence or, more rarely, distant metastases.

INTERPRETATION. In this study, 369 women were randomized to receive either concurrent single agent cisplatin (40 mg/m^2 weekly for 6 weeks) and radiotherapy, or radiotherapy alone. The median duration of treatment was 50 days.

This study differed to the GOG 120 trial in that a control group receiving only radiotherapy was used. The median duration of follow-up was 36 months in over half the patients.

Survival at the end of this period was 74% in the radiation-only group and 83% in the group receiving radiation therapy and cisplatin ($P = 0.008$). The rate of progression-free survival was significantly higher in the patients receiving chemoradiation ($P = 0.001$). The relative risks of progression of disease and death in the combined chemoradiation group were 0.51 and 0.54, respectively, as compared with the radiotherapy alone group. Acute toxicity was more marked in the combination group (35% compared with 13%).

Comment

The total dose of radiation to point A was 75 Gy, lower than in the Rose *et al.* study, because all patients proceeded to an extrafascial hysterectomy 3–6 weeks after completion of radiotherapy. This radiation dose would be thought suboptimal by many clinicians. Surgery was undertaken because previous studies have shown higher rates of pelvic recurrence after radiotherapy alone for treatment of stage IB tumours. However, a subsequent GOG study assessing the value of a completion hysterectomy after radiotherapy found that while there was a significant reduction in the rate of local recurrence, the overall risk of recurrence was not reduced by hysterectomy and there was no significant difference in survival. This led Keys *et al.* to conclude that the combination of cisplatin and radiotherapy was adequate treatment for stage IB cancers.

This study confirms the findings in the Rose *et al.* trial that cisplatin is effective in combination with radiotherapy in the treatment of cervical cancer. A lively debate continues as to the best form of treatment of stage IB cancers between radical surgery and radiotherapy. This is often influenced by the availability of specialties, the age of the patient and perceived toxicities. Thirty-five per cent of patients receiving cisplatin and radiation therapy in this study experienced grade 3 or 4 adverse effects, mainly haematological or gastrointestinal. The addition of chemotherapy obviously leads to the patient experiencing side-effects from both treatment modalities, and the optimum level of each still needs to be refined.

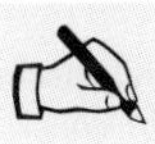

Pelvic radiation with concurrent chemotherapy compared with pelvic and para-aortic radiation for high-risk cervical cancer: a randomised Radiation Therapy Oncology Group clinical trial.

M Morris, PJ Eifel, J Lu, *et al. New Engl J Med* 1999; **340**: 1137–43.

BACKGROUND. **A previous study had reported increased survival among women with locally advanced cervical cancer who received prophylactic radiation to the para-aortic nodes as well as traditional radical pelvic radiotherapy. This trial studied this as the control arm against concurrent chemoradiation, in an attempt to evaluate the ability of chemotherapy to improve local control and eradicate distant micrometastases.**

INTERPRETATION. Women with disease ranging from stage IIB through to stage IVA, or stage IB or IIA with a tumour diameter of at least 5 cm, or with pelvic lymph node involvement were eligible. A total of 388 patients were randomized to receive either radiotherapy to the pelvic and para-aortic lymph nodes, or concurrent radiotherapy to the pelvis and cisplatin (75 mg/m^2 over 4 h) followed by fluorouracil (4 g/m^2 over 96 h) from days 1 to 5. The total dose of radiation was the highest of all three studies, with a median dose of 85 Gy to point A and a median length of treatment of 58 days.

Five-year survival was 73% for patients receiving radiotherapy with cisplatin and fluorouracil compared with 58% for the radiation-only group ($P = 0.004$). Sixty-seven per cent of the combined treatment group were free of disease at 5 years compared with 40% of patients treated with radiotherapy alone ($P = 0.001$). There were lower rates of both local pelvic recurrence ($P < 0.001$) and distant metastases ($P < 0.001$) in the combined group. Toxicity was similar in the two groups.

Comment

Studies have demonstrated that local tumour control is proportional to the total dose of radiation. This study confirms the findings of both GOG trials that survival with a combination of pelvic radiotherapy and cisplatin-based chemotherapy is superior to extended-field radiotherapy in the treatment of advanced cervical cancer. The rate of local recurrence in the radiotherapy-only group was 33% compared with 13% for the combination therapy group ($P < 0.001$). Similarly, the rate for distant metastases was less for the chemoradiation group (19% versus 35% for the radiotherapy-only group, $P < 0.001$).

The dose of cisplatin was almost double that in the two previous studies, but fewer cycles were given, so the cumulative dose was similar. Although grade 3 and 4 haematological effects were frequent with the chemotherapy group, these were acute and reversible. As the follow-up was longer for this group of patients, late complications of radiotherapy were reported, which may be expected to be significant as this study utilized the highest radiation dose of the three studies. The most common were grade 3 and 4 bowel complications, but these occurred in less than 1% of patients, with similar rates in both treatment arms. This demonstrates that

Table 10.2 Summary of trials in concurrent chemoradiation in cervical carcinoma

Trial	No. of women	Stage	Control group	Comparison group	Reduction in RR of death
GOG 120	526	IIB–IVA	RT + hydroxyurea	RT + cisplatin or RT + cisplatin, 5FU, hydroxyurea	0.61
GOG 123	369	Bulky IB	RT	RT + cisplatin	0.54
RTOG	388	IIB–IVA or IB/IIA >5 cm or positive pelvic nodes	Extended-field RT	RT + cisplatin	0.52

RR = relative risk; RT = radiotherapy; 5FU = 5-fluorouracil.
Source: Morris *et al.* (1999).

this radiation dose is well tolerated even when used in conjunction with cytotoxic therapy. Table 10.2 summarizes the results of trials in concurrent chemoradiation in cervical carcinoma.

Summary

Initial phase I/II trials showed promising results using chemotherapy as an adjunct to radiotherapy, although they were criticized as they lacked a control group. As radiotherapy alone gives such good response rates, it was necessary to conduct these formal phase III trials in order to establish whether the combination of chemotherapy and radiation therapy would be superior to radiotherapy alone. The major problem with advanced local cervical cancer is pelvic recurrence. Although radiotherapy doses are increased proportional to tumour size, there is an absolute maximum level due to the amount normal tissues are able to withstand in order for long-term toxicity to be avoided. Therefore it is advantageous to add another treatment modality to increase the effectiveness of treatment. These studies demonstrated an increased survival with chemoradiation incorporating a cisplatin-containing regimen, with toxicity being moderate and generally well tolerated. Chemotherapy has the added advantage of reducing distant metastases.

Conclusion

The mortality from ovarian cancer has been unchanged over recent years. Thus, the prospect of ovarian cancer screening is very attractive. Trials into ultrasound and CA125 screening techniques have advanced enough to justify a randomized trial, UKCTOCS, which should determine the potential effectiveness of a screening programme. Meanwhile efforts continue to improve the treatment for stage III ovarian cancer. In the absence of major new breakthroughs in ovarian chemotherapy, the best surgical strategies continue to be explored. Interval debulking has been reported to improve survival and this may lead to primary chemotherapy and interval surgery in more advanced cases.

Radical trachelectomy offers the hope of fertility for young women with small early stage cervical cancer. The treatment of late stage cervical cancer has been reported to be significantly improved by the addition of concurrent chemotherapy to radiotherapy.

The increasing complexity of differing options in gynaecological malignancies has led to recent national cancer guidelines from the National Health Service Executive, stating that all cases of ovarian cancer and all cases of cervical cancer above stage IA2 should be treated in dedicated gynaecological cancer centres. It is hoped that this concentration of clinical work will lead to improved entry of women into clinical trials. Randomized trials will hopefully be the means to improve the efficacy of treatments in the future.

11

Infertility

Introduction

Reproductive technology moves on apace. The development of in vitro fertilization (IVF) remains the biggest milestone in the field of fertility treatment, but this opened the gates to many further advances. There is an exponential increase in the published literature in this field and it is a difficult task to select the key papers for discussion.

Diagnosis comes before treatment, and laparoscopy is widely regarded as the gold standard in assessment of the uterus and Fallopian tubes. There is currently great interest in less invasive 'office procedures' and 'one-stop' investigations. Two papers have been selected which present new methods of assessing the uterine cavity and pelvis.

Laparoscopy is increasingly used for treatment as well as diagnosis, and 'minimally invasive surgery' conducted endoscopically has almost replaced traditional open surgery in reproductive medicine. The treatment of endometriosis, pelvic adhesions and adnexal pathology is particularly suited to laparoscopic surgery. Even procedures such as myomectomy and reversal of sterilization may be conducted laparoscopically, although they require appropriate training and high levels of skill. Endometriosis remains a controversial area and is discussed below.

IVF is now commonplace, with more than 20 000 cycles conducted in the UK each year (and the number continues to grow annually). Attention has recently been focused on the risks of IVF to the children born of it. By far the greatest risk of mortality and morbidity in these pregnancies is the outcome of multiple birth, and three papers are presented which recommend restriction of numbers of embryos transferred to prevent multiple pregnancy.

Intrauterine insemination (IUI) is a simpler technique than IVF and deserves consideration because it can offer acceptable pregnancy rates with very little risk. Because the treatment is less demanding, it can be repeated to yield a cumulative pregnancy rate that may rival IVF. Multiple pregnancy remains a concern here too. The publications presented here on IUI lead into a discussion of cost-effectiveness of treatment. Cost is often the determining factor in patients' access to fertility treatment. Cost-effectiveness analysis is surprisingly uncommon, even in a publicly funded health system.

Finally, for the future there are great hopes that cryopreservation may enable us to store oocytes and ovarian tissue as easily as we can now bank sperm. This will be gratefully received by young patients with cancer, who are now surviving in increasing numbers, but often face sterility as a result of chemotherapy or radiotherapy. Oocyte or ovarian cryopreservation also raises the possibility that women will overcome the biological barrier of ovarian ageing by storing gametes for later use.

New diagnostic techniques—uterine assessment

The hysterosalpingogram is the traditional method of assessment of tubal patency. However, the value of the hysterosalpingogram in assessment of the uterine cavity is often overlooked. Uterine abnormalities may be the underlying cause of infertility in up to 15% of cases. The success of IVF treatment depends on implantation of the embryo into the endometrium and the integrity of the uterine cavity is vital. The presence of an abnormal uterine cavity can be found in approximately 34–62% of infertile women and therefore evaluation of the uterine cavity is an integral part of infertility management.

The hysterosalpingogram remains the most commonly used diagnostic technique for evaluation of the uterine cavity. Once pathology has been identified, further assessment and treatment is carried out with operative hysteroscopy under general anaesthesia. Newer out-patient procedures are: (a) hysteroscopy with saline distension and direct visualization of the uterine cavity and (b) hysterosonography which utilizes fluid distension of the cavity visualized by vaginal ultrasonography.

Evaluation of outpatient hysteroscopy, saline infusion hysterosonography and hysterosalpingography in infertile women: a prospective, randomised study.

S Brown, C Coddington, J Schnorr, J Toner, W Gibbons, S Oehninger.
Fertil Steril 2000; **74**: 1029–34.

BACKGROUND. Three out-patient procedures can be used to perform uterine cavity assessment: hysterosalpingography, hysteroscopy and hysterosonography. This prospective randomized study compared the diagnostic accuracy, pain scores and procedure length in women undergoing these investigations.

A total of 46 patients were included in this study and randomly assigned to each of the three out-patient procedures. For women identified with a uterine abnormality, an operative hysteroscopy was performed under general anaesthesia. The mean age of the patients was 34.1 years, the mean body mass index was 27.8 kg/m^2 and the mean duration of infertility was 4.8 years. All but four of the women completed all three investigations.

INTERPRETATION. Twenty-five (59%) of the women were found to have an abnormal result on at least one of the three out-patient uterine evaluations and 17 women had a normal uterine cavity after all three tests. No difference was found in the detection rate

INTERPRETATION. The chances of a live birth among women undergoing IVF were related to the number of eggs fertilized and thus the number of embryos available for transfer. When more than four embryos were fertilized and available, transfer of only two embryos did not reduce the woman's chance of becoming pregnant, but it did reduce her chance of multiple pregnancy. This was true for women of all ages, including those of around 40 years.

Comment

Older age, tubal infertility, longer duration of infertility and a higher number of previous attempts at IVF were all associated with a significantly decreased chance of a birth and of multiple births. Previous live birth was associated with an increased chance of a birth but not multiple births.

The higher the number of eggs fertilized, the higher the likelihood of a live birth. When more than four eggs were fertilized, there was no increase in the birth rate for women receiving three transferred embryos compared with those receiving two, but there was a considerable increase in the rate of multiple births when three were transferred (odds ratio 1.6; 95% CI 1.5–1.8). Table 11.1 shows the factors affecting the results of IVF.

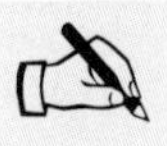

External validation of the Templeton model for predicting success after IVF.

JM Smeenk, AM Stolwijk, JA Kremer, DD Braat. *Hum Reprod* 2000; **15**: 1065–8.

BACKGROUND. The aim of this study was to validate externally the model presented by Templeton. Data were used from the University Hospital, Nijmegen, the Netherlands from March 1991 to January 1999. The data of 1253 couples and 2674 IVF cycles were used in the validation.

INTERPRETATION. The Templeton model was able to identify the women with a low chance and the women with a high chance of achieving a live birth, but it is not applicable or usable in daily clinical practice, because the model did not give more information about the prognosis for the vast majority of the patients.

Comment

Assisted reproduction is more and more concerned with making choices from seemingly unlimited options. As a part of the decision-making for each individual, the physical, psychological, as well as the financial costs should be weighed against the probability of success. Prognostic models can help predict the chance of a live birth objectively, although it is practically impossible to predict accurately the individual chance of a live birth for an individual couple.

The development of a better model may be possible by increasing the predictive value by including other promising predictive factors such as basal follicle stimulating hormone (FSH), day 3 oestradiol or inhibin rather than age alone.

Table 11.1 Factors affecting the results of in vitro fertilization (IVF)

Variable	Odds of a birth (95% CI)	*P* value	Odds of multiple births (95% CI)	*P* value
Maternal factors				
Age (per additional year)	0.9 (0.9–1.0)	<0.001	0.97 (0.95–0.99)	0.013
Tubal infertility (versus no tubal infertility)	0.7 (0.7–0.8)	<0.001	0.8 (0.7–0.9)	<0.001
Number of previous attempts at IVF (versus none)				
1–3	0.8 (0.8–0.9)	<0.001	1.0 (0.9–1.1)	0.85
4 or more	0.6 (0.5–0.7)	<0.001	0.6 (0.4–0.8)	<0.001
Duration of infertility (per additional year)	0.98 (0.98–0.99)	<0.001	0.98 (0.97–0.99)	0.02
Previous live birth (versus none)				
Not IVF	1.1 (1.0–1.2)	<0.001	Not included in model	
IVF	1.6 (1.4–1.8)	<0.001	Not included in model	
Number of eggs fertilized and embryos transferred				
2 eggs, 2 embryos	0.5 (0.4–0.5)	<0.001	0.5 (0.4–0.7)	<0.001
3 or 4 eggs, 2 embryos	0.6 (0.5–0.7)	<0.001	0.7 (0.6–0.9)	0.008
3 or 4 eggs, 3 embryos	0.7 (0.7–0.8)	<0.001	1.3 (1.1–1.4)	0.008
>4 eggs, 2 embryos	1.01 (0.9–1.1)	–	1.0 (0.9–1.1)	–
>4 eggs, 3 embryos	1.0 (0.9–1.1)	0.78	1.6 (1.5–1.8)	<0.001

CI = confidence interval.

Source: Templeton *et al.* (1998).

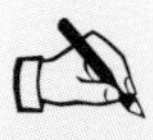

Elective transfer of one embryo results in an acceptable pregnancy rate and eliminates the risk of multiple birth.

S Vilska, A Tiitinene, C Hyden-Granskog, O Hovatta. *Hum Reprod* 1999; **14**: 2392–5.

BACKGROUND. Pregnancy results among 74 elective one-embryo transfers were compared with 94 transfers where only one embryo was available. All the fresh embryo cycles during 1997 in two clinics in Helsinki were analysed and cumulative pregnancy rates among these couples after frozen–thawed embryo transfers up to June 1998 were counted.

INTERPRETATION. Where at least two embryos were available for transfer and elective one-embryo transfer was carried out on day 2 or 3, the pregnancy rate per embryo transfer was 29.7%. Where only one embryo was available for transfer, the pregnancy rate per embryo transfer was 20.2%. During the same period, 742 two-embryo transfers were carried out. The pregnancy rate per embryo transfer was 29.4%, but 23.9% of the pregnancies were twins.

If only one embryo was available the pregnancy rate did not relate to the age of the woman (20.4% in women younger than 35 years and 20.0% in women older than 35 years). Young women from whom only one embryo can be obtained appear to be in a group with an overall poor prognosis. In elective one-embryo transfers, the pregnancy rate was higher in women younger than 36 years (32.8%). For older women the figure was 18.8%.

The implantation rates, as well as the pregnancy rates, were highest when the embryos were transferred at the four to five cell stage on day 2 (35.8% versus 9.7% compared with the two to three cell stage; $P < 0.001$) or at the six to eight cell stage on day 3 (45.5%). The pregnancy rate per embryo transfer was higher when a grade 1 or 2 embryo was transferred compared with a grade 3 embryo (34.0 and 26.7% versus 8.8%, respectively, $P < 0.05$). No pregnancies were achieved with transfer of grade 4 embryos.

Blastocyst transfer has been suggested as a means of facilitating higher pregnancy rates when the number of embryos is limited. The implantation rate of 35.8% achieved when day 2 embryos at the four cell stage are transferred suggests that it may not be necessary to culture embryos to the blastocyst stage in order to obtain acceptable implantation rates. A delay from 48 to 72 h after oocyte retrieval improved the clinical outcome with an implantation rate of 45.5% when six to eight cell embryos were transferred on day 3.

Embryo transfer of cryopreserved and thawed embryos resulted in pregnancy rates of 14.3% per single frozen–thawed embryo transfer and 17.9% per double frozen–thawed embryo transfer. After transfers of two frozen–thawed embryos, two of seven pregnancies were twins. Elective one-embryo transfer should be considered in selected cases for frozen–thawed as well as fresh embryo transfer.

Comment

On the basis of these results, elective one-embryo transfer can be highly recommended, at least in women who are younger than 35 years of age, and who have grade 1 or 2 embryos available for transfer.

IUI

IUI with prepared semen samples in conjunction with ovarian stimulation is a relatively simple assisted reproductive technique, and inexpensive compared with IVF. It may be the first-line treatment of choice for most cases of subfertility in women with patent tubes.

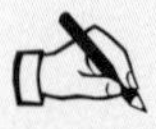

Intrauterine insemination treatment in subfertility: an analysis of factors affecting outcome.

S Nuojua-Huttunen, C Tomas, R Bloigu, L Tuomivaara, II Martikainen.
Hum Reprod 1999; **14**: 698–703.

BACKGROUND. IUI with ovarian stimulation carries reported pregnancy rates per cycle of between 8 and 22%. This retrospective study examined the variables contributing to success of treatment. A total of 831 treatment cycles were performed between January 1992 and December 1996, using a clomiphene citrate/human menopausal gonadotrophin (HMG) stimulation protocol in conjunction with a standard IUI technique with the partner's spermatozoa. Ovarian stimulation involved the use of clomiphene citrate 50 or 100 mg for days 3–7 of the menstrual cycle followed by HMG 75–150 IU daily until human chorionic gonadotrophin (hCG) was administered when at least one dominant follicle was greater than 16 mm diameter. IUI was performed 36 h after hCG administration.

INTERPRETATION. All couples studied had at least 1 year of infertility, median duration 3 (range 1–15) years. The median female age at the time of treatment was 32 (range 20–46) years. The causes of infertility included: unexplained (51%), male factor (28%), minimal (stage I) to mild (stage II) endometriosis (17%) and ovulatory disorders excluding polycystic ovarian syndrome (4%).

The average pregnancy rate per cycle was 12.6%. Of the 102 pregnancies, 70.6% were viable, 23.5% resulted in spontaneous miscarriage and 5% were ectopic. The multiple pregnancy rate was 13.7%, with 12 pairs of twins and two sets of triplets.

Five variables were identified as predictive of treatment success:

- duration of infertility less than 6 years;
- female age less than 40 years;
- treatment cycle number (97% of pregnancies occurred in the first four cycles);
- number of pre-ovulatory follicles (the highest pregnancy rate was seen in those cycles with three follicles); and
- aetiology of infertility (endometriosis conferred a significantly lower pregnancy rate per cycle).

Comment

The outcome of ovarian stimulation and IUI makes it a useful and cost-effective treatment for subfertile couples with a range of diagnoses. It should be considered a first-line treatment option in women less than 40 years of age with a duration of infertility of less than 6 years and who do not suffer from endometriosis. Courses of treatment should not be continued beyond four cycles.

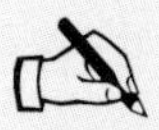

Efficacy of double intrauterine insemination in controlled ovarian hyperstimulation cycles.

G Ragni, P Maggioni, E Guermandi, *et al. Fertil Steril* 1999; **72**: 619–22.

BACKGROUND. IUI is commonly used in the treatment of moderate male factor and unexplained infertility. It is often combined with controlled ovarian hyperstimulation with a significant improvement in pregnancy rate. It is unclear, however, whether 'double IUI' (two timed treatment procedures) confers any benefit compared with standard IUI. This study compared standard single peri-ovulatory IUI with two regimens of 'double IUI' performed at different times around ovulation.

This prospective randomized study included 273 patients (112 patients with male factor infertility and 161 patients with unexplained infertility of at least 24 months' duration). In total, the patients underwent 449 treatment cycles with clomiphene citrate and gonadotrophins. Each patient was randomly assigned to one of three groups. Group A, 90 patients (156 cycles), underwent a single IUI 34 h after hCG administration; group B, 92 patients (144 cycles), underwent a double IUI 12 and 34 h after hCG administration; and group C, 91 patients (149 cycles), underwent a double IUI 34 and 60 h after hCG administration.

INTERPRETATION. There were no statistically significant differences among the three groups with respect to patient age, mean number of follicles >15 mm diameter on the day of hCG administration or the mean number of motile sperm inseminated.

The overall pregnancy rate was 18.7% per patient and 11.3% per cycle. The pregnancy rates for each group were as follows: group A, 14.4% per patient and 8.3% per cycle; group B, 30.4% per patient and 19.4% per cycle; and group C, 10.9% per patient and 6.7% per cycle. There was a statistically significant difference ($P < 0.05$) between groups A and B and a statistically significant difference ($P < 0.01$) between groups B and C.

Comment

This study supports the hypothesis that 'double IUI' is more effective than a single procedure. Timing of IUI treatment is important and it appears that delayed IUI reduces pregnancy rates. Consecutive IUIs performed 12 and 34 h after hCG administration is the most effective treatment regimen.

Cost-effective fertility treatment

The validity of spending health service money on fertility treatment has been questioned; subfertile couples are not ill, and in a cash-limited public health system in Great Britain it is not surprising that fertility treatment receives a low priority. It is difficult to assess the 'value' of fertility treatment compared with other medical procedures. To a childless couple, the birth of their much-wanted baby is priceless, but how does it compare with the benefit to an elderly person regaining mobility after a hip replacement operation or a 50-year-old returning to work after a coronary bypass graft? These are sometimes measured in quality of life years, but fertility treatment cannot be measured in this way—perhaps the potential life of a child should be 'virtual' quality of life years!

It is much more straightforward to compare the value of different fertility treatments in terms of their outcome and their relative costs. Outcome should be defined as the likelihood of a live birth; success rates may be quoted as pregnancy rates on the basis of positive pregnancy tests, but these need to be confirmed by ultrasound (clinical pregnancy rate) and pregnancy outcome (live birth rate). It is then possible to calculate, for each type of treatment, the financial cost to achieve a birth. This analysis of 'cost-effectiveness' may be used by policy-makers and purchasers of health care to determine the best use of their resources.

It must be remembered that this comparison may not take account of risks or complications of treatment. Multiple pregnancies are likely to deliver prematurely and preterm babies require neonatal care with the risk of death or handicap |7, 9|. Thus, fertility treatment carries substantial additional costs in terms of perinatal care.

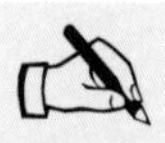

Cost-effective treatment of the infertile couple.

BJ Van Voorhis, DW Stovall, BD Allen, CH Syrop. *Fertil Steril* 1998; **70**: 995–1005.

BACKGROUND. **The literature on the economics and cost-effectiveness of fertility treatment was reviewed. Studies were identified through MEDLINE searching.**

INTERPRETATION. In the absence of tubal blockage and severe male factor, the use of IUI and super-ovulation with IUI was more cost-effective than IVF. IVF was at least as cost-effective as tubal surgery.

Comment

Few studies on the cost-effectiveness of fertility treatment have been published. This review indicates that relatively simple treatment with IUI, and IUI with fertility drug stimulation, is more cost-effective than IVF for a substantial group of patients who have 'unexplained infertility' or a mild reduction in semen quality. These conclusions are encouraging for the many couples who are reluctant to undergo the complex procedures involved in IVF, and for those who cannot afford or are not government funded for IVF.

For women with Fallopian tube blockage, IUI is not an option, and in the past most patients would have been treated with tubal surgery. There is now a trend towards IVF for all but the mildest cases of tubal damage. This is supported by this review, which shows that IVF is at least as cost-effective as tubal surgery. This should be noted by organizations involved in purchasing health care. In the USA, insurance plans may exclude IVF but allow tubal surgery, and this has been shown to result in social and ethnic differences in access to treatment, with more white women of high socio-economic status able to self-fund IVF treatment and a higher proportion of African-American and Hispanic women undergoing tubal surgery |10|; a substantial proportion of the American population is denied access to specialist fertility services |11|. In the UK, within the National Health Service, in most areas there is no restriction on tubal surgery because this falls within the funding arrangements for gynaecological surgery, whereas IVF funding is severely restricted. The imbalance in funding should be reconsidered in light of this review.

Successful tubal surgery may allow the patient to achieve several pregnancies following one procedure, greatly increasing its cost-effectiveness. Cryopreservation of 'spare' embryos following IVF, with subsequent replacement in a natural or supplemented menstrual cycle, increases the effectiveness of IVF (additional pregnancies per cycle initiated).

The comparison between the cost-effectiveness of IVF and tubal surgery can be extended to include complications of treatment. Multiple pregnancies and ovarian hyperstimulation syndrome increase the costs associated with IVF. However, there is an increased risk of ectopic pregnancy following tubal surgery, resulting in hospital admissions for emergency surgery.

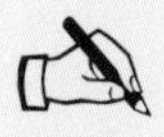

Intra-uterine insemination or in-vitro fertilisation in idiopathic subfertility and male subfertility: a randomised trial and cost-effectiveness analysis.

AJ Goverde, J McDonnell, JPW Vermeiden, R Schats, FFH Rutten, J Schoemaker. *Lancet* 2000; **335**: 1318.

BACKGROUND. This study randomized 258 couples with idiopathic (unexplained) subfertility or male subfertility to treatment with IUI in spontaneous cycles, IUI after mild ovarian stimulation, or IVF. Outcome was studied prospectively up to a maximum of six cycles of treatment.

INTERPRETATION. IUI offered the same likelihood of a successful pregnancy as IVF, and was a more cost-effective approach. Although the pregnancy rate per cycle was higher with IVF than IUI or stimulated IUI (12.2, 7.4, 8.7%, respectively), the cumulative pregnancy rate was not significantly better. More couples dropped out of the IVF group. The cost per live birth was approximately three-fold higher with IVF than IUI.

Comment

This is one of the few randomized comparative studies of subfertility treatments to include a cost analysis. The authors concluded that couples with unexplained or male infertility 'should be counselled that IUI offers the same likelihood of successful pregnancy as IVF'. This conclusion should be modified because the likelihood per cycle was greater with IVF. The cumulative pregnancy rate was, however, not different. This study offered six cycles of the allocated treatment and this limits its applicability to the 'real world' where most couples only undertake one or two treatment cycles. However, their conclusion emphasizes an important principle, that repeated cycles of treatment have a cumulative effect, and thus treatment with a relatively low success rate per cycle may still be effective.

This study included treatment by IUI in a natural cycle, and because it carries fewer health risks than IUI with hormonal stimulation they considered it first-choice treatment. There may be a trade-off between efficacy and risk of treatment.

Acceptability of treatment is important; in this study 47% of couples dropped out of the IVF group, whereas 84% of the IUI groups continued up to the maximum of six attempts. Clearly IVF is more physically and emotionally demanding. Repeated attempts, even of a low-key treatment such as natural cycle IUI, may be extremely demoralizing for the patient.

Couples with severe male factor infertility may be treated with IVF with intracytoplasmic sperm injection (ICSI) with pregnancy and live birth rates equivalent to IVF for other indications. Alternatively pregnancy can be achieved with insemination with donor sperm. Pregnancy rates are around 9% per cycle |12|, but this is a simple treatment which can be repeated to achieve good cumulative conception rates. Comparison with ICSI shows that donor insemination is the more cost-effective treatment (costs per delivery 50% lower). However, the child born will be genetically unrelated to the male partner and this may be unacceptable to the couple. ICSI allows the man to become a genetic father, and the value placed on this may make the additional cost of ICSI treatment well worthwhile.

Cryopreservation and fertility

Cryopreservation facilitates the long-term storage of oocytes from women in danger of losing ovarian function and allows greater flexibility in fertility services for other women. Cryopreservation of women's own oocytes was originally reported more than 10 years ago |13, 14|, but success has been limited to a few case reports world-wide. However, with the combination of cryopreservation and ICSI, the results in terms of fertilization, embryo cleavage and implantation approach those obtained with fresh oocytes |15|. Oocyte survival rates are poor and one of the main problems in the cryopreservation of mature oocytes arises from the sensitivity of the microtubular spindle to low temperatures and cryoprotectants. One way of avoiding these problems would be to preserve oocytes at the germinal vesicle stage when no microtubular spindle is present. The use of immature oocytes would mean that women could receive less hormonal stimulation but with the disadvantage that an additional maturation process is required. Pregnancies following immature oocyte retrieval from unstimulated ovaries of women with polycystic ovary syndrome have been reported |**16**|.

The most plentiful source of oocytes is ovarian tissue itself, containing many thousands of primordial follicles in healthy cortical tissue. Fertility has been restored in sheep, following cryopreservation of ovarian cortex and autografting |**17**| and this seems the most likely clinical model for restoration of fertility in women who are at risk of losing their ovarian function. This may include not only women about to undergo cancer therapy, but also women who have a family history of early menopause, and those with non-malignant diseases such as thalassaemia or certain autoimmune conditions which may be treated by high-dose chemotherapy. In vitro culture of ovarian tissue itself following cryopreservation |**18**| may prove to be an effective means to reconstitute a woman's fertility after successful cancer therapy, for example, without the need to autograft ovarian tissue with its risk of reseeding the woman's body with cancerous cells |**19**|.

Earlier successful work with cryopreservation of rat ovarian tissue has led the way to cryopreservation of both sheep and human ovarian tissue. Up to 80% survival of follicles has been reported, but such tissue may contain malignant cells if removed from a woman about to undergo cancer therapy and may not be suitable for auto-grafting to such a woman if she was to survive. The tissue may be screened before or after thawing for the presence of malignant cells to enable some assessment of the safety of such an approach, or it may be grown in a host animal (e.g. SCID mouse) until such a time as in vitro maturation could be undertaken more effectively |**20**|. Successful in vitro culture of small follicles isolated from frozen–thawed ovary to produce mature oocytes has been reported in the mouse |**21**| and grafting of cryopre-served ovary has restored a normal reproductive life span in the mouse |**22**|.

Results from animal studies must be extrapolated to the human with caution as there are differences between the oocytes of different species. Human oocytes are almost double the size of mouse oocytes resulting in a difference in the surface area to volume ratio. However, Oktay and Karlikaya |**23**| have reported successful autologous transplantation of frozen–thawed human ovarian tissue with follicular development and ovulation in response to stimulation by HMG and hCG.

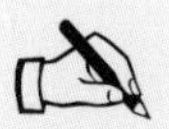

Ovarian function after transplantation of frozen, banked autologous ovarian tissue.

K Oktay, G Karlikaya. *New Engl J Med* 1999; **342**: 1919.

BACKGROUND. **A 29-year-old woman had undergone right salpingo-oophorectomy and wedge resection of the left ovary at 17 years of age in order to remove dermoid cysts. A left salpingo-oophorectomy was performed aged 28 years because of intractable menometrorrhagia. At that time, multiple pieces of ovarian cortex were cryopreserved. She was treated with oestrogen and cyclic progestogen. Six months later she requested transplantation of her ovarian tissue because of persistent menopausal symptoms. Eight pieces of tissue were thawed and sutured to an**

absorbable cellulose membrane which was then laparoscopically sutured beneath the left pelvic peritoneum.

Fifteen weeks after transplantation, daily administration of menopausal gonadotrophins resulted in follicular development. A dominant follicle appeared and ovulation was triggered by hCG. Ovulation was confirmed by ultrasound demonstration of a corpus luteum, free fluid in the cul de sac and endometrial thickening with luteal pattern. Cyclic oestrogen and progestogen was then resumed. Six months later, ultrasonographic studies showed follicular development in response to gonadotrophin stimulation, confirming the long-term survival of the graft.

INTERPRETATION. Cryopreserved human ovarian tissue can be transplanted successfully with follicular development and ovulation stimulated by FSH and hCG.

Comment

Many cancers in young women are curable with surgery, radiotherapy or combination treatment. However, treatment commonly results in premature menopause and may also affect the ability to carry a pregnancy. Cryopreservation as an option for preserving fertility remains experimental. Spontaneous ovulation is not seen and in addition surgical transplantation may cause pelvic adhesions and tubal factor infertility.

This cryopreserved ovary was removed from a young healthy woman for a benign indication and, presumably, uncompromised ovarian reserve. Cancer itself can affect ovarian function as menstrual cycle disturbance is common before the diagnosis is made. Chemotherapy commenced before ovarian biopsy can result in progressive damage to ovarian follicles with increasing FSH and temporary oligo- or amenorrhoea. This effect is age related so that women over 30 years have a greater reduction in ovarian reserve. Radiotherapy causes severe dose-related damage and in a high-dose field of 44–60 Gy, it is unlikely that a pregnancy will be sustained, even if fertility was restored. At lower doses there is evidence of increased spontaneous miscarriage. There is also the theoretical risk that transplantation of cryopreserved ovary reintroduces cancerous cells |**19**|.

Cryopreservation and transplantation of human ovary has not resulted in pregnancy and for preserving fertility is experimental. In practical terms, however, it often offers the only option for future fertility, as treatment for cancer needs to be started urgently and there is often insufficient time for the pituitary down-regulation and ovarian stimulation required for oocyte collection.

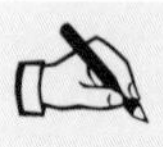

Cycles of human oocyte cryopreservation and intracytoplasmic sperm injection of cryopreserved human oocytes.

E Porcu, R Fabbri, PM Ciotti. *Fertil Steril* 1999; **72**(S1): S2.

BACKGROUND. Only a few live births have been achieved from immature oocytes cultured in vitro because of low survival, fertilization and cleavage rates. However,

with the combination of cryopreservation and ICSI, the results in terms of fertilization, embryo cleavage and implantation approach those obtained with fresh oocytes. The only limiting step seems to be oocyte survival.

INTERPRETATION. Ninety-six women underwent 112 IVF cycles with oocyte cryopreservation. A total of 1769 oocytes were frozen and 1502 were thawed. The survival rate was 54.1% and the cleavage rate was 91.2%. Sixteen pregnancies were achieved. Nine pregnancies (seven singletons and two twins) ended with the birth of 11 healthy children, eight girls and three boys.

Comment

ICSI will overcome problems of sperm penetration if cryopreservation alters the structure of the zona pellucida. Oocyte survival should be improved further. However, it may be unrealistic to expect more than 70% survival of oocytes, as unlike embryos, oocytes have not been preselected by the process of fertilization.

Conclusion

The publications discussed in this chapter have been selected to highlight areas of development and controversy, but they can only give an outline of the field of reproductive medicine. There is an exponential increase in the published literature in this field.

Much basic clinical research remains to be done in reproductive medicine—there is a lack of randomized trials in many areas—and this applies particularly to surgical treatment. However, the scientific developments will continue to drive forward the clinical frontiers. In the future we will see much research work in the areas of in vitro culture and maturation of human eggs, which could allow us to undertake IVF without drug stimulation by harvesting immature eggs, and may lead to the use of stored ovarian tissue for IVF. This could allow women to beat the biological clock and choose to have families later in life by utilizing reproductive technology. This area of medicine will continue to raise ethical questions for debate.

References

1. Harkki-Siren P, Sjoberg J, Kurki T. Major complications of laparoscopy: a follow-up Finnish study. *Obstet Gynecol* 1999; **94**: 94–8.

2. Mahmood TA, Templeton A. Prevalence and genesis of endometriosis. *Hum Reprod* 1991; **6**: 544–9.

3. Hughes E, Fedorkow D, Collins J, Vandekeckhove P. Ovulation suppression vs. placebo in the treatment of endometriosis (Cochrane Review). In: *The Cochrane Library*, Issue 3. Update Software, Oxford, 1999.

4. Adamson GD, Pasta DJ. Surgical treatment of endometriosis-associated infertility: meta-analysis compared with survival analysis. *Am J Obstet Gynecol* 1994; **171**: 1488–504.

5. Parazzini F. Ablation of lesions or no treatment in minimal–mild endometriosis in infertile women: a randomized trial. Gruppo Italiano per lo studio dell'Endometriosi. *Hum Reprod* 1999; **14**: 1332–4.

6. Human Fertilisation and Embryology Authority. *The Patients' Guide to IVF Clinics.* Human Fertilisation and Embryology Authority, London, 2000.

7. Bryan EM. *Twins and Higher Order Births. A Guide to their Nature and Nurture.* Edward Arnold, London, 1992.

8. Office for National Statistics. *Mortality Statistics: Childhood, Infant and Perinatal Series PH3, no. 27.* HMSO, London, 1996.

9. Petterson B, Nelson K, Watson L, Stanley F. Twins, triplets and cerebral palsy in births in Western Australia in the 1980s. *Br Med J* 1993; **307**: 1239–43.

10. Copperman AB, Mukherjee T, Shaer J, *et al.* A cost analysis of in vitro fertilization versus tubal surgery within an institution under two payment systems. *J Women's Health* 1996; **5**: 335–41.

11. Wilcox LS, Mosher WD. Use of infertility services in the United States. *Obstet Gynecol* 1993; **82**: 122–7.

12. Granberg M, Wikland M, Hamberger L. Cost-effectiveness of intra-cytoplasmic sperm injection in comparison with donor insemination. *Acta Obstet Gynecol Scand* 1996; **75**: 734–7.

13. Chen C. Pregnancy after human oocyte cryopreservation. *Lancet* 1986; **i**: 884–6.

14. Van Uem JF, Siebzehnrubl ER, Schuh B, Koch R, Trotnow S, Lang N. Birth after cryopreservation of unfertilized oocytes. *Lancet* 1987; **ii**: 752–3.

15. Porcu E, Fabbri R, Ciotti PM, *et al.* Cycles of human oocyte cryopreservation and intracytoplasmic sperm injection of cryopreserved human oocytes. *Fertil Steril* 1999; **72**(S1): S2.

16. Cha KY, Han SY, Chung HM, *et al.* Pregnancies and deliveries after culture followed by in vitro fertilization and embryo transfer without stimulation in women with polycystic ovary syndrome. *Fertil Steril* 2000; **73**: 978–83.

17. Gosden RG, Baird DT, Wade JC, Webb R. Restoration of fertility to oophorectomised sheep by ovarian autografts stored at −196 degrees centigrade. *Hum Reprod* 1994; **9**: 597–603.

18. Oktay K, Newton H, Aubard Y, Salha O, Gosden RG. Cryopreservation of immature oocytes and ovarian tissue: an emerging technology? *Fertil Steril* 1998; **69**: 1–7.

19. Gosden RG, Rutherford AJ, Norfolk DR. Transmission of malignant cells in ovarian grafts. *Hum Reprod* 1997; **12**: 403.

20. Oktay K, Newton H, Gosden RG. Transplantation of cryopreserved human ovarian tissue results in follicle growth initiation in SCID mice. *Fertil Steril* 2000; **73**: 599–603.

21. Newton H, Illingworth P. In-vitro growth of murine pre-antral follicles after isolation from cryopreserved ovarian tissue. *Hum Reprod* 2001; **16**: 423–9.

22. Candy CJ, Wood MJ, Whittingham DG. Restoration of a normal reproductive lifespan after grafting of cryopreserved mouse ovaries. *Hum Reprod* 2000; **15**: 1300–4.

23. Oktay K, Karlikaya G. Ovarian function after transplantation of frozen, banked autologous ova. *New Engl J Med* 2000; **342**: 1919.

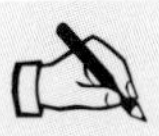

Correlation of intraurethral ultrasonography and needle electromyography of the urethra.

JR Fischer, MH Heit, MH Clark, JT Benson. *Obstet Gynecol* 2000; **95**: 156–9.

BACKGROUND. There is great interest in imaging the urethral sphincter as this may be the cause of genuine stress incontinence. One of the methods of imaging the urethral sphincter would be ultrasound, but the images obtained have not been validated in vivo. This study attempted to correlate the image seen with the electrical activity measured using a needle electrode to define the extent of the urethral sphincter.

INTERPRETATION. Intraurethral ultrasound has been used to image the urethral sphincter in the past. The main problem with these ultrasound probes is that the ultrasound frequency is greater than 10 MHz which means that the depth of penetration of the ultrasound waves is no more than 1–2 cm, thus not imaging the whole urethral sphincter. The second problem of the intraurethral ultrasound probe is that it can change orientation travelling along the urethra. The urethra is not a straight tube and the orientation changes. Using a concentric needle to localize the striated urethral sphincter, with intraurethral ultrasound three layers were seen, a mildly hyperechoic inner, a hypoechoic middle layer and a hyperechoic outer layer. The concentric needle tip was seen in all subjects and motor unit action potentials were located in the outer hyperechoic layer. Interestingly, the mean thickness of the outer hyperechoic layer was 2.6 mm. The authors suggested that because motor unit action potentials were found in the striated muscle it indicates that the outer hyperechoic layer on intraurethral ultrasound contained striated muscle.

Comment

The authors recognized that the ultrasound probe might distort the sonographic appearance of the urethral sphincter and thus alter any circumference or area measurements of periurethral structures. They also indicated that sonographic images remain hyperechoic where muscle has largely been replaced by fibrous tissue. The authors warned against using sphincter volume to indicate a functional urethral sphincter.

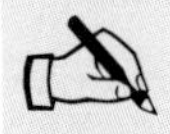

Voiding cystourethrography findings in elderly women with urge incontinence.

JR Fielding, JH Lee, CE Dubueau, KH Zou, NM Resnick. *J Urol* 2000; **163**: 1216–8.

BACKGROUND. Voiding cystourethrography is the introduction of contrast into the bladder while imaging it radiologically. It has been used in association with urodynamics to diagnose the causes of urge incontinence. In spite of this technique

being available for 30 years it has not been described in the literature in particular association with symptoms of urge incontinence.

INTERPRETATION. Fifty elderly women had their voiding cystourethrograms reviewed and additional urodynamic testing was carried out. Bladder wall trabeculation and bladder diverticula, cystocoele and vesicoureteric reflux were all noted. The maximum bladder capacity, postvoid residual and history of previous continence surgery and hysterectomy were noted from clinical records. Of the women who had incontinence, 70% (35) had trabeculation, which was regarded as mild in 30 and moderate in five, and 82% (41) had a cystocoele which was mild in over half the cases. The maximum bladder capacity ranged from less than 100 ml to more than 900 ml. The continent women appeared to have smooth bladders. The authors then proceeded to use these cystographic findings as a predictor for urge incontinence. Diverticula had a remarkable specificity as did trabeculation, cystocoele and bladder capacities greater than 500 ml and large postvoid residuals did not appear to correlate well. Even though the idea of imaging the bladder may appear attractive there is no reason to feel that this replaces urodynamics in any way and certainly the patient would describe urge incontinence.

Comment

A useful study documenting the appearance of the bladder in urge incontinence. Unfortunately there is very little reason to diagnose urge incontinence from a cystogram.

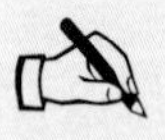

Differential effects of cough, Valsalva, and continence status on vesical neck movement.

D Howard, JM Miller, JOL Delancey, JA Ashton-Miller. *Obstet Gynecol* 2000; **95**: 535–40.

BACKGROUND. Valsalva and cough have been used as methods of determining the leak point pressure and in turn attempting to quantify urinary incontinence. This group wished to test the hypothesis that vesical neck descent was the same during Valsalva manoeuvres.

INTERPRETATION. Three groups of women were studied: 17 nulliparous continent women, 18 primiparous continent women and 23 primiparous stress incontinent women. The vesical neck positions at rest and during displacement were obtained by ultrasound. Abdominal pressures were recorded simultaneously using an intravaginal microtransducer catheter. To control for different abdominal pressures, the stiffness of the vesical neck support was calculated by dividing the the bladder neck excursion by the intra-abdominal pressure which was recorded simultaneously using an intravaginal microtransducer catheter.

Interestingly, the primiparous stress incontinent women displayed the same vesical neck mobility during cough effort and Valsalva manoeuvre as nulliparous continent women, and primiparous continent women displayed less mobility during a cough than during a Valsalva manoeuvre, despite greater abdominal pressures generated during a cough. Nulliparous women displayed greater floor stiffness during a cough compared with incontinent primiparous women. This suggests that the pelvic floor and other supporting structures to the bladder neck act differently during cough and Valsalva.

Comment

This may be the reason for differences in the leak point pressures that have been found in previous studies. Vaginal delivery appeared to alter the amount of movement of the bladder neck in response to an increasing intra-abdominal pressure. It was noticeable that there was greater mobility after vaginal delivery. Unfortunately, the use of stiffness factor cannot be truly validated until it has been compared at different pressures as there may not be a linear relationship between bladder neck movement and an increase in pressure.

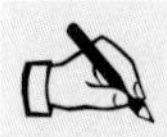

Bladder outlet obstruction in women: definition and characteristics.

A Groutz, J Blaivas, D Chaikin. *Neurourol Urodynam* 2000; **19**: 213–20.

BACKGROUND. **The prevalence of bladder outlet obstruction is unknown in women and most probably has been underestimated. There are also no standard definitions of a diagnosis. This study attempted to define the clinical and urodynamic characteristics of bladder outlet obstruction among women referred for the evaluation of voiding symptoms.**

INTERPRETATION. In this study, bladder outlet obstruction was defined as a persistent, low, maximum free flow rate of <12 ml/sec in repeated, non-invasive uroflow studies, combined with high detrusor pressure at a maximum flow >20 cm of water. Out of a urodynamic database of 587 consecutive women, 38 were diagnosed as having bladder outlet obstruction. The mean age of these women was 64 years, with the mean maximum free flow rate being 9 ml/sec, with the postvoid residual urinary volume of 86 ml. The pressure at maximum flow was 37 cm of water. Previous anti-incontinence surgery and severe genital prolapse were the most common aetiologies, accounting for half the cases. Less commonly, urethral stricture, primary bladder neck obstruction, learned voiding dysfunction, as well as detrusor sphincter dyssynergia. Symptomatology did not really diagnose these problems as a third had isolated irritative symptoms and only 8% had isolated obstructive symptoms.

Comment

From this study it appears that bladder outlet obstruction is more common that we have supposed and that symptoms are not a good way of diagnosing these problems. This study probably required a much larger number of women, as 38 is a small number on which to make such wide sweeping statements.

Treatment of incontinence

Treatment success is defined differently after conservative or surgical therapy. Conservative treatment is considered a 'success' if cure or improvement result. Surgical treatment is only considered a success if total continence is demonstrated objectively.

Conservative therapy

Simple measures

All women with urinary incontinence can be helped even if a 'cure' is not possible. General advice regarding lifestyle should include moderating fluid intake to 1–1.5 litres a day, avoiding caffeine- or alcohol-containing drinks. Evening fluid intake is thought to be related to nocturia and the nocturnal voided volume. However, evening fluid restriction does not improve nocturia significantly. There is a weaker relationship between diurnal fluid intake and voiding. Nocturnal polyuria appears to be related to subclinical heart failure when fluid pools in the limbs during the day and returns to the intravascular space at night to produce a diuresis. Frusemide taken 6 h before sleep has been shown to reduce nocturia in a randomized placebo-controlled trial |5|.

Losing weight has been thought to improve urinary incontinence, but there are no prospective randomized trials. However, two prospective cohort studies have investigated this, one involved using objective tests. Incontinence was found to resolve when massive weight loss occurred in morbidly obese women after stomach stapling and morbid obesity appears to be an independent risk factor in the prevalence of urinary incontinence, having an increased odds ratio of 1.6 per 5 body mass index units |6|. It has been argued that women who suffer from urinary incontinence cannot exercise, thus they become overweight. Unfortunately there is no information regarding weight loss in moderately overweight women and any improvement in urinary incontinence. There is no evidence that strenuous exercise causes incontinence, but exercise does exacerbate it.

Pelvic floor exercises

Pelvic floor exercises were first advocated by Kegel in 1948 for the treatment of genuine stress incontinence and mixed incontinence. Four prospective randomized studies have compared pelvic floor exercises with no treatment. All these studies have described significant improvements in those groups undergoing pelvic floor exercises compared with the control group. Improvement and cure rates of 68–74% have been reported compared with 3–5% in the control groups. Burns *et al.* |7| reported a 68% cure/improvement rate compared with 18% in controls.

Henalla *et al.* |8| used an objective outcome measure (pad test) and found that 65% of the treatment group were cured/improved compared with 0% of the control group. O'Brien *et al.* |9| described 68% of the women being cured/improved

that 90% of the treatment group were continent compared with 23% of the control group. Fantl *et al.* |24| included women with genuine stress incontinence, detrusor instability and mixed incontinence. They found that 12% of the treatment group were continent and 76% had reduced incontinence episodes by 50%. Bladder retraining is an effective treatment for urge, stress and mixed incontinence.

Bladder retraining has been compared with anticholinergic therapy in two randomized controlled trials. The first used flavoxate hydrochloride and imipramine and the second used oxybutynin. Unfortunately, these women only had 6 weeks of follow-up |25, 26| (see Table 12.5).

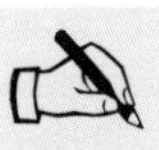

Conservative treatment of urge urinary incontinence in women: a systematic review of randomized clinical trials.

LCM Berghmans, HJM Hendriks, RA De Bie, ESC van Waalwijk, KB van Doorn, PHEV van Kerrebroek. *Br J Urol Int* 2000; **85**: 254–63.

BACKGROUND. **Conservative therapies have been reported in a non-standard manner and need the same detailed assessment as surgical treatments have had.**

INTERPRETATION. This was a review of randomized clinical trials between 1980 and 1999 using the key words physical therapies of bladder retraining, pelvic floor muscle exercises, biofeedback and electrical stimulation. Fifteen randomized controlled trials were identified. The quality of the studies was moderate and eight were considered sufficient quality to be included for further analysis. The results of these studies showed weak evidence to suggest that bladder retraining is more effective than no treatment and that bladder retraining is better than drug therapy. Electrical stimulation studies were heterogenous in both their content and their methods and there was insufficient evidence that electrical stimulation was more effective than sham electrical stimulation. There were too few studies to show that the effects of the pelvic floor muscle exercises with or without biofeedback or toilet training were of any value in women with urge urinary incontinence.

Comment

This paper shows the paucity of real evidence behind the use of conservative methods of treatment for urge urinary incontinence and more studies need to be carried out.

Table 12.5 Cure/improvement rates (%) of randomized trials of anticholinergic drug therapy versus bladder retraining

Authors	Bladder retraining	Anticholinergics
Jarvis 1981 |27|	84	56
Columbo *et al.* 1995 |25|	74	42

Drug therapy

There are many drugs available to treat an overactive detrusor (Table 12.6), few have been tested in placebo-controlled clinical trials. This is important as treatment of detrusor instability has a large placebo response.

Anticholinergic drugs

Voluntary and involuntary detrusor contractions are mediated through muscarinic receptors which are suppressed by anticholinergic drugs. The most widely used drugs in this group are propantheline bromide and emepronium which produce a competitive blockade of acetylcholine receptors at postganglionic parasympathetic receptor sites. These drugs have a low bioavailability (5–10%) and this often results in 'treatment failure' when blood levels are inadequate for treatment. The drug dose should be titrated against the improvement in urinary symptoms and the anticholinergic side-effects such as dry mouth, constipation, blurred vision, tachycardia and drowsiness. Propantheline bromide has a recommended adult dose of 15–30 mg four times a day (qid). This is often inadequate and doses of 60 mg qid or more may be needed. The side-effects can be minimized by starting the drug at a low dose and gradually increasing the dose.

Table 12.6 Drug treatment for detrusor instability

Anticholinergic drugs	Tricyclic antidepressants
Propantheline bromide	Imipramine
Emepronium bromide/carrageenate	Doxepin
Tolterodine	
Darifenacin	Beta adrenoceptor agonists
Trospium	Terbutaline
	Salbutamol
Musculotrophic drugs	Isoprenaline
Oxybutynin chloride	
Dicyclomine chloride	Alpha adrenoceptor antagonists
Flavoxate hydrochloride	Phenoxybenzamine
	Prazosin
Anticholinergic/calcium antagonists	
Propiverine	Prostaglandin synthetase inhibitors
	Flurbiprofen
Calcium antagonists	Indomethacin
Nifedipine	
Flunarizine	Neurotoxins
	Capsaicin
Potassium channel openers	Resiniferatoxin
Cromakalim	
Nicorandil	Other drugs
Pinacidil	Desmopressin

Tolterodine

Tolterodine is a competitive muscarinic receptor antagonist with relative functional selectivity for bladder muscarinic receptors and whilst it shows no specificity for receptor subtypes, it does appear to target the bladder over the salivary glands. It is completely absorbed from the gastrointestinal tract, having a short half-life of 2–3 h, and is metabolized in the liver to an active metabolite DD01 which has similar properties. Tolterodine has greater affinity for bladder muscarinic receptors than salivary gland receptors, the opposite of oxybutynin. A dose of 2 mg twice a day (bid) has been found to have greater efficacy than 1 mg bid, although both are superior to placebo. Effects of the drug are seen after 4 weeks of treatment and a maximum effect is seen after 5–8 weeks of treatment.

Several randomized, double-blind, placebo-controlled trials on patients with idiopathic detrusor instability and detrusor hyperreflexia have demonstrated a significant reduction in incontinent episodes and micturition frequency. Further studies have confirmed the safety of tolterodine and at the recommended daily dosage the incidence of adverse events was no different to that in patients taking placebo.

In addition, the safety and efficacy of tolterodine has also been compared with that of oxybutynin. A randomized, double-blind, placebo-controlled, parallel group study of 293 patients reported that the clinical efficacy of the two drugs was comparable, although oxybutynin was associated with higher withdrawal rates and a higher incidence of adverse events, notably dry mouth [28]. A pooled analysis of the safety, efficacy and acceptability of tolterodine in 1120 patients in four randomized, double-blind, parallel, multicentre trials found that both tolterodine and oxybutynin significantly decreased incontinent episodes, although tolterodine was associated with fewer adverse events, dose reductions and patient withdrawals than oxybutynin [29].

In summary, the evidence would suggest that tolterodine is as effective as oxybutynin. However, as it has fewer adverse effects, tolerability and patient compliance is improved and in this respect it may represent an advance in anticholinergic therapy.

Trospium

Trospium chloride is a quaternary ammonium compound which is non-selective for muscarinic receptor subtypes and shows low biological availability. At present it is not available in the UK. In a recent placebo-controlled, randomized, double-blind, multicentre trial, trospium chloride produced significant improvements in maximum cystometric capacity and bladder volume at first unstable contraction [30]. Clinical improvement was significantly greater in the group receiving trospium and the frequency of adverse events was similar in both groups. Trospium chloride has also been compared with oxybutynin in a randomized, double-blind, multicentre trial [31]. With both agents there was a significant increase in bladder capacity, a decrease in maximum voiding detrusor pressure and a significant increase in compliance, although there were no statistically significant differences between the two treatment groups. Those taking trospium had a lower incidence of dry mouth (4 versus 23%) and were also less likely to withdraw (6 versus 16%) when compared with the group receiving oxybutynin. On balance the evidence would suggest that trospium chloride is effective in suppressing uninhibited detrusor contractions and may be associated with fewer side-effects than oxybutynin.

Musculotrophic agents

Oxybutynin chloride is the most commonly used drug for the treatment of detrusor instability. It has local anaesthetic, direct muscle relaxant effect, anticholinergic action and antihistaminic properties. Oral oxybutynin has been shown to be effective in both neuropathic and non-neuropathic bladder dysfunction, but causes severe systemic anticholinergic side-effects. Intravesical instillation of oxybutynin has recently been shown to be efficacious in the treatment of severe detrusor instability and detrusor hyperreflexia without the problem of distressing systemic anticholinergic side-effects, particularly where voiding difficulties are associated with detrusor instability.

Double-blind, placebo-controlled trials have shown symptomatic as well as cystometric improvements with oxybutynin |32–34|. Reduced compliance in taking the drug has been found because of severe anticholinergic side-effects. This is the reason why 10–23% of women discontinue oxybutynin. Compliance has been improved by increasing the dose from a small starting level. This is particularly important in the elderly where therapeutic blood levels occur with low oral doses due to altered metabolism with increasing age. Another method of increasing compliance is prescribing the medication when necessary rather than regularly |35|. In addition, to try and minimize the troublesome side-effects, other methods of administration have been developed, such as the rectal route.

More recently, controlled release oxybutynin preparations using an osmotic system have been developed which have been shown to have comparable efficacy when compared with immediate release oxybutynin, but are associated with fewer adverse effects. These findings are in agreement with a further study of controlled release oxybutynin (Ditropan XL) which reported the incidence of moderate to severe dry mouth to be 23% and only 1.6% of participants discontinued the medication due to adverse effects |36|.

In summary, the efficacy of oxybutynin is well documented although very often the clinical usefulness is limited by adverse effects. Alternative routes of administration and the development of slow release preparations may lead to an improved side-effect profile producing better patient acceptability and compliance. Oxybutynin is one of the most useful drugs in the treatment of detrusor instability, but usefulness is limited by side-effects.

Propiverine

Propiverine has been shown to combine anticholinergic and calcium channel blocking actions and is the most popular drug for detrusor instability in Germany,

Austria and Japan. Open studies in patients with detrusor overactivity have demonstrated a beneficial effect and in a double-blind, placebo-controlled trial of its use in detrusor hyperreflexia it has been shown to increase bladder capacity and compliance significantly in comparison with placebo. Dry mouth was experienced by 37% in the treatment group as opposed to 8% in the placebo group with dropout rates being 7 and 4.5%, respectively. The evidence would suggest that propiverine will have a role in the management of women with detrusor instability, although at present there is a need for further long-term studies to evaluate its efficacy and safety profile fully.

Flavoxate hydrochloride

This compound has direct smooth muscle relaxant properties through calcium antagonistic activity, local anaesthetic properties and an ability to inhibit phosphodiesterase. There are no or mild anticholinergic effects. In a double-blind crossover study on women with detrusor instability comparing emepronium bromide and flavoxate hydrochloride administered at 200 mg three times a day (tds), improvement rates of 66 and 83% were reported. No beneficial effect was found at a dose of 100–200 mg three to four times a day. Few side-effects have been reported with flavoxate, but efficacy compared with placebo has not been established and its use cannot be recommended.

Tricyclic antidepressants

Imipramine has been used in the elderly with detrusor instability starting at a dose of 25 mg at night and increasing this by 25 mg every third day, until the patient is continent or has marked side-effects, to a maximum dose of 150 mg. Six of the 10 patients treated became continent and in those who underwent repeat cystometry bladder capacity was increased and the maximum urethral closure pressure increased |37|.

Imipramine has also been used for childhood nocturnal enuresis at doses of 10–50 mg before bedtime. Imipramine produces continence within a few days of starting drug therapy; the effect is unrelated to the antidepressant effect of the drug which takes at least a fortnight to occur.

Doxepin has been found to be more potent in its musculotropic relaxant and antimuscarinic activity than other tricyclic antidepressants. Women with detrusor instability were studied in a randomized, double-blind, placebo-controlled crossover trial using doxepin 50 mg at night or 25 mg twice daily. There was a significant decrease in nocturia and night time incontinence. Cystometrically an increase in first sensation to void and maximum bladder capacity occurred |38|.

At therapeutic levels, tricyclic drugs used to treat depression can cause orthostatic hypotension and ventricular arrhythmias. As children are particularly sensitive to the cardiotoxic action, care must be taken in their use. Allergic reactions such as rashes, hepatic dysfunction, obstructive jaundice and agranulocytosis may also occur. Stopping drug treatment should be done gradually as side-effects of nausea, abdominal discomfort, vomiting, headache, lethargy and irritability have been reported on discontinuing medication after having taken high doses.

Capsaicin

This is the pungent ingredient found in the chilli pepper. It is a neurotoxin of substance P containing (C) nerve fibres. These fibres are usually involved in the sensation of pain. Patients with detrusor hyperreflexia secondary to multiple sclerosis appear to have abnormal C fibre sensory innervation of the detrusor which leads to premature activation of the voiding reflex arc during bladder filling. Intravesical application of capsaicin dissolved in a 30% alcohol solution to patients with detrusor hyperreflexia appears to act for up to 6 months. The effects can be variable and the long-term safety of this substance has not been evaluated. Resiniferatoxin, a substance isolated from a cactus, is a stronger analogue of capsaicin and appears to have a similar efficacy but with fewer of the acute side-effects such as pain and burning during instillation. It has been shown to be 1000 times more potent than capsaicin in stimulating bladder activity, although to date studies have produced contradictory findings when used in patients with detrusor overactivity. An increase in bladder capacity has been demonstrated in patients with detrusor overactivity which was short lived and occurred in only 30% of patients. Other authorities have shown no significant effect. At present the available evidence does not support the routine clinical use of these agents, although further studies may establish their role as an intravesical agent in neurological patients with detrusor hyperreflexia.

Oestrogens

There have been many subjective uncontrolled studies on the effects of oestrogen on the lower urinary tract. However, objective studies are important because of the large placebo effect associated with the drug treatment of urinary incontinence. In a double-blind, multicentre study of women with the 'urge syndrome', 64 postmenopausal women were treated with oral oestriol 3 mg daily or placebo for 3 months. Compliance was confirmed by an increase in the maturation index of the vaginal epithelial cells in the active treatment group. Oestriol produced subjective and objective improvements in urinary symptoms but this was not significantly better than placebo.

It appears that oestrogens may improve irritative symptoms, but there is no proven benefit in the treatment of detrusor instability.

Desmopressin

Desmopressin (1-desamino-8-D-arginine vasopressin; DDAVP) is a synthetic vasopressin analogue. It has strong antidiuretic effects without altering blood pressure. The drug has been used primarily in the treatment of nocturia and nocturnal enuresis in children and adults. It is administered as an intranasal spray at a dose of 10–40 μg and this reduces urine production for 7–10 h. This approach is more effective than fluid restriction which appears to indicate that there is an abnormality in the circadian peak of antidiuretic hormone at night in these patients. Desmopressin is safe for long-term use. However, the drug should be used with care in the elderly. Nocturnal frequency and urinary incontinence can be reduced by the use of DDAVP. A significant decrease from 3.2 to 2.5 in voids 6 h after

postoperative Q-tip values were 42 and 31°, respectively. Twelve of the women had a Q-tip test greater than 30° after surgery and 11 of these women were cured.

Comment

This study indicates that urethral hypermobility has no place in the assessment of women who have stress incontinence as correction of this hypermobility was not necessary for the cure of stress incontinence.

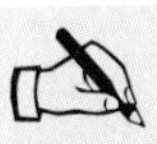

Incisionless cystourethropexy—the Intac device—an initial experience.

A Macgibbon, G Brieger, A Korda. *N Z J Obstet Gynecol* 2000; **40**: 59–61.

BACKGROUND. **Many new devices have been introduced to treat genuine stress incontinence. There is a question about all these devices and whether they do produce an objective cure and long-term outcome.**

INTERPRETATION. This was a study of 15 women with type 1 and type II urinary stress incontinence who were treated with a new per vaginal bone anchor device designed to fix periurethral tissues to the pubic bone. None of the patients had significant operative morbidity and they were followed up for 6–13 months using a follow-up questionnaire and repeat urodynamic testing. Subjectively 73% of the women stated that they had an improvement in their urinary symptoms, but only 40% reported cure of their stress incontinence. On urodynamic testing only 53% of the women were cured.

Comment

This paper clearly shows that the Intac procedure has a greatly reduced success rate compared with the gold standard of colposuspension and this is with relatively short follow-up. The second important message of this paper is that subjective findings do not correlate well with objective findings and it is important to have both modalities to test whether or not a treatment is effective.

Laparoscopic surgery

A laparoscopic approach has been used to perform colposuspensions and has been compared with open procedures in two randomized studies. Burton |**48, 49**| randomized 60 women and reported objective continence rates of 97 and 73% at 1 year follow-up. After 3 years the objective continence rate had dropped to 93 and 60%, respectively. Su *et al.* |**50**| reported a 96% open colposuspension objective cure rate compared with 80% after laparoscopic surgery at 3 months. Laparoscopic colposuspension produces significantly inferior results to open colposuspension. However, both studies did suffer from the operator starting the study while still on their 'learning curve'. A multicentre Medical Research Council-funded study is underway and should help to clarify this contentious issue.

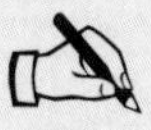

Laparoscopic colposuspension: a short term urodynamic follow-up and a three-year questionnaire study.

J Persson, T Bossmar, P Wolner-Hanssen. *Acta Obstet Gynecol Scand* 2000; **79**: 414–20.

BACKGROUND. Laparoscopic colposuspension is still a relatively new procedure and from all the randomized studies it appears to have a lower rate of cure than the open procedure, but it is important to look at reported series to determine if something can be learned and applied to randomized studies.

INTERPRETATION. Eighty-five consecutive women with genuine stress incontinence were included in this prospective non-controlled study. The surgeons introduced two polytetrafluoroethylene sutures on each side of the urethra and fixed them to Cooper's ligaments. Pre- and postoperative clinical and urodynamic evaluations were performed, including the pad test, and a mailed questionnaire was used to evaluate cure and complication rates 3 years after surgery. At follow-up, 62 of 76 women were cured, 10 were improved and four were regarded as failure. Questionnaires were returned by 80 women: 41 (51%) considered themselves cured, 31 (39%) considered themselves improved and eight (10%) considered themselves unimproved or minimally improved. Clinical outcome was not associated with alterations in urethral functional length or in urethral closing pressure, but short pre-operative urethral functional length was associated with failure. The incidence of new onset symptoms of urgency were 13% and entero/rectocele was 9%.

Comment

From this study it appears that the success of laparoscopic colposuspension still appears to be less than that reported for open colposuspension. However, it is interesting that the complications of open colposuspension also occur in laparoscopic procedures.

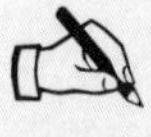

Periurethral collagen injection for stress incontinence with and without urethral hypermobility.

AC Steele, N Kohli, MM Karram. *Obstet Gynecol* 2000; **95**: 327–31.

BACKGROUND. Injectables have been used for treating the infirm or those who do not wish to have a major continence.

INTERPRETATION. A series of 40 women who underwent periurethral collagen injections was reviewed. Nine (23%) had urethral hypermobility on Q-tip testing and these were compared with women without hypermobility. Comparing the two groups of patients, a similar number of procedures was required with a mean of 1.9 in the urethral hypermobility group compared with 1.4 in the women without hypermobility. Additionally, similar amounts of collagen were required on the first injection, 5.6 ml compared with 5.3 ml. Pre-operative urodynamic parameters were similar and the rates of subjective dryness were equivalent in patients with and without hypermobility at 1 month (76 and 46%) and also at 6 months (71 and 32%).

Comment

There are great concerns about this paper as there were only nine patients with urethral hypermobility, this impaired the power of the study. A post hoc power analysis by the authors revealed that the sample size would be sufficient to detect a 2.5-fold difference. This is a massive difference to be detected and the authors stated that co-existing urethral hypermobility should not preclude the use of collagen injections. It is interesting that in this study the women who did have urethral hypermobility actually achieved higher cure rates than those without hypermobility, but this may indicate that they had more severe incontinence than the group without increased bladder neck mobility.

Prolapse and genuine stress incontinence

Vaginal prolapse and genuine stress incontinence can co-exist as they have a common aetiology. Continent women sometimes become incontinent once a prolapse has been reduced. One approach is to repair the prolapse and perform a continence procedure at the same time to treat occult genuine stress incontinence. Thirty women with severe uterovaginal prolapse and occult genuine stress incontinence underwent vaginal repair and a Kelly bladder neck plication. Fifteen (50%) women developed postoperative stress incontinence and this was confirmed as genuine stress incontinence on urodynamics. An additional 11 (37%) women had objective evidence of genuine stress incontinence but no symptoms. Bump |51| performed a prospective randomized trial of 29 women with both severe uterovaginal prolapse and occult genuine stress incontinence who were randomized to needle suspension or bladder neck endopelvic fascia plication. Only 7% of the women developed stress incontinence compared with the 67% predicted by pre-operative urodynamics. Sze *et al.* |52| reported the results of sacrospinous ligament fixation with a transvaginal needle suspension. Of 54 women, 18 (33%) developed recurrent prolapse beyond the hymenal ring and five (9%) developed recurrent stress incontinence.

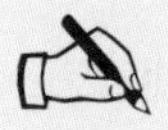

Randomised comparison of Burch colposuspension versus anterior colporrhaphy in women with stress urinary incontinence and anterior vaginal wall prolapse.

M Colombo, D Vitobello, F Proietti, R Milani. *Br J Obstet Gynaecol* 2000; **107**: 544–51.

BACKGROUND. The problem of genuine stress incontinence and anterior wall prolapse is a difficult one as both problems need treating concurrently.

INTERPRETATION. Seventy-one women with genuine stress incontinence and a cystocoele descending to or beyond the vaginal introitus were randomized to colposuspension or anterior colporrhaphy. They were then followed for 8–17 years. Eighty-six per cent of the 35 evaluable women who had a Burch colposuspension were subjectively cured compared with 52% of the 33 evaluable women who had anterior colporrhaphy. Objective cure rates were 74% for the women who underwent Burch colposuspension and 42% for the women who underwent anterior colporrhaphy. Recurrent cystocoele with or without vaginal prolapse at other sites with 34% of women who underwent Burch colposuspension compared with 3% of the women who underwent anterior colporrhaphy.

Comment

This study appears to show that Burch colposuspension is better at controlling stress incontinence but there is a higher rate of vaginal prolapse. This paper highlighted the difficulties treating vaginal prolapse and genuine stress incontinence and it does not appear from this paper that either form of problem is adequately treated by one operation. This certainly has not been the experience quoted in the literature of others using the Burch colposuspension for anterior vaginal wall prolapse.

Vaginal prolapse

The assessment and evaluation of treatment for vaginal prolapse have been difficult as methods of examination have not been reproducible. The International Continence Society (ICS) prolapse score is simple to perform and has good inter- and intra-observer variability. This will allow an accurate assessment of treatment and the outcome of treatment. There has been only one randomized study using two different methods of treating recurrent anterior vaginal wall prolapse. This study compared the use of a marlex mesh and a routine fascial defect repair. After 2 years there were significantly more failures in the fascial repair group |53|. There are inadequate data in this area and further randomized studies need to be carried out.

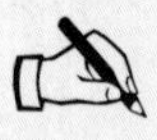

Use of the pelvic organ prolapse staging system of the International Continence Society, American Urogynecologic Society, and Society of Gynecologic Surgeons in perimenopausal women.

D Bland, B Earle, M Vitolins, G Burke. *Am J Obstet Gynecol* 1999; **181**: 1324–8.

BACKGROUND. The pelvic organ prolapse system is a logical method of recording vaginal prolapse. However, there have been no long-term measurement studies to determine changes over time or normal values.

INTERPRETATION. This study used the ICS prolapse staging system in perimenopausal women to determine its reproducibility over time and also to obtain some general values for women. Unfortunately, it was not clear whether these women were screened for symptoms of prolapse. Thus, whether these were normal values for asymptomatic women or merely a range of values for women in the general population cannot be determined. A total of 241 women were studied, 28% of them had previously had a hysterectomy and 66% complained of urinary incontinence at enrolment. It was interesting that the mean prolapse score that described the position of the cervix, posterior fornix and total vaginal length changed over a 1-year period, reflecting increased vaginal prolapse, and there appeared to be no factor correlated with change over a year.

Comment

It is questioned whether the changes measured are the effect of examining the women on a second occasion or that the women underwent some form of intervention which altered the measurements. This study underlines the importance of always having a control group when evaluating vaginal prolapse.

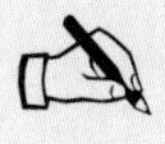

Female pelvic organ prolapse: a comparison of triphasic dynamic MR imaging and triphasic fluoroscopic cystocolpoproctography.

F Kelvin, DDT Maglinte, DS Hale, JT Benson. *Am J Radiol* 2000; **174**: 81–8.

BACKGROUND. Imaging of vaginal prolapse is not very advanced and the optimal method has not been determined. It is felt that by imaging vaginal prolapse accurately the treatment of vaginal prolapse will improve.

INTERPRETATION. This study involved 10 patients with vaginal prolapse who underwent triphasic dynamic magnetic resonance imaging in the supine position and triphasic fluoroscopic cystocolpoproctography which involved using contrast to opacify the bladder, vagina and rectum. Both techniques appear to be equally good at visualizing rectoceles and cystoceles. However, both techniques appear to have deficiencies in identifying enteroceles and sigmoidoceles. Interestingly, the enteroceles were less protuberant on dynamic magnetic resonance imaging which may indicate that the supine position in magnetic resonance imaging alters the visualization of pelvic organ prolapse. There was no preference by the patients for either imaging technique.

Comment

This study unfortunately did not really compare the imaging techniques, but discriminated between the different positions of the patients during imaging.

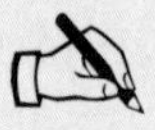

Dynamic MR imaging of the pelvic floor in asymptomatic subjects.

V Goh, S Halligan, G Kaplan, JC Healy, CI Bartram. *Am J Radiol* 2000; **174**: 661–6.

BACKGROUND. Determination of the normal values of dynamic imaging of the pelvic floor has not been carried out. These are required for the test to have any validity in the treatment of vaginal prolapse.

INTERPRETATION. Fifty healthy adult volunteers, 25 men and 25 women, were prospectively recruited and examined using dynamic magnetic resonance imaging. All subjects were interviewed and established as healthy using a validated questionnaire. Axial, coronal and sagittal magnetic resonance imaging was performed at rest during maximum pelvic strain which they practised prior to imaging the pelvic floor, even though it was noted that the bladder, uterus and anorectal junction all descended somewhat on straining. The anorectal angle did not change on straining nor did the levator plate angle. Interestingly, the pelvic floor hiatus area did increase on straining as did the perimeter. It was interesting in this carefully selected group that seven volunteers did indeed have pelvic prolapse in spite of not having any symptoms.

Comment

This study underlines the importance of studying normal asymptomatic controls to evaluate any new test as the level of abnormality in asymptomatic volunteers may be high.

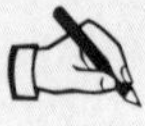

MR-based three-dimensional modelling of the normal pelvic floor in women: quantification of muscle mass.

JR Field, H Dumanli, AG Schreyer, *et al. Am J Radiol* 2000; **174**: 657–60.

BACKGROUND. The pelvic floor is thought to become damaged during childbirth and this is felt to be the possible trigger for vaginal prolapse later in life. By quantifying the various parameters of the pelvic floor it is hoped that the missing component which leads to vaginal prolapse will be discovered.

INTERPRETATION. Ten healthy nulliparous female volunteers underwent magnetic resonance imaging of the pelvis and three-dimensional colour-coded models of pelvic bones, organs and three major components of the levator ani were created and source images were used to measure muscle width, signal intensity and to identify ligamentous structures. Using a three-dimensional model the volume of the levator ani muscle, the angle of the levator plate, posterior urethrovesical angle and the distance of the bladder neck from the symphysis pubis and the pubococcygeal line were calculated. The average volume of the levator ani muscle was 46.6 ml, the average width of the levator hiatus was 41.7 mm and the average posterior urethrovesical angle was 143.5°. The muscle morphology, signal intensity and volume were relatively uniform in healthy young women.

Comment

It was interesting that the authors commented on the levator ani hiatus being much smaller than has been quoted as occurring with pelvic organ prolapse. This method of imaging will lead to some very interesting findings in the treatment of patients with pelvic organ prolapse and urinary incontinence.

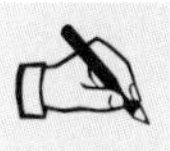

Diagnosis of anal sphincter tears by postpartum endosonography to predict fecal incontinence.

DL Faltin, M Boulvain, O Irion, S Bretones, C Stan, A Weil. *Obstet Gynecol* 2000; **95**: 643–7.

BACKGROUND. **Anal sphincter defects have been found to be associated with faecal incontinence later in life. There is a question about whether the defects are present immediately after childbirth or develop later in life.**

INTERPRETATION. This group studied women immediately after vaginal delivery and those who were thought not to have any anal sphincter defects. To determine whether any defects could be seen with endosonography the sonographer was blind to the delivery and the obstetricians and the women were not informed of any results of the endosonography. Three months after delivery, the investigators assessed the women for faecal incontinence using self-administered questionnaires. Clinically undetected tears of the anal sphincter were diagnosed by anal endosonography in 42 of 150 women (28%). The external anal sphincter alone was involved in 30 women (20%) and the internal anal sphincter alone was involved in two (1.3%), with both being involved in 10 women (7%). The postal questionnaire was returned by the majority of women (144) and faecal incontinence was reported by 22 women (15%). This mainly consisted of incontinence to flatus alone. Clinically undetected anal sphincter tears diagnosed on endosonography were associated with faecal incontinence 3 months after delivery, having an odds ratio of 8.8. The sensitivity of anal endosonography was 68% with a positive predictive value of 37%.

Comment

This raises the whole issue of anal endosonography being a very poor method of screening for anal sphincter defects.

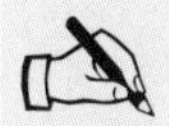

Are sphincter defects the cause of anal incontinence after vaginal delivery?

L Abramowitz, I Sobhani, R Ganansia, *et al. Dis Colon Rectum* 2000; **43**: 590–6.

BACKGROUND. **It is being questioned as to whether anal sphincter defects are the actual cause of faecal incontinence.**

INTERPRETATION. In this study, 259 women were studied 6 weeks before and 8 weeks after delivery. They filled in a questionnaire to assess faecal incontinence and underwent endoanal ultrasound. The internal and external anal sphincters were analysed by two independent observers: a total of 233 patients (90%) were assessed, of whom 31 underwent Caesarean section. De novo sphincter defects were observed in 17% in the postpartum period only after vaginal delivery. These disruptions occurred with the same incidence in first and second childbirth. Independent risk factors for sphincter defects were forceps (12), perineal tears (16), episiotomy (6.6) and parity (8.8). The overall rate of anal incontinence was 9%, but among those women only 45% had sphincter defects. Anal incontinence appears to be multifactorial and anal sphincter defects account for only 45% of these problems.

Comment

This study shows that anal endosonography has revolutionized the understanding of the pathogenesis of urinary incontinence and has reduced the importance of pelvic neuropathy as a cause but, undoubtedly, vaginal childbirth remains the major contributory factor to anal sphincter damage. This study is interesting in that it shows that sphincter defects may not be the only cause and there may also be other factors which are, as yet, undiscovered.

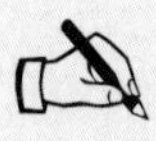

Anal sphincter electromyography after vaginal delivery: neuropathic insufficiency or normal wear and tear?

S Podnar, A Lukanovi, D Voduek. *Neurourol Urodynam* 2000; **19**: 249–57.

BACKGROUND. This study was performed to evaluate the potential role of vaginal delivery on innervation of the external anal sphincter.

INTERPRETATION. Forty-four women, 18 nulliparous and 26 of varying parity, without vaginal prolapse, urogynaecological, anorectal or neurological dysfunction were included. Using concentric needle electromyography in all the patients' anal sphincters, the motor unit potentials and interference pattern for the sphincter muscles were analysed and there were no differences between the measured unit potentials between the groups, other than some difference in the interference patterns. Interestingly, parous women with slight stress incontinence had less pathological parameters than those without stress incontinence.

Comment

This study is interesting as it shows how misleading electromyography can be and how difficult it can be to show that there has been any damage when there may have been catastrophic problems occurring with the anal sphincter. This test in not only painful but probably clinically still awaits a place.

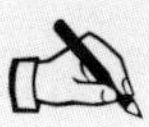

Anatomy of pelvic arteries adjacent to the sacrospinous ligament: importance of the coccygeal branch of the inferior gluteal artery.

J Thompson, J Gibb, R Genadry, L Burrows, N Lambrou, J Buller. *Am J Obstet Gynecol* 1999; **94**: 973–7.

B ACKGROUND . **The surgical anatomy around the sacrospinous ligament has not been fully investigated and may help prevent complications.**

I NTERPRETATION . Twenty-three cadavers were dissected and the sacrospinous ligament examined to disclose the pudendal vessels and nerves passing medial and inferior to the ischial spine. It was noted that the pudendal artery ran anterior to the sacrotuberous ligament which passed behind the ischial spine. The inferior gluteal artery passed between the sciatic nerve and sacrospinous ligament. There was a 3–5 mm window where the inferior gluteal vessel was left uncovered above the superior edge of the sacrospinous ligament and below the lower edge of the main body of the sciatic nerve plexus. Additionally the coccygeal branch of the inferior gluteal artery passed immediately behind the mid-portion of the sacrospinous ligament and pierced the sacrotuberous ligament in multiple sites.

Comment

The safe zone along the sacrospinous ligament is 2.5 cm medial to the ischial spine where there were no major vessels apart from a few twigs of the coccygeal branch. Additionally, it is important that the entire thickness of the sacrospinous ligament should not be used as there are vessels behind the ligament which may be damaged.

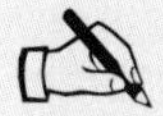

The anatomic and functional outcomes of defect-specific rectocele repairs.

W Porter, A Steele, P Walsh, N Kohli, M Karram. *Am J Obstet Gynecol* 1999; **181**: 1353–9.

B ACKGROUND . **Fascial defect repairs of vaginal prolapse are thought to be an improvement on previous methods of performing vaginal prolapse repairs.**

I NTERPRETATION . This was a retrospective observational study of 125 women who underwent site-specific posterior vaginal repair which was performed with or without other pelvic procedures. A physical examination was performed 6 months after the operation to determine anatomical success. The women were examined at maximum Valsalva in the supine position which is known to be unreliable. Eighty-two per cent of the women were followed up using quality of life, sexual function and bowel function questionnaires. All aspects of living had improved significantly, sexual function did not appear to be affected. Dyspareunia was significantly cured after the operation in 73% of the women and worsened in 19%. Bowel symptoms appeared to be significantly improved.

Comment

This study suggests that defect-specific posterior colporrhaphy is equal or superior to traditional posterior colporrhaphy. Unfortunately this study group did not use a prolapse quality of life questionnaire so it is very difficult to determine if this is a real finding or merely a finding with a significant placebo effect as the patients have just been operated on.

Conclusion

There have been many new articles in the past year reflecting changing views on the aetiology and treatment of both urinary incontinence and vaginal prolapse.

References

1. Thomas TM, Egan M, Walgrove A, Meade TW. The prevalence of faecal and double incontinence. *Comm Med* 1984; **6**: 216–20.

2. Brocklehurst JC. Urinary incontinence in the community—analysis of a MORI poll. *Br Med J* 1993; **306**: 832–4.

3. James MC, Jackson SL, Shepherd AM, *et al.* Can detrusor instability really be discounted with a history of pure stress urinary incontinence? *Int Urogyne J* 1997; **8**: S53.

4. Salvatore S, Khullar V, Cardozo LD, *et al.* Ambulatory urodynamics: do we need it? *Neurourol Urodynam* 1999; **18**: 321–1.

5. Reynard JM, Cannon A, Yang Q, Abrams P. A novel therapy for nocturnal polyuria: a double-blind randomized trial of frusemide against placebo. *Br J Urol* 1998; **81**: 215–8.

6. Bump RC, Sugerman HJ, Fantl JA, McClish DK. Obesity and lower urinary tract function in women: effect of surgically induced weight loss. *Am J Obstet Gynecol* 1993; **167**: 392–7.

7. Burns PA, Pranikoff K, Nochajksi TH, Hadley EC, Levy KJ. A comparison of effectiveness of biofeedback and pelvic muscle exercise treatment of stress incontinence in older community-dwelling women. *J Gerontol* 1993; **48**: M167–74.

8. Henalla SM, Hutchins CJ, Robinson P, Macvicar J. Non-operative methods in the treatment of female genuine stress incontinence of urine. *J Obstet Gynaecol* 1989; **9**: 222–5.

9. O'Brien J, Austin M, Sethi P, O'Boyle P. Urinary incontinence: prevalence, need for treatment and effectiveness of intervention by nurse. *Br Med J* 1991; **303**: 1308–12.

10. Hahn I, Sommar S, Fall M. A comparative study of pelvic floor training and electrical stimulation for the treatment of genuine stress urinary incontinence. *Neurourol Urodynam* 1991; **10**: 545–54.

11. Hofbauer VJ, Preisinger F, Nurnberger N. Der stellenwert der physiokotherapie bei der weiblichen genuinen stress-inkontinenz. *Z Urol Nephrol* 1990; **83**: 249–54.

12. Laycock J, Jerwood D. Does pre-modulated interferential cure genuine stress incontinence? *Physiotherapy* 1993; **79**: 553–60.

13. Smith JJ. Intravaginal stimulation randomized trial. *J Urol* 1996; **155**: 127–30.

14. Klarskov P, Belving D, Bischoff N, Dorph S, Gerstenberg TC. Pelvic floor exercise versus surgery for female urinary stress incontinence. *Urol Int* 1986; **41**: 129–32.

15. Tapp A, Hills B, Cardozo LD. Randomised study comparing pelvic floor physiotherapy with the Burch colposuspension [Abstract]. *Neurourol Urodynam* 1989; **8**: 356–7.

16. Lose G, Jorgensen L, Thunedborg P. 24 hour home pad weighing test versus 1 hour ward test in the assessment of mild stress incontinence. *Acta Obstet Gynecol Scand* 1989; **68**: 211–5.

17. Davila GW. Introl bladder neck support prosthesis: a nonsurgical urethropexy. *J Endourol* 1996; **10**: 293–6.

18. Boos K, Anders K, Hextall A, Toozs-Hobson P, Cardozo L. Randomised trial of Reliance versus Femassist devices in the management of genuine stress incontinence. *Neurourol Urodynam* 1998; **17**: 455–6.

19. Blowman C, Pickles C, Emery S, Creates V, Towell L. Prospective double blind controlled trial of intensive physiotherapy with and without stimulation of the pelvic floor in the treatment of genuine stress incontinence. *Physiotherapy* 1991; **77**: 727.

20. Luber KM, Wolde-Tsadik G. Efficacy of functional electrical stimulation in treating genuine stress incontinence: a randomized clinical trial. *Neurourol Urodynam* 1997; **16**: 132–3.

21. Sand PK, Richardson DA, Staskin DR, Swift SE, Appell RA. Pelvic floor electrical stimulation in the treatment of genuine stress incontinence: a multicenter, placebo-controlled trial. *Am J Obstet Gynecol* 1995; **173**: 72–9.

22. Brubaker L, Benson JT, Bent A, Clark A, Shott S. Transvaginal electrical stimulation for female urinary incontinence. *Am J Obstet Gynecol* 1997; **177**: 334–8.

23. Jarvis GJ, Millar DR. Controlled trial of bladder drill for detrusor instability. *Br Med J* 1980; **281**: 1322–3.

24. Fantl JA, Wyman JF, McClish DK, *et al.* Efficacy of bladder training in older women with urinary incontinence. *J Am Med Assoc* 1991; **265**: 609–13.

25. Colombo M, Zanetta G, Scalambrino S, Milani R. Oxybutynin and bladder retraining in the management of female urinary urge incontinence. *Int Urogynecol J* 1995; **6**: 63–7.

26. Szonyi G, Collas DM, Ding YY, Malone Lee JG. Oxybutynin with bladder retraining for detrusor instability in elderly people: a randomized controlled trial. *Age Ageing* 1995; **24**: 287–91.

27. Jarvis GJ. A controlled trial of bladder drill and drug therapy in the management of detrusor instability. *Br J Urol* 1981; **53**: 565–7.

28. Abrams P, Freeman RN, Anderstrom C, Mattiasson A. Efficacy and tolerability of tolterodine vs. oxybutynin and placebo in patients with detrusor instability. *J Urol* 1997; **157**(Suppl.): 103.

29. Appell RA. Clinical efficacy and safety of tolterodine in the treatment of overactive bladder: a pooled analysis. *Urology* 1997; **50**: 90–6.

30. Stohrer M, Bauer P, Giannetti BM, Richter R, Burgdorfer H, Murtz G. Effect of trospium chloride on urodynamic parameters in patients with detrusor hyperreflexia due

to spinal cord injuries: a multicenter placebo controlled double-blind trial. *Urol Int* 1991; **47**: 138–43.

31.   Madersbacher H, Stohrer M, Richter R, Burgdorfer H, Hachen HJ, Murtz G. Trospium chloride versus oxybutynin: a randomized, double-blind, multicentre trial in the treatment of detrusor hyper-reflexia. *Br J Urol* 1995; **75**: 452–6.

32.   Moore KH, Hay DM, Imrie AE, Watson A, Goldstein M. Oxybutynin hydrochloride (3 mg) in the treatment of women with idiopathic detrusor instability. *Br J Urol* 1990; **66**: 479–85.

33.   Tapp AJ, Cardozo LD, Versi E, Cooper D. The treatment of detrusor instability in postmenopausal women with oxybutynin chloride: a double blind placebo controlled study [see comments]. *Br J Obstet Gynaecol* 1990; **97**: 521–6.

34.   Thuroff J, Bunke B, Ebner A, *et al.* Randomised double-blind multicentre trial on treatment of frequency, urgency and incontinence related to detrusor hyperactivity: oxybutynin vs. propantheline vs. placebo. *J Urol* 1991; **145**: 813–7.

35.   Burton G. A randomised cross over trial comparing oxybutynin taken three times a day or taken 'when needed'. *Neurourol Urodynam* 1994; **13**: 351–2.

36.   Nilsson CG, Lukkari E, Haarala M, Kivela A, Hakonen T, Kiilholma P. Comparison of a 10-mg controlled release oxybutynin tablet with a 5-mg oxybutynin tablet in urge incontinent patients. *Neurourol Urodynam* 1997; **16**: 533–42.

37.   Castelden CM, George CF, Benwick AJ. Imipramine: a possible alternative to current therapy for urinary incontinence in the elderly. *J Urol* 1981; **125**: 318–20.

38.   Lose G, Jorgensen L, Thunedborg P. Doxepin in the treatment of female detrusor overactivity: a randomised double-blind crossover study. *J Urol* 1989; **142**: 1024–7.

39.   Hilton P, Stanton SL. The use of desmopressin (DDAVP) in nocturnal urine frequency in the female. *Br J Urol* 1982; **54**: 252–5.

40.   Jarvis GJ. Surgery for genuine stress incontinence. *Br J Obstet Gynaecol* 1994; **101**: 371–4.

41.   Stanton SL, Chamberlain GVP, Holmes DM. Randomised study of the anterior repair and colposuspension operation in the control of genuine stress incontinence [Abstract]. *Proceedings of the International Continence Society* 1986, pp. 236–7.

42.   Bergman A, Ballard CA, Koonings PP. Comparison of three different surgical procedures for genuine stress incontinence: prospective randomized study [see comments]. *Am J Obstet Gynecol* 1989; **160**: 1102–6.

43.   Colombo M, Scalambrino S, Maggioni A, Milani R. Burch colposuspension versus modified Marshall–Marchetti–Krantz urethropexy for primary genuine stress urinary incontinence: a prospective, randomized clinical trial. *Am J Obstet Gynecol* 1994; **171**: 1573–9.

44.   Milani R, Scalambrino S, Quadri G, Algeri M, Marchesin A. Marshall–Marchetti–Krantz procedure and Burch colposuspension in the surgical treatment of female urinary incontinence. *Br J Obstet Gynaecol* 1985; **92**: 1050–3.

45.   Milani R, Magsoni A, Colombo M, *et al.* Burch colposuspension versus modified Marshall–Marchetti–Krantz for stress urinary incontinence [Abstract]. *Neurourol Urodynam* 1991; **10**: 454–5.

46.   Colombo M, Milani R, Vitobello D, Maggioni A. A randomized comparison of Burch colposuspension and abdominal paravaginal defect repair for female stress urinary incontinence [see comments]. *Am J Obstet Gynecol* 1996; **175**: 78–84.

47. Richmond DH, Sutherst JR. Burch colposuspension or sling for stress incontinence? A prospective study using transrectal ultrasound. *Br J Urol* 1989; **64**: 600–3.

48. Burton G. A randomised comparison of laparoscopic and open colposuspension [Abstract]. *Neurourol Urodynam* 1994; **7**: 497–8.

49. Burton G. A three year prospective randomised urodynamic study comparing open and laparoscopic colposuspension [Abstract]. *Neurourol Urodynam* 1997; **16**: 353–4.

50. Su TH, Wang KG, Hsu CY, Wei HJ, Hong BK. Prospective comparison of laparoscopic and traditional colposuspensions in the treatment of genuine stress incontinence [Review]. *Acta Obstet Gynecol Scand* 1997; **76**: 576–82.

51. Bump RC. Racial comparisons and contrasts in urinary incontinence and pelvic organ prolapse. *Obstet Gynecol* 1993; **81**: 421–5.

52. Sze EHM, Miklos JR, Partoli L, Roat TW, Karam MM. Sacrospinous ligament fixation with transvaginal needle suspension for advanced pelvic organ prolapse and stress incontinence. *Obstet Gynecol* 1997; **89**: 94–6.

53. Julian TM. The efficacy of Marlex mesh in the repair of severe, recurrent vaginal prolapse of the anterior midvaginal wall. *Am J Obstet Gynecol* 1996; **175**: 1472–5.

13

Screening for chromosomal and structural fetal anomalies in early pregnancy

Introduction

First trimester ultrasonography was initially introduced to confirm fetal viability and to date the pregnancy accurately. With the improved resolution of ultrasound and the development of transvaginal probes, it has become feasible to examine the fetal anatomy in the first trimester of pregnancy.

Screening for chromosomal abnormalities can now be performed by the measurement of a subcutaneous collection of fluid in the fetal nuchal region that can be visualized by ultrasonography as nuchal translucency (NT) at 10–14 weeks of gestation. Since the 1990s, a series of studies has reported that increased NT is associated with chromosomal defects and a wide range of fetal abnormalities and genetic syndromes. In addition, first trimester ultrasound has a role in the detection of structural anomalies. The sonographic features may be similar to those described in the second and third trimester, but in some conditions there are characteristic sonographic features confined to the first trimester.

Recently, the emphasis of maternal serum screening for trisomy 21 has moved from the second to the first trimester of pregnancy. Two serum markers, free β human chorionic gonadotrophin (β-hCG) and pregnancy-associated plasma protein-A (PAPP-A), are particularly useful at this gestation. Screening in the first trimester will provide early reassurance for the majority of patients. In those cases where an abnormality is detected the parents will have the option of early prenatal diagnosis.

One of the most exciting areas of current research is aimed at the development of a non-invasive method for prenatal diagnosis based on the isolation and examination of fetal cells found in the maternal circulation. A variety of nucleated fetal cells have been demonstrated in the maternal circulation, including erythrocytes, lymphocytes and trophoblasts. The number of fetal cells within the maternal circulation is extremely small and therefore a process of cell enrichment is required prior to analysis. At present, this complex process is being developed with the aim of ultimately replacing invasive prenatal diagnosis.

Screening for chromosomal defects

Screening for trisomy 21 is nowadays a well-established part of routine antenatal care in the UK. However, there continues to be debate over the most practical and cost-effective method (Table 13.1). Current screening strategies are based on various combinations of parameters including maternal age, NT and serum biochemical markers.

Maternal age

The risks for trisomies 21, 18 and 13 increase with advancing maternal age and therefore screening is based on the detection of all three trisomies, even though trisomy 21 has the highest birth prevalence. The prevalence of trisomy 21 in the UK has been estimated at 1.4 per 1000 live births in the UK.

Despite 20 years of screening for fetal trisomies by advanced maternal age, there has not been a notable effect on the birth incidence of trisomy 21. There are several reasons for this. First, the great majority of affected babies are born to women less than 35 years of age, by virtue of the much larger number of babies born to women of this age. Women who are 35 years and over contribute only 20–30% of the babies with trisomy 21. Second, the uptake of invasive fetal karyotyping in the 'high-risk' group is generally less than 50%. Third, an expected fall in the birth prevalence of

Table 13.1 Summary table of current screening tests for trisomy 21

Screening test	Advantages	Disadvantages
Maternal age	Simple, cheap	Low sensitivity
Nuchal translucency (10–14 weeks)	Early Association with structural anomalies and genetic syndromes Applicable in multiple pregnancy	Detection of affected fetuses destined to miscarry
First trimester serum screening	Improved detection rate when combined with nuchal translucency Rapid results allowing one-stop counselling session	Availability
Second trimester serum screening	Screening for neural tube and anterior abdominal wall defects Assessment of placental function	Second trimester termination of pregnancy Not applicable to multiple pregnancies

trisomy 21 may have been reversed by the mean maternal age increasing from 26.1 years in 1970 to 29 years now.

The poor performance of screening for trisomy 21 on the basis of advanced maternal age is now universally accepted and this has necessitated the introduction of newer screening modalities.

NT

During the last decade, there have been a number of studies that have shown an association between increased NT and chromosomal defects, fetal structural abnormalities and genetic syndromes. However, the majority of these studies were either performed in high-risk populations (e.g. women undergoing fetal karyotyping for advanced maternal age) or were too small in size to comment on the effectiveness of screening based on NT. The studies from these high-risk populations have reported a mean prevalence of chromosomal defects of 29%, ranging from 11 to 88% [1]. Consistent with this are reports from other series with detection rates of 29–91% [2].

In an unselected population of 20 804 pregnancies, the risk for fetal trisomies 21, 18 and 13 was derived by multiplying the maternal age-related risk by a likelihood ratio, which depended on the degree of deviation in NT from the normal median for crown–rump length (CRL) [3]. The detection rate for trisomy 21 in this study was 77% and 78% for the other chromosomal defects, with a false-positive rate of 5%.

The only other study with sufficient numbers to allow assessment of effectiveness of screening by NT is that of Taipale *et al.* [4] with 10 010 pregnancies. The sensitivity of screening at 10–14 weeks was 66% for a screen-positive rate of 0.9%. The largest study to date on NT screening for trisomy 21 is the multicentre study reported by Snijders *et al.* [5].

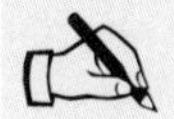

UK multicentre project on assessment of risk of trisomy 21 by maternal age and fetal nuchal translucency thickness at 10–14 weeks of gestation.
RJM Snijders, P Noble, N Sebire, A Souka, KH Nicolaides. *Lancet* 1998; **352:** 343–6.

BACKGROUND. Prenatal diagnosis of trisomy 21 currently relies on invasive testing in pregnancies considered to be at high risk based on maternal age, second trimester biochemical or ultrasound screening and family history. This large study involving 22 centres in the UK investigated the assessment of risk for trisomy 21 by a combination of age and fetal NT, measured by ultrasound at 10–14 weeks of gestation.

INTERPRETATION. The ultrasound scans were performed by a total of 306 appropriately trained sonographers. Strict sonographic criteria (Table 13.2), as defined by the Fetal Medicine Foundation, were used to achieve uniformity of results from different operators. In each pregnancy, the fetal CRL and NT were measured and the risk

Table 13.2 Ultrasonographic criteria for measurement of crown–rump length and nuchal translucency

Good mid-sagittal section of fetus
The fetus should occupy at least 75% of image
Neutral position
Clear distinction between fetal skin and amnion
Exclude nuchal umbilical cord
Measurement of maximum thickness of subcutaneous translucency between skin and soft
   tissue overlying cervical spine

Source: Fetal Medicine Foundation, London.

for trisomy 21 was calculated from the maternal age and gestational age-related prevalence, multiplied by a likelihood ratio depending on the deviation from normal in NT for CRL. The calculation of risk was based on a model devised from the first 20 804 pregnancies |3|.

100 311 singleton pregnancies with live fetuses were examined by ultrasonography at 10–14 weeks of gestation. Of these, 4184 (4.2%) were excluded from analysis as a result of loss to follow-up or change of address or because the pregnancy resulted in a miscarriage and no fetal karyotyping was undertaken. The study group therefore consisted of 96 127 singleton pregnancies, including 326 cases of trisomy 21. The median gestation at the time of screening was 12 weeks (range 10–14 weeks) and the median maternal age was 31 years (range 14–49 years). In 13 315 (13.3%) cases, the maternal age was at least 37 years. The fetal NT was above the 95th centile for CRL in 4767 (4.8%) pregnancies including 234 (71.8%) with trisomy 21. The estimated risk for trisomy 21 based on maternal age and fetal NT was greater than 1 in 300 in 8651 (8.6%) pregnancies including 268 (82.2%) with trisomy 21. For a screen-positive rate of 5%, the sensitivity was 77% (95% CI 72–82%).

This study also addressed the issue of intrauterine lethality of fetuses with trisomy 21 between the 10–14-week scan and term. Trisomy 21 was diagnosed in 326 pregnancies, either antenatally or postnatally. On the basis of the maternal age distribution of the 96 127 pregnancies and the maternal age-related prevalence of trisomy 21 in live births, it was estimated that 266 babies with trisomy 21 would have been live born had there not been any antenatal testing and selective termination of affected pregnancies. On the extreme assumption that all intrauterine deaths would have been from the group with increased NT, the number of trisomy 21 live births in this group would have been 58 (22%) of the total 266 potential live births with trisomy 21. Consequently, assessment of risk by a combination of maternal age and fetal NT, followed by invasive diagnostic testing for those with a risk of 1 in 300 or higher and selective termination of affected fetuses, would have reduced the potential live birth prevalence of trisomy 21 by 78%.

The authors concluded that, because of a relatively low prevalence of trisomy 21, even with this method of risk assessment, about 30 invasive tests are required to identify one affected fetus.

Comment

This study shows that, for a cut-off risk of 1 in 300, the sensitivity of this method of screening was 82.2% with a false-positive rate of 8.3%. The positive predictive value was 3.2% and the negative predictive value was 99.9%. Alternatively, at a 5% false-positive rate, approximately 80% of fetuses with trisomy 21 were detected.

To date, this is the largest multicentre study on antenatal detection of trisomy 21 by an assessment of risk based on maternal age and NT thickness at 10–14 weeks of gestation. The study clearly defines the criteria for measurement of NT to achieve uniformity of results. In addition, all 306 sonographers had attended theoretical and practical courses and submitted 50 NT images that were reviewed prior to recruiting patients. The large number of sonographers and centres that participated in this study suggest that the results are applicable to routine practice.

Because this was an interventional study, women with fetuses with an increased NT thickness were offered the option of fetal karyotyping. The concern is that those fetuses with an increased NT may be destined to miscarry spontaneously and by implication a spontaneous miscarriage is 'converted' into a termination of pregnancy. The study addressed this issue by calculating the expected number of live births based on the maternal age distribution of the women. From their calculation, screening based on NT with a false-positive rate of 5% would have reduced the live birth prevalence of trisomy 21 by 78%.

There has been no cost–benefit analysis of NT screening compared with serum screening to date. It has been suggested that automated assays for biochemical analysis provide cheap and reproducible results, while first trimester ultrasound requires expensive equipment and increased manpower. However, a prerequisite to the analysis of any biochemical marker requires accurate dating of the pregnancy and this is done by ultrasound. With ultrasound machines that are presently used in routine practice, all appropriately trained sonographers can date the pregnancy and measure the NT at the same time |**3**|.

Maternal serum biochemistry

The discovery in the early 1980s that maternal serum α-fetoprotein (AFP) levels were reduced on average in trisomy 21 pregnancies resulted in a radically different approach to antenatal screening. Initially, a low serum AFP level *per se* was regarded as justification for prenatal diagnosis regardless of maternal age. However, it soon became obvious that it was more efficient to integrate all the available information by calculating an individual's risk of trisomy 21 given the AFP level and maternal age.

Throughout the 1990s, additional maternal serum markers were found to be associated with trisomy 21 including free α-hCG, free β-hCG, PAPP-A, inhibin A, unconjugated oestriol (uE3) and neutrophil alkaline phosphatase. This resulted in a steady increase in the extent and complexity of trisomy 21 screening. Many of the serum markers were subsequently shown to be effective in both first and second trimester screening |**6**|.

Second trimester

In 1988, Wald *et al.* |**7**| analysed maternal serum samples from 77 trisomy 21 pregnancies and 385 normal controls at 16 weeks of gestation. Using a combination of maternal age with serum hCG, AFP and uE3, this method of screening for trisomy 21 yielded a detection rate of 59% for a false-positive rate of 5%.

However, the most effective combination of serum markers remains contentious, as screening performance varies according to the choice of markers used and whether ultrasound is used to estimate the gestational age. On the basis of results from prospective screening studies (demonstration projects), it appears that for a screen-positive rate of 5%, the detection rate for trisomy 21 after revision of gestation by ultrasound is about 60%. This detection rate is similar both for the combination of maternal age with hCG, AFP and uE3 as well as the combination of maternal age with AFP and free β-hCG.

With the 'quadruple' test, based on a combination of maternal age with hCG, AFP, uE3 and inhibin A, the estimated detection rate for trisomy 21 is about 76% for a 5% screen-positive rate. However, these predictions are yet to be confirmed in prospective screening research. Recently, studies have reported on the value of first trimester biochemical screening.

First trimester

The markers free β-hCG (which is elevated in trisomy 21) and PAPP-A (which is lower) are particularly useful in the first trimester. It has been estimated that the combination of these markers with maternal age would identify about 60–65% of trisomy 21 pregnancies for a screen-positive rate of 5% |8|, which is similar to second trimester biochemical screening.

Recent interest in prenatal screening for trisomy 21 has focused on the combination of fetal NT and maternal serum biochemistry in the first trimester of pregnancy.

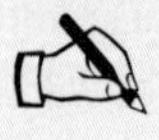

A screening program for trisomy 21 at 10–14 weeks using fetal nuchal translucency, maternal serum free beta-human chorionic gonadotrophin and pregnancy-associated plasma protein-A.

K Spencer, V Souter, N Tul, R Snijders, KH Nicolaides. *Ultrasound Obstet Gynecol* 1999; **13**: 231–7.

BACKGROUND. Of the serum markers that have been investigated for first trimester screening, only free β-hCG and PAPP-A have been shown to have any value. The aim of this study was to examine the potential impact of combining these markers with maternal age and fetal NT in screening for trisomy 21 at 10–14 weeks of gestation.

INTERPRETATION. The study population was derived from two groups of women. The first group comprised women with singleton pregnancies who had been referred for fetal karyotyping because screening, by a combination of maternal age and fetal NT, had identified them as being at high risk for trisomy 21. The second group consisted of self-referred women for assessment of risk.

This retrospective study assessed 210 singleton pregnancies with trisomy 21 and 946 chromosomally normal controls, matched for maternal age, gestational age and sample storage time. Maternal blood was collected at the time of the scan and serum free β-hCG and PAPP-A were measured with a random access immunoassay analyser based on cryptate emission technology. Reproducible measurements were obtained within 30 min of sample collection.

Regression analysis was performed to derive the relationship between free β-hCG and PAPP-A in multiples of the median (MoM) with gestational age. Correction of each MoM for maternal weight was also performed using a reciprocal linear regression weight correction procedure. Assessment of the performance of various marker combinations was examined using standard statistical modelling techniques. The measured parameters (corrected for maternal weight) for free β-hCG and PAPP-A and the reported parameters for NT from 95 476 normal and 326 trisomy 21 pregnancies were used. A series of 15 000 random MoM values were selected for each marker from within the distributions of the affected and unaffected pregnancies. These values were used to calculate likelihood ratios for the various marker combinations. The likelihood ratios were then used together with the age-related risk for trisomy 21 in the first trimester to calculate the expected detection rate of affected pregnancies, at a fixed false-positive rate, in a population with the maternal age distribution of pregnancies in England and Wales. The distribution of each parameter was thus determined both in the trisomy 21 group and in the controls.

There was no significant correlation between maternal age either in the control or the trisomy 21 pregnancies for free β-hCG, PAPP-A or NT thickness. When individual marker levels (as MoM) were compared against each other, there was no significant correlation between NT (as MoM) either in the control or in the trisomy 21 pregnancies for free β-hCG and PAPP-A. However, there was a small but significant correlation between free β-hCG in MoM and PAPP-A in MoM.

In the trisomy 21 pregnancies, free β-hCG was above the 95th centile of the controls in 70 (33%) cases and PAPP-A was below the fifth centile in 79 (38%) cases. Using the observed statistical parameters in the previously described mathematical model, the estimated detection rates using various marker combinations with maternal age, at a fixed false-positive rate of 5%, varied from 46% with maternal age and free β-hCG to 89% with maternal age and all three markers (maternal age, NT and serum biochemistry).

Alternatively, at a fixed detection rate of 70%, the false-positive rate was 6% with maternal age and serum biochemistry (free β-hCG and PAPP-A) compared with 1% with maternal age, fetal NT, free β-hCG and PAPP-A. The inclusion of biochemical parameters appeared to add an additional 16% to the detection rate obtained using maternal age and NT alone.

Comment

An important advantage of NT screening over serum screening is the ability to discuss the findings with the patient at the same time. The new technology for biochemical analysis provides rapid measurement of serum markers, thus allowing combined biochemical and sonographic testing with counselling in one-stop clinics for early fetal assessment. Such interdisciplinary clinics would have the advantage of providing a more efficient service.

Wald *et al.* |9| recently reviewed several data sets |7, **10**| to conclude that first trimester screening for trisomy 21 with a combination of NT and serum biochemistry (80% detection rate for a 5% false-positive rate) may be a more effective method of screening than second trimester serum screening alone (76% for a 5% false-positive rate). However, these estimates need verification in large prospective trials. In addition, they do not take into account any association between the markers and spontaneous fetal loss, an issue that would require non-interventional studies.

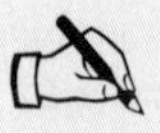

Integrated screening for Down's syndrome based on tests performed during the first and second trimesters.

NJ Wald, HC Watt, AK Hackshaw. *New Engl J Med* 1999; **341**: 521–2.

BACKGROUND. With screening tests for trisomy 21 in the first or second trimester, 5% of women need to undergo amniocentesis in order to detect 60–80% of affected fetuses. The majority of women with screen-positive results have unaffected pregnancies. Not only do false-positive results cause considerable anxiety; diagnostic prenatal diagnosis such as amniocentesis is associated with a 1% risk of miscarriage. A screening test that has a rate of detection similar to those of the current tests but a markedly reduced rate of false-positive results would be of great benefit. An 'integrated' test is proposed whereby measurements of various markers obtained during both first and second trimesters are integrated to provide a single estimated risk for trisomy 21 in the second trimester.

INTERPRETATION. In this study, the performance of antenatal screening for trisomy 21 was estimated on the basis of maternal age combined with published data on the distribution of several first and second trimester markers in pregnancies affected by and those not affected by trisomy 21. The estimates of the performance of first trimester screening (at 10–13 weeks) were based on measurements of NT in 326 affected fetuses and 95 476 unaffected fetuses |5| as well as on measurements of serum PAPP-A and free β-hCG in 77 affected pregnancies and 383 unaffected pregnancies |11|.

The estimates of the performance of second trimester screening (at 14–22 weeks) were based on measurements of serum hCG, AFP, uE3 and inhibin A in a different study on 77 pregnancies affected by trisomy 21 and 385 unaffected pregnancies |10|. The integrated test combined markers measured during both of the first two trimesters. All markers were expressed as MoM for women with unaffected pregnancies at a given gestational age. A multivariate Gaussian model was fitted to the data on first and second trimester markers in the affected and unaffected pregnancies and the likelihood ratio was calculated. This ratio was used to adjust the risk of having a pregnancy at a particular maternal age that, in the absence of screening, would result in a live born infant with trisomy 21.

The performance of the integrated test in screening for trisomy 21 was compared with that of the first and second trimester screening tests by examining the detection rates for specified false-positive rates and the false-positive rates for specified detection rates of each test. Estimates of the number of unaffected fetuses that were lost as a result of invasive testing were obtained from a review of randomized trials |9|.

At a 5% false-positive rate, the estimated rate of detection with the integrated test was 94%, greater than that with the most effective second trimester test (quadruple test, 76%) or first trimester test (combined test, 85%). At a 1% false-positive rate, the estimated rate of detection for the integrated test was 85% (54 and 72% for the quadruple and combined tests, respectively). The integrated test detected at least as many affected pregnancies at a 1% false-positive rate as either first or second trimester screening alone at a 5% false-positive rate. At a 1% false-positive rate, the rate of detection was 85%, as compared with 46% for the triple test. The steep early rise in the rate of detection reflects both high rates of detection and low rates of false-positive results.

Furthermore, even if some centres were not to perform measurement of NT or serum inhibin A, it would still be of benefit to integrate first and second trimester markers into a single screening test. If it was not possible to measure NT, ultrasound would nevertheless be essential to date the pregnancy accurately (by measurement of CRL).

The odds of being affected given a positive result for the integrated test was 1 in 9 (i.e. for every nine invasive procedures performed one pregnancy would be affected with trisomy 21), much lower than that for the first trimester test (1 in 45) or for the best second trimester test (1 in 88). This would result in a substantial reduction in the number of unaffected fetuses lost as a result of invasive testing. Eight fetuses would have been lost per 100 pregnancies found by the integrated test to be affected, as compared with 61 per 100 and 70 per 100 with the best first and second trimester tests, respectively.

To achieve a detection rate of 85% with the integrated test, the risk cut-off would be set at 1 in 120, a level at which the false-positive rate would be 0.9%. Using the second trimester quadruple test or first trimester combined test, a much lower cut-off (1 in 630 or 1 in 540, respectively) would be needed to achieve a similar detection rate and the false-positive rates would be much higher (9.8 and 4.9%). At a 5% false-positive rate, the detection rate of the integrated test would be 95%, but the risk cut-off required to achieve this rate (1 in 940) may be regarded as too low to be clinically acceptable. The reduction of the false-positive rate with the integrated test is particularly evident for older women. For every 100 000 women 35 years of age or older who were screened, only 30 unaffected fetuses would be lost due to diagnostic invasive procedures with the integrated test, as compared with 171 with the triple test.

Comment

The strength of integrated screening is that it may be feasible to maintain a high detection rate with a lower false-positive rate. This should result in fewer amniocenteses and therefore a reduction in the number of normal pregnancies miscarrying. The authors concluded that, for a detection rate of trisomy 21 of about 85%, current screening tests based on either combined first trimester screening or second trimester biochemical screening would have higher false-positive rates of 5 or 10%, respectively, in comparison with 1% with the integrated test. For example, if integrated testing was to replace the widely used triple test, the detection rate would be 85% instead of 65%, with a reduction in invasive diagnostic procedures from 5 to 1%.

However, several critical comments need to be made. First, this study was based on a mathematical model and the figures have yet to be confirmed in prospective studies. Second, increased NT is currently the best single marker for chromosomal abnormality. It therefore seems inappropriate to conceal an abnormal result for up to 4 weeks before discussing the option of fetal karyotyping and further investigation. This is particularly relevant when the NT is above the 99th centile. In this group of fetuses, not only is the risk of chromosomal abnormality increased, but NT is also a marker of structural anomalies and genetic syndromes.

It is important to be aware that the worst scenario is first trimester NT screening with its incumbent false-positive rate followed by second trimester serum screening with an additional false-positive rate (sequential screening). Without appropriate adjustment for previous screening, the invasive karyotyping rate is significantly higher without improving the detection rate for trisomy 21 |**12, 13**|. The majority of fetuses affected by trisomy 21 are detected by NT screening. Consequently, these fetuses are removed from the population, which significantly affects the likelihood ratio for subsequent second trimester screening. It is therefore imperative that the results of NT screening are taken into account if women subsequently request second trimester biochemical screening.

Which tests to use?

It is widely accepted that maternal age alone has a low sensitivity and is no longer valuable as a screening test for trisomy 21. Second trimester serum screening can be applied to all pregnant women and achieves detection rates far superior to maternal age alone. However, second trimester screening is unattractive to many women because of the late stage at which affected pregnancies are identified, when termination of pregnancy is less desirable and more traumatic. This disadvantage also applies to the ultrasound examination at 18–20 weeks of gestation. However, it should be borne in mind that ultrasound has more value than just the detection of markers of chromosomal abnormality.

The ideal method of comparison of NT screening and maternal serum screening would be through randomized studies. On the assumption that the prevalence of trisomy 21 is 1 in 500, the sensitivity of screening with maternal age and NT is about 78% and the sensitivity of screening by maternal age and the quadruple test is about 76%, then in order to prove that 78% is significantly different from 76%, it would be necessary to recruit 9 million patients into a randomized study.

Given the fact that there are either real or perceived major differences in the implications for patients between NT screening [chorionic villous sampling (CVS) at 12 weeks for the screen positive followed by first trimester termination of pregnancy for those who request this] and biochemical screening at 16–17 weeks (amniocentesis at 16 weeks for the screen positive followed by termination after 17 weeks for the affected pregnancies), it is very unlikely that such a study will ever be undertaken. Even if it was carried out, the results would almost certainly become irrelevant because there are many new sonographic and biochemical markers that are rapidly being developed, which would make the results of such a randomized study obsolete.

In the future, if the results of integrated first and second trimester screening are validated, it may be appropriate to combine the results. While there are many advantages of first trimester screening, earlier is not always better. It is important that parents do not feel rushed. The two-stage integrated test, e.g. at 12 and 16 weeks of gestation, gives parents some time to assimilate information, allows spontaneous losses to occur and thus avoids the need to make a decision whether to terminate or not. If the false-positive rate is kept down to 1%, there will be fewer invasive tests and fewer losses of healthy fetuses as well as considerable financial savings.

What is more likely to happen is that sonographic and biochemical markers will be combined in the first trimester of pregnancy. The first trimester has many theoretical advantages and would be the most attractive gestation to perform screening. At present, this would entail the measurement of fetal NT in conjunction with β-hCG and PAPP-A. However, in the future this may entail a detailed anomaly scan and newer biochemical markers in the first trimester.

Ultimately, the decisions that parents make are based on intensely personal values. Some place a premium on early diagnosis enabling them to have the option of early termination of pregnancy. Others may decide that termination is not an option and they may wish to wait for prenatal diagnosis in the second or third trimester to allow appropriate management of labour and referral to a tertiary paediatric unit. The role of those involved in antenatal care is to provide objective information and support to enable the parents to make their own choice.

Screening for structural fetal anomalies and genetic syndromes

At present, the standard of care in the majority of units within the UK is an ultrasound examination at 18–20 weeks of gestation. One of the aims of this examination is to detect structural fetal anomalies. However, during the last decade, advances in ultrasound resolution and the introduction of transvaginal sonography have made it possible to describe the normal anatomy of the fetus and to diagnose or suspect the presence of a wide range of fetal defects in the first trimester of pregnancy. In some conditions, the sonographic features are similar to those described in the second and third trimesters of pregnancy, but in others there are characteristic sonographic features confined to the first trimester.

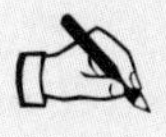

Defects and syndromes in chromosomally normal fetuses with increased nuchal translucency thickness at 10–14 weeks of gestation.

AP Souka, RJ Snijders, A Novakov, W Soares, KH Nicolaides. *Ultrasound Obstet Gynecol* 1998; **11**: 391–400.

B A C K G R O U N D . Increased fetal NT at 10–14 weeks of gestation is a common phenotypic expression of trisomy 21 and other chromosomal defects. Several case reports and small series have also suggested that there may be an association between increased NT and a wide range of fetal abnormalities and genetic syndromes. This large study involving 22 centres in the UK investigated the prevalence of fetal defects and syndromes in 4116 chromosomally normal singleton fetuses with NT thickness above the 95th centile at 10–14 weeks of gestation.

INTERPRETATION. The ultrasound scans were performed by 306 sonographers each of whom had received the Fetal Medicine Foundation certificate of competence in the theory and practice of the 10–14-week scan. Measurements of CRL and NT were carried out according to previously described criteria. Demographic details, ultrasound findings, karyotype results and details of pregnancy outcome were entered into a computer database.

The patients were subdivided into five groups according to NT thickness: 95th centile to 3.4 mm, 3.5–4.4 mm, 4.5–5.4 mm, 5.5–6.4 mm and greater than 6.5 mm. NT normally increases with CRL and the 95th centile was 2.2 mm for a CRL of 38 mm and 2.8 mm for a CRL of 84 mm. The 99th centile did not change significantly with CRL and was about 3.5 mm.

In the 4116 pregnancies, there were 3885 live births that survived the neonatal period, 38 neonatal deaths, 74 spontaneous abortions or intrauterine deaths and 77 terminations at the request of the parents. There was a wide range of structural defects and genetic syndromes and the prevalence of these increased with NT thickness.

The observed prevalence for some of the abnormalities, such as anencephaly, holoprosencephaly, microcephaly, facial cleft, gastroschisis, renal abnormalities, bowel obstruction and spina bifida, may not be different from that in the general population. However, the prevalence of major cardiac defects, diaphragmatic hernia, exomphalos, body stalk anomaly and fetal akinesia deformation sequence appeared to be substantially higher than in the general population and it is therefore likely that there is an association between these abnormalities and increased NT thickness.

Similarly, there may well be an association between increased NT and a wide range of rare skeletal dysplasias and genetic syndromes that are usually found in less than 1 in 10 000 pregnancies. However, the number of affected cases both in the present and previous series of fetuses with increased NT was too small for definite conclusions to be drawn. In addition, the rates of miscarriage and perinatal death increase with fetal NT thickness.

Comment

This study suggests that a correlation exists between increased NT and unfavourable pregnancy outcome such as fetal abnormality and pregnancy loss. However, it is emphasized that NT thickness *per se* does not constitute a fetal abnormality. Indeed, once chromosomal defects have been excluded, about 90% of pregnancies with a NT thickness below 4.5 mm result in healthy live births; the rates for NT of 4.5–6.4 mm and greater than 6.5 mm are about 80 and 45%, respectively.

The authors have also suggested a variety of mechanisms to explain subcutaneous nuchal oedema, including cardiac failure, venous congestion in head and neck, failure of lymphatic drainage, abnormal or delayed development of the lymphatic system and altered composition of subcutaneous connective tissue.

Screening for cardiac defects

Cardiac defects are the most common congenital abnormalities with a birth prevalence of 3–8 per 1000; about half are classified as major because they are either lethal or require surgery and half are asymptomatic. Specialist echocardiography at around 20 weeks of gestation can identify most of the major cardiac defects, but the main challenge in prenatal diagnosis is to identify the high-risk group for referral to specialist centres. Currently, screening is based on examination of the four-chamber view of the heart at the 18–20-week scan, but this identifies only 26% of the major cardiac defects |**14**|.

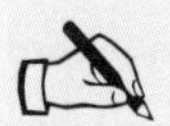

Using fetal nuchal translucency to screen for major congenital cardiac defects at 10–14 weeks of gestation: population based cohort study.

JA Hyett, M Perdu, GK Sharland, RJM Snijders, KH Nicolaides. *Br Med J* 1999; **318**: 81–5.

BACKGROUND. Presently, screening for fetal cardiac abnormalities is based on examination of the four-chamber view and out-flow tracts of the heart during routine ultrasonography at 18–20 weeks of gestation. Studies involving pathological examination in both chromosomally abnormal and normal fetuses with increased NT at 10–14 weeks of gestation have demonstrated a high prevalence of cardiac defects |15|. This retrospective study examined the utility of measuring fetal NT thickness in screening for major defects of the heart and great arteries at 10–14 weeks of gestation.

INTERPRETATION. In this study, 29 154 singleton pregnancies with presumed chromosomally normal fetuses were investigated. The prevalence of major defects of the heart and great arteries was 1.7 per 1000 (50/29 154) cases. This included 18 pregnancies that were diagnosed antenatally by scan at 16–31 weeks of gestation, 13 diagnosed at pathological examination after intrauterine death or termination of pregnancy for conditions other than cardiac defects and 19 diagnosed in live births. There were essentially six groups of cardiac defects: tetralogy of Fallot, hypoplastic left heart, transposition of the great arteries, ventricular and atrio-ventricular septal defects and a group of other complex defects.

The prevalence of major abnormalities of the heart and great arteries increased exponentially with NT thickness from about four per 1000 for NT of 3.4 mm (95th centile), 27 per 1000 for NT of 3.5–4.4 mm, 43 per 1000 for NT of 4.5–5.4 mm, 63 per 1000 for NT of 5.5–6.4 mm, to 169 per 1000 for NT above 6.5 mm.

Of the 50 cases of major cardiac defects, 56% were in the subgroup of 1822 pregnancies with fetal NT thickness above the 95th centile of the normal range. The positive and negative predictive values for this cut-off point of NT thickness were 1.5 and 99.9%, respectively.

Comment

The subgroup of chromosomally normal fetuses with NT above the 95th centile of the normal range may contain more than 50% of all cases with major abnormalities of the heart and great arteries. The clinical implication of the findings in this study is that increased NT in the first trimester constitutes an indication for specialist fetal echocardiography, traditionally performed at around 20 weeks of gestation. Although this identifies most of the major cardiac defects, it is an expensive and time-consuming resource.

At present, there may be insufficient facilities for specialist fetal echocardiography to accommodate the potential increase in demand if the 95th centile is used as the cut-off point for referral. Alternatively, a cut-off point of the 99th centile would result in a small increase in workload and in this population the prevalence of major cardiac defects would be very high (about 6%).

Improvements in the resolution of ultrasound machines have made it possible to perform detailed fetal cardiac ultrasound examinations from as early as 14 weeks of gestation. This will reassure the majority of patients that there is no major cardiac defect and in those cases with a major defect, the early scan can either lead to the correct diagnosis or at least raise suspicions so that follow-up scans can be arranged. However, until more prospective data are available, the majority of cases would require a repeat ultrasound examination at 20–22 weeks of gestation.

In summary, increased NT at 10–14 weeks of gestation is associated with a wide range of fetal abnormalities and it is imperative that these abnormalities are searched for at subsequent scans.

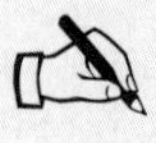

The value of sonography in early pregnancy for the detection of fetal abnormalities in an unselected population.

BJ Whitlow, IK Chatzipapas, ML Lazanakis, RA Kadir, DL Economides.
Br J Obstet Gynaecol 1999; **106:** 926–36.

BACKGROUND. Limited evidence is available regarding the ability to detect structural anomalies between 11 and 14 weeks of gestation. This prospective cross-sectional study aimed to determine the value of early pregnancy ultrasound in the detection of fetal abnormalities in an unselected obstetric population and to ascertain the cost implications of such a screening procedure.

INTERPRETATION. The population studied included 6634 sequential unselected women (mean maternal age 29.9 years) carrying a total of 6443 live fetuses. Prenatal invasive diagnostic testing was performed in 9.3% of the women and the indications were: NT measurement above the 99th centile or structural abnormality (0.9%), abnormal second trimester serum biochemistry (3.6%), maternal age above 37 years (4.1%) and maternal request or family history (0.7%).

The incidence of anomalous fetuses was 1.4% (92/6443) including 43 chromosomal abnormalities. Overall, 78% of chromosomal abnormalities were diagnosed at

11–14 weeks, either due to NT measurement above the 99th centile (43%) or due to the presence of structural abnormalities (35%). Twenty-three of the 43 chromosomal abnormalities were trisomy 21 and of these, 15 (65%) were diagnosed at 11–14 weeks.

The detection rate for structural abnormalities was 59% (37/63) with a specificity of 99.9% in early pregnancy. When the first and second trimester scans were combined, the sensitivity for detection of structural abnormalities was 81% (51/63). The commonest structural defects diagnosed in the first trimester were central nervous system defects (43%) and cystic hygroma (35%). Forty-five per cent (5/11) of fetuses with cardiac abnormalities had NT measurements above the 95th centile.

The authors concluded that the majority of fetal structural and chromosomal abnormalities can be detected by sonographic screening at 11–14 weeks, but that the second trimester scan should not be abandoned. The estimated cost of diagnosing one anomalous fetus was calculated at £4453.

Comment

This is the only recent publication evaluating routine first trimester ultrasound examination in a low-risk population. Certain fetal abnormalities such as central nervous system defects, neck anomalies, gastrointestinal and renal defects can be detected at 11–14 weeks of gestation. While it is more difficult to detect spina bifida, heart anomalies and limb defects at this early stage, it must be remembered that these are the abnormalities that are also difficult to diagnose in the second trimester. It is interesting to note that even in a low-risk population, the overall invasive karyotyping rate was almost 10%. This is in part explained by the fact that a significant number of women above the age of 37 years requested invasive testing (264/554, 48%) after presumably a normal first trimester scan.

The combination of first and second trimester ultrasound detected 81% of the structural anomalies. This detection rate compares favourably with randomized studies reporting routine ultrasound examination in the second trimester, which have reported detection of abnormalities from 16.6 to 76.9%. These figures should now be validated in a large prospective study.

Trisomy 21 screening in twin pregnancy

The past decade has seen a rise in mean maternal age as well as an increase in the use of assisted reproduction techniques. This has resulted in a higher incidence of twin pregnancies at increased risk of aneuploidy. With a maximum detection rate of 40%, second trimester serum screening for trisomy 21 in twin pregnancies has little value. In addition, even if aneuploidy is suspected with serum screening, it is impossible to identify the affected twin.

Ultrasound examination has the advantage of examining the fetuses individually and screening for trisomy 21 can be performed on the basis of NT thickness, as performed in singleton pregnancies [16]. However, biochemical screening may have a role to play in twin pregnancies when combined with first trimester NT.

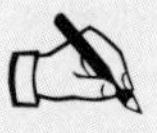

Screening for trisomy 21 in twin pregnancies in the first trimester using free beta-hCG and PAPP-A, combined with fetal nuchal translucency thickness.

K Spencer. *Prenat Diagn* 2000; **20:** 91–5.

BACKGROUND. Few data are available on the behaviour of biochemical markers in twin pregnancies in the first trimester. This study aimed to identify those patterns and to predict the likely detection rates when combined with NT in situations when both twins are affected and in situations when only one twin is affected.

INTERPRETATION. Maternal serum β-hCG and PAPP-A were measured with the previously described random access immunoassay analyser. The marker distribution was analysed in 159 twin pregnancies and compared with 3466 singleton pregnancies.

The average free β-hCG values were 2.1 times higher in twins than in singletons and PAPP-A was 1.86 times higher. Using statistical modelling techniques, it was predicted that, at a false-positive rate of 5%, the detection rate by biochemical markers in twins discordant for trisomy 21 would be 52%, whereas in twins concordant for trisomy 21 this would be 55%. Although this detection rate is lower than that estimated by NT alone in twins (75%), the use of both modalities would yield a detection rate of approximately 80%.

It was concluded that the addition of first trimester maternal serum biochemistry to NT screening could be expected to increase the detection rate by a further 5–6%.

Comparison of nuchal translucency measurement and second trimester triple serum screening in twin versus singleton pregnancies.

R Maymon, E Dreazen, S Rozinsky, I Bukovsky, Z Weinraub, A Herman. *Prenat Diagn* 1999; **19:** 727–31.

BACKGROUND. The aim of this study was to compare NT and second trimester biochemical screening for trisomy 21 in twin pregnancies with these tests in matched control singletons.

INTERPRETATION. The study group included 60 twin pregnancies of which three were monochorionic. Each co-twin was matched with a singleton fetus for CRL and maternal age and, thus, there were 120 fetuses in the control group. All women underwent first trimester NT measurement and second trimester measurement of AFP, hCG and uE3. In either analysis, a risk of 1 in 380 or higher for trisomy 21 was considered screen positive, the equivalent risk to that of a 35-year-old gravida in the population.

The median NT measurement, expressed as MoM for CRL, was similar in the study group (0.85) and the control group (0.88). Based on NT measurement, there was a non-significant difference in false-positive rates between the study group (5%) and the control group (2.5%). In contrast, biochemical screening showed a significant difference with 15% (9/60) of twin pregnancies found to be screen positive compared with 6%

(7/120) of controls. This high false-positive rate resulted in an 18% amniocentesis rate in the study group compared with 7.5% in the control group.

Comment

Serum screening for trisomy 21 in twin pregnancies has a relatively poor detection rate, presumably because altered biochemical markers in the aneuploid fetus are masked by normal levels in the euploid co-twin. In contrast, first trimester ultrasound in twin pregnancy offers important advantages including accurate dating, determination of chorionicity and assessment of individual fetal NT, thus allowing identification of the fetus at increased risk of trisomy 21.

In twins, the sensitivity of NT screening to detect trisomy 21 is similar to that in singletons, but the false-positive rate is higher because NT is increased in 8% of euploid monochorionic fetuses [16]. The increased NT in monochorionic fetuses may be an early manifestation of twin-to-twin transfusion syndrome. This explains why the false-positive rate in this study was higher in the twin group than in singleton fetuses.

Furthermore, NT may be useful in choosing the appropriate invasive test. In pregnancies where the risk of trisomy is greater than 1 in 50, CVS (with its inherent problems) should be the technique of choice, otherwise amniocentesis is preferable. Whilst NT is currently the best marker to screen for trisomy 21 in twin pregnancies, in the future consideration should be given to its use in combination with first trimester biochemistry.

Other imaging modalities

Two-dimensional ultrasound has become the standard technique for fetal imaging. However, with the improvement in image quality, the limitations of two-dimensional ultrasound have become clearer. The position of the fetus in the uterus and the reduced mobility of the transducer, in particular during transvaginal examination, may not always allow an optimal section through the fetus. Furthermore, because two-dimensional ultrasound cannot provide images of the fetal surface, the evaluation of complex structures such as the fetal face and limbs is limited.

The first three-dimensional image of a fetus was presented in 1974 by using 15 tomograms recorded at intervals of 1 cm each [17]. With further development of computed visualization techniques, it has become possible to create sections by processing a block of volume data (anyplane slicing) [18]. This method allows visualization of the surface of an object (surface shading) as well as its internal structures (transparency mode). In addition, the possibility of volume calculation using three dimensions may have significant applications.

In the early 1990s, the first three-dimensional images of early pregnancies were presented [19]. Subsequently, these techniques have been used in the diagnosis of fetal anomalies.

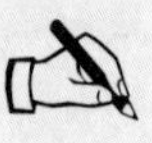

The detection of spina bifida before 10 gestational weeks using two- and three-dimensional ultrasound.

HG Blaas, SH Eik-Nes, CV Isaksen. *Ultrasound Obstet Gynecol* 2000; **16:** 25–9.

B ACKGROUND. In 1964, the first sonographic diagnosis of a neural tube defect was made. In the mid-1980s, Nicolaides *et al.* [20] reported the characteristic 'lemon' and 'banana' signs, which have become diagnostic keys in the detection of spina bifida in the second trimester. With the improvements in ultrasound, embryonic (below 10 weeks of gestation) diagnosis of anomalies has become possible.

I NTERPRETATION. In this study from Trondheim in Norway, three cases of spina bifida in embryos less than 10 weeks of gestation were presented. Two women were suffering from epilepsy and used sodium valproate and the third woman had previously undergone termination of pregnancy for a fetus affected with a myelomeningocele. All three were offered targeted vaginal ultrasound examination of the embryonic spine between 9 and 10 weeks of gestation. With informed consent, the pregnancies continued until 12–13 weeks to confirm the diagnosis by ultrasound, followed by termination.

Using a 7.5 MHz transducer, an irregularity at the caudal part of the spine was demonstrated in all three cases. With three-dimensional imaging, it was possible to visualize the defects from different angles, but this did not alter the diagnosis. The earliest appearance of the 'lemon' sign, scalloping of frontal bones, was at 12 weeks of gestation. The 'banana' sign, part of the Arnold–Chiari malformation, was not seen in any case.

Ultrasound performed to detect fetal structural anomalies at less than 10 weeks of gestation requires knowledge of normal embryonic development for correct interpretation of the ultrasound findings.

Comment

At present, the majority of fetuses with a neural tube defect are not detected until the second trimester, either as a result of raised maternal serum AFP or on routine examination at the 18–20-week scan. This study illustrates that early diagnosis at less than 10 weeks of gestation is feasible. However, it does not necessarily change the outcome of the pregnancy. It is important to bear in mind that this study was reported in a highly preselected population by a group of experts in embryonic ultrasound. They emphasized that detailed knowledge of fetal embryology is essential to differentiate normal from abnormal fetal structures. Besides difficulties in two-dimensional sonographic interpretation at such an early gestation, the diagnosis of spina bifida can easily be missed in the absence of the typical cranial signs. However, fetuses with major neural tube defects such as acrania (failure of formation of the calvarium), will be detected during the routine 10–14-week scan.

In this study, the use of three-dimensional imaging did not contribute towards the diagnosis. Nonetheless, for cases where surface shading or volume calculation of internal organs is required, three-dimensional imaging may be useful as an additional tool. At present, three-dimensional imaging is still in its infancy and most diagnoses made by three-dimensional ultrasound can also be made by two-dimensional ultrasound.

Another new method of fetal imaging is by magnetic resonance imaging (MRI) and again, this is likely to find its use mainly in conjunction with conventional ultrasound. The technique of fast MRI can be performed either in two or three dimensions. Fast MRI is increasingly being used as a correlative imaging modality in pregnancy because it uses no ionizing radiation, provides excellent soft tissue contrast and has multiple planes for reconstruction and a large field of view |21|. However, two-dimensional sonographic evaluation of the fetus is required to select the appropriate fetuses for MRI and to guide the protocol of the examination.

Currently, the best application for fast MRI is the demonstration of normal fetal brain development and the further definition of suspected brain abnormalities found on ultrasound |22|. MRI differentiates well between the various types of fetal ventriculomegaly and allows, for example, differentiation of Dandy–Walker malformation from a large cisterna magna. MRI is also valuable in the evaluation of fetal neck masses for planning delivery of the baby and surgery for life-threatening airway obstruction. In the chest, MRI differentiates masses such as diaphragmatic hernia, cystic adenomatoid malformation and sequestration, and aids in planning fetal surgery because MRI directly visualizes the position of the lung, liver and bowel.

Fetal cells in maternal blood

During the last three decades, there has been an extensive search for a non-invasive method of prenatal diagnosis based on examination of a variety of fetal nucleated cells in the maternal circulation. An estimated one in 10^7 nucleated cells in pregnant maternal blood is fetal in origin |23|. Although complete separation of fetal from maternal cells is not yet possible, the proportion of fetal cells can be enriched by centrifugation and techniques such as magnetic- or fluorescence-activated cell sorting after attachment of magnetically labelled or fluorescent antibodies on to a specific fetal cell surface marker. However, the resulting sample is unsuitable for traditional cytogenetic analysis because of contamination with maternal cells. Preliminary reports suggest that chromosomal abnormalities can be diagnosed using fluorescence in situ hybridization (FISH) on maternal blood enriched for fetal cells |24|.

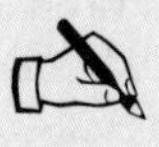

Investigation of maternal blood enriched for fetal cells: role in screening and diagnosis of fetal trisomies.

R Al-Mufti, H Hambley, F Farzaneh, KH Nicolaides. *Am J Med Genet* 1999; **85**: 66–75.

B ACKGROUND. With the use of techniques such as chromosome-specific DNA probes and FISH, normal disomic cells contain two signals for a particular chromosome. It is possible to suspect fetal trisomy by the presence of three-signal nuclei in some of the fetal cells in the enriched cell population |24|. This study examined the potential role of the use of these techniques in the detection of fetal trisomies at 10–14 weeks of gestation.

I NTERPRETATION. The study population included 230 women assessed to be at high risk for trisomy 21 based on maternal age and NT measurement at 10–14 weeks of gestation. Just prior to invasive testing, 20 ml of maternal blood was obtained from all 230 women and the samples were processed before the results of the invasive testing became available. Triple-density gradient centrifugation was carried out and the middle layer containing nucleated erythrocytes and neutrophilic granulocytes was separated. These cells were then isolated and incubated with magnetically labelled CD71 antibody to the transferrin receptor antigen.

Following fetal cell enrichment by magnetic cell sorting |25|, the cells were cytospun on to slides, stained and examined by light microscopy. Fetal haemoglobin-positive cells were detected in 222 (97%) samples. The cells in these samples were then re-centrifuged, incubated and kept frozen. For FISH, the cells were transferred to glass slides and hybridization was performed using multicolour probes for chromosomes 21, 18, 13, X and Y. Subsequently, using a fluorescence microscrope, the proportion of cells with positive signals in the chromosomally normal and abnormal samples was determined. The distribution of cells with positive signals in the chromosomally normal and abnormal groups was compared and the sensitivity and false-positive rates for different cut-off percentages of positive cells were calculated.

Fetal NT was above the 95th centile of the normal range for CRL in 97 (68%) of the chromosomally normal group and in 79 (99%) of the abnormal group. In the 222 pregnancies with fetal haemoglobin-positive cells, the fetal karyotype was normal in 142 (64%) cases and abnormal in 80 (36%) cases, including 36 with trisomy 21. Using a chromosome 21-specific probe, three-signal nuclei were present in at least 5% of the enriched cells from 61% of the trisomy 21 pregnancies and in none of the normal pregnancies. There was no significant association between NT thickness and the percentage of cells with three signals in either the chromosomally normal or abnormal group.

It was calculated that, for a cut-off point of 3% of three-signal nuclei, the sensitivity for trisomy 21 was 97% for a false-positive rate of 13%. Similar values were obtained in trisomies 13 and 18 using the appropriate chromosome-specific probes. The authors concluded that with this method in combination with maternal age and fetal NT, the detection rate of trisomy 21 could remain at 80%, but the need for invasive testing may be reduced from 5% to less than 1%.

Comment

This study provides evidence on the feasibility of screening for fetal chromosomal abnormalities by the application of FISH in maternal blood enriched for fetal cells. The results are not diagnostic because the enriched population of cells is contaminated with maternal cells and therefore precludes accurate determination of chromosomal number. The results of this study confirm those of previous studies |24|. Therefore, this non-invasive method of screening for trisomy 21 could potentially identify 60% of affected pregnancies.

While the population in this study was preselected, the data may be applicable to a low-risk population, as no correlation was found between NT and the percentage of cells with three-signal nuclei. Furthermore, this finding suggests that the data from NT thickness and the percentage of cells with three-signal nuclei can be combined to improve the effectiveness of screening for trisomy 21 (sensitivity 80%) at a lower (1%) false-positive rate.

However, the main disadvantages of this screening method are that the techniques involved are time-consuming, requiring expensive equipment with highly skilled operators to carry out the tests. Until cheaper automated systems are devised using a process that will enrich or ideally provide a sample of pure fetal cells, this technique cannot be implemented into routine care. At present, it seems more likely that examination of fetal cells in maternal blood may find an application as a method for assessment of risk, rather than for non-invasive prenatal diagnosis of chromosomal defects.

Conclusion

The last decade has seen a significant shift from second to first trimester screening for fetal trisomies and structural anomalies. Among the many currently available biochemical and ultrasound markers for trisomy 21 screening, NT thickness has emerged as the single most powerful marker. Paramount in the process of trisomy 21 risk estimation is the appropriate integration of the different screening modalities, in particular ultrasound examination of the fetus and maternal serum biochemical markers. The 'ideal' screening test should be efficient, cost-effective and enable parents to have individual choice.

Cuckle |6| recently reviewed the screening efficiency for trisomy 21 for a variety of combined modalities:

- NT and serum screening performed at the same time ('concurrent');
- two or more modalities at different times with results not reported until all are complete ('non-disclosure');
- intermediate results reported as they are ready ('sequential');
- subsequent modalities only used if the earlier modality has a positive result ('contingent').

Cuckle concluded that the most effective policy is that of 'concurrent' first trimester NT and maternal serum screening, which offers a detection rate of 89% at a 5% false-positive rate, or alternatively a 70% detection rate at a 1% false-positive rate |6|.

Whilst a routine first trimester screening programme for fetal abnormalities appears to offer many advantages, several important issues must be taken into account. Pregnant women need to be referred and seen prior to 14 weeks of gestation. Ultrasound departments may need to perform transvaginal ultrasound examinations in about 20% of patients |26|. Furthermore, expectant management may allow for spontaneous miscarriage to occur and avoid the need to make a decision whether to terminate a pregnancy or not. If prenatal diagnosis was to be performed in the first trimester, this would necessitate CVS because of the increased risk of fetal loss with amniocentesis at this gestation. At present, CVS is only performed in referral centres and this may limit availability. In addition, the commonly used method of suction termination of pregnancy in the first trimester often makes pathological examination impossible thereby depriving parents the chance to have the diagnosis confirmed or even explained.

In the foreseeable future, two-dimensional ultrasound will continue to provide the mainstay in diagnosis of fetal abnormalities. It is likely that the examination of the fetal anatomy will be performed at an earlier gestation than the routine 18–20-week scan, possibly at 11–14 weeks. In the future, screening may involve the use of new techniques such as analysis of fetal cells in maternal blood, three-dimensional ultrasound and fetal MRI.

References

1. Pandya PP. The 11–14 week scan: the diagnosis of fetal abnormalities. In: Nicolaides KH, Sebire NJ, Snijders RJM (eds): *Diploma in Fetal Medicine Series*. Parthenon, London, 1999, pp. 3–33.

2. Snijders RJ, Johnson S, Sebire NJ, Brizot M, Nicolaides KH. First trimester ultrasound screening for chromosomal defects. *Ultrasound Obstet Gynecol* 1996; 7: 216–26.

3. Pandya PP, Snijders RJM, Johnson SJ, Brizot M, Nicolaides KH. Screening for fetal trisomies by maternal age and fetal nuchal translucency thickness at 10 to 14 weeks of gestation. *Br J Obstet Gynaecol* 1995; 102: 957–62.

4. Taipale P, Hiilesmaa V, Salonen R, Ylostalo P. Increased nuchal translucency as a marker for fetal chromosomal defects. *New Engl J Med* 1997; 337: 1654–8.

5. Snijders RJM, Noble P, Sebire N, Souka A, Nicolaides KH. UK multicentre project on assessment of risk of trisomy 21 by maternal age and fetal nuchal translucency thickness at 10–14 weeks of gestation. *Lancet* 1998; 352: 343–6.

6. Cuckle H. Integrating antenatal trisomy 21 screening. *Curr Opin Obstet Gynecol* 2001; **13**: 175–81.

7. Wald NJ, Cuckle HS, Densem JW, *et al.* Maternal serum screening for trisomy 21 in early pregnancy. *Br Med J* 1988; **297**: 883–7.

8. Wald NJ, George L, Smith D, Densem JW, Petterson K. Serum screening for trisomy 21 between 8 and 14 weeks of pregnancy. *Br J Obstet Gynaecol* 1996; **103**: 407–12.

9. Wald NJ, Kennard A, Hackshaw A, McGuire A. Antenatal screening for trisomy 21. *J Med Screen* 1997; **4**: 181–246.

10. Wald NJ, Densem JW, Smith D, Klee GG. Four-marker serum screening for trisomy 21. *Prenat Diagn* 1994; **14**: 707–16.

11. Wald NJ, Hackshaw AK. Combining ultrasound and biochemistry in first trimester screening for trisomy 21. *Prenat Diagn* 1997; **17**: 821–9.

12. Kadir RA, Economides DL. The effect of nuchal translucency measurement on second trimester biochemical screening for trisomy 21. *Ultrasound Obstet Gynecol* 1997; **9**: 461–7.

13. Thilaganathan B, Slack A, Wathen NC. Effect of first trimester increased nuchal translucency on second trimester maternal serum biochemical screening for trisomy 21. *Ultrasound Obstet Gynecol* 1997; **10**: 261–4.

14. Tegnander E, Eik-Nes SH, Johanson OJ, Linker DT. Prenatal detection of heart defects at the routine fetal examination at 18 weeks in a non-selected population. *Ultrasound Obstet Gynecol* 1995; **5**: 372–80.

15. Hyett JA, Perdu M, Sharland GK, Snijders RJM, Nicolaides KH. Increased nuchal translucency at 10–14 weeks of gestation as a marker for major cardiac defects. *Ultrasound Obstet Gynecol* 1997; **10**: 242–6.

16. Sebire NJ, Snijders RJM, Hughes K, Sepulveda W, Nicolaides KH. Screening for trisomy 21 in twin pregnancies by maternal age and fetal nuchal translucency thickness at 10–14 weeks of gestation. *Br J Obstet Gynaecol* 1996; **103**: 999–1003.

17. Szilard J. An improved three-dimensional display system. *Ultrasonics* 1974; **76**: 273–6.

18. Baba K, Satoh K, Sakamoto S, *et al.* Development of an ultrasonic system for three-dimensional reconstruction of the fetus. *J Perinat Med* 1989; **17**: 19–24.

19. Kelly IMG, Gardener JE, Lees WR. Three-dimensional fetal ultrasound. *Lancet* 1992; **339**: 1062–4.

20. Nicolaides KH, Gabbe SG, Campbell S, Guidetti R. Ultrasound screening for spina bifida: cranial and cerebellar signs. *Lancet* 1986; **2**: 72–4.

21. Levine D. Ultrasound versus magnetic resonance imaging in fetal evaluation. *Top Magn Reson Imaging* 2001; **12**: 25–38.

22. Hubbard AM, Harty MP. MRI for the assessment of the malformed fetus. *Baillieres Best Pract Res Clin Obstet Gynaecol* 2000; **14**: 629–50.

23. Bianchi DW, Flint AF, Pizzimenti MF, Knoll JHM, Latt SA. Isolation of fetal DNA from nucleated erythrocytes in maternal blood. *Proc Natl Acad Sci USA* 1990; **87**: 3279–83.

24. Bianchi DW, Mahr A, Zickwolf GK, Houseal TW, Flint AF, Klinger KW. Detection of fetal cells with 47, XY, +21 karyotype in maternal peripheral blood. *Human Genet* 1992; **90**: 368–70.

25. Ganshirt-Ahlert D, Borjesson-Stoll R, Burschyk M, *et al.* Detection of fetal trisomies 21 and 18 from maternal blood using triple gradient and magnetic cell sorting. *Am J Reprod Immunol* 1993; **30**: 194–201.

26. Whitlow BJ, Chatzipapas IK, Lazanakis ML, Kadir RA, Economides DL. The value of sonography in early pregnancy for the detection of fetal abnormalities in an unselected population. *Br J Obstet Gynaecol* 1999; **106**: 926–36.

List of Abbreviations

AD	Alzheimer's disease
AFP	α-fetoprotein
AMI	acute myocardial infarction
APC	activated protein C
APOE	apolipoprotein E gene
APP	amyloid precursor protein
bid	twice a day
BMC	bone mineral content
BMD	bone mineral density
CDR	Clinical Dementia Rating
CEE	conjugated equine oestrogen
CGHFBC	Collaborative Group for Hormonal Factors in Breast Cancer
CGIC	Clinical Global Impression of Change
CHD	coronary heart disease
CI	confidence interval
COC	combined oral contraceptive
CRL	crown–rump length
CSA	cross-sectional area
CVD	cardiovascular disease
CVS	chorionic villous sampling
DDAVP	1-desamino-8-D-arginine vasopressin
DEXA	dual-energy X-ray absorptiometry
DMPA	depot medroxyprogesterone acetate
EBCTCG	Early Breast Cancer Trialists' Collaborative Group
ENG	etonogestrel
EORTC	European Organization for Research and Treatment of Cancer
ER	oestrogen receptor
ERA	oestrogen replacement in atherosclerosis
FACT-B	Functional Assessment of Cancer Treatment
FIGO	Fédération Internationale Gynécologie Obstetrique
FISH	fluorescence in situ hybridization
FSH	follicle stimulating hormone
GOG	Gynaecologic Oncology Group
GP	general practitioner
GPRD	General Practice Research Database
h	hour
hCG	human chorionic gonadotrophin
HDL	high-density lipoprotein
HERS	Heart and Estrogen/progestin Replacement Study
HMG	human menopausal gonadotrophin
HRT	hormone replacement therapy
ICS	International Continence Society
ICSI	intra-cytoplasmic sperm injection
IGF	insulin-like growth factor
IGFBP	insulin-like growth factor-binding protein
IUD	intrauterine device
IUI	intrauterine insemination
IVF	in vitro fertilization
LDL	low-density lipoprotein
LH	luteinizing hormone
LNG-IUS	Levonorgestrel-releasing Intrauterine System
MBL	menstrual blood loss
MI	myocardial infarction
min	minute

MMSE	Mini Mental State Examination
MoM	multiples of the median
MORE	Multiple Outcomes of Raloxifene Evaluation
MP	micronized progesterone
MPA	medroxyprogesterone acetate
MRC	Medical Research Council
MRI	magnetic resonance imaging
MVF	maximum voluntary force
NT	nuchal translucency
PAPP-A	pregnancy-associated plasma protein-A
PCP	postcoital contraceptive pills
PEPI	Postmenopausal Estrogen/Progestin Interventions
PgR	progesterone receptor
PID	pelvic inflammatory disease
POP	progestogen-only pill
pp	post partum
PTH	parathyroid hormone
qid	four times a day
RTOG	Radiation Therapy Oncology Group
SD	standard deviation
SE	standard error
SEER	National Surveillance, Epidemiology and End Results
SERM	selective oestrogen receptor modulator
STAR	Study of Tamoxifen and Raloxifene trial
STI	sexually transmitted infection
TCRE	transcervical resection of the endometrium
tds	three times a day
uE3	unconjugated oestriol
UK	United Kingdom
UKCTOCS	UK Collaborative Trial of Ovarian Cancer Screening
UNDP	United Nations Development Programme
UNFPA	United Nations Family Planning Association
USA	United States of America
VTE	venous thromboembolism
WHO	World Health Organization

Index of Papers Reviewed

B Gbolade, S Ellis, B Murby, S Randall, R Kirkman. Bone density in long term users of depot medroxyprogesterone acetate. *Br J Obstet Gynaecol* 1998; **105**: 790–4. **66**

A Glasier, D Baird. The effects of self-administering emergency contraception. *New Eng J Med* 1998; **339**(1): 1–4. **110**

AF Gordon, P Owen. Emergency contraception: change in knowledge of women attending for termination of pregnancy from 1984 to 1996. *Br J Fam Plann* 1999; **24**: 121–2. **106**

J Huber. Pharmacokinetics of Implanon®. An integrated analysis. *Contraception* 1998; **58**: 85S–90S. **87**

GA Irvine, MB Campbell-Brown, MA Lumsden, A Heikkila, JJ Walker, IT Cameron. Randomised comparative trial of the levonorgestrel intrauterine system and norethisterone for treatment of idiopathic menorrhagia. *Br J Obstet Gynaecol* 1998; **105**: 592–8. **30**

H Jick, A James, JA Kaye, C Vasilakis-Scaramozza, SS Jick. Risk of venous thromboembolism among users of third generation oral contraceptives compared with users of oral contraceptives with levonorgestrel before and after 1995: cohort and case–control analysis. *Br Med J* 2000; **321**: 1190–5. **43**

N Kittelsen, O Istre. A randomised study comparing levonorgestrel intrauterine system (LNG-IUS) and transcervical resection of the endometrium (TCRE) in the treatment of menorrhagia: preliminary results. *Gynaecol Endosc* 1998; **7**: 61–5. **34**

E Kosunen, A Vikat, M Rimpela, A Rimpela, H Huhtala. Questionnaire study of use of emergency contraception among teenagers. *Br Med J* 1999; **319**: 91. **108**

P Lahteenmaki, M Haukkamaa, J Puolakka, U Riikonen, S Sainio, J Suvisaari, CG Nilsson. Open randomised study of use of levonorgestrel releasing intrauterine system as alternative to hysterectomy. *Br Med J* 1998; **316**: 1122–6. **32**

I Martinelli, E Taioli, P Bucciarelli, S Akhavan, PM Mannucci. Interaction between the G20210A mutation of the prothrombin gene and oral contraceptive use in deep vein thrombosis. *Arterioscl Thromb Vasc Biol* 1999; **19**: 700–3. **52**

L Mascarenhas. Insertion and removal of Implanon®. *Contraception* 1998; **58**: 79S–83S. **85**

S Middledorp, J Meijers, A van den Ende, A van Enk, B Bouma, G Tans, J Curvers, J Rosing, M Prins, H Buller. Effects on coagulation of levonorgestrel and desogestrel containing low dose oral contraceptive: a cross over study. *Thromb Haemost* 2000; **84**: 4–8. **47**

NR Poulter, CL Chang, TM Farley, MG Marmot, O Meirik. Effect on stroke of different progestagens in low oestrogen dose oral contraceptives. WHO Collaborative Study of Cardiovascular Disease and Steroid Hormone Contraception. *Lancet* 1999; **354**: 301–3. **50**

T Raine, C Harper, K Leon, P Darney. Emergency contraception: advance provision in a young, high-risk clinic population. *Obstet Gynaecol* 2000; **96**(1): 1–7. **110**

EG Raymond, MD Creinin, KT Barnhart, AE Lovvorn, RW Rountree, J Trussell. Meclizine for prevention of nausea associated with use of emergency contraceptive pillsÑa randomised trial. *Obstet Gynecol* 2000; **95**(2): 271–7. **105**

S Reuter. Barriers to the use of IUDs as emergency contraception. *Br J Fam Plann* 1999; **25**: 63–8. **109**

C Rice, S Killick, D Hickling, H Coelingh Bennink. Ovarian activity and vaginal bleeding patterns with a desogestrel-only preparation at three different doses. *Hum Reprod* 1996; **11**(4): 737–40. **58**

C Vasilakis, SS Jick, H Jick. The risk of venous thromboembolism in users of post-coital contraceptive pills. *Contraception* 1999; **59**(2): 79–83. **44**

P Vercellini, G Aimi, S Panazza, O De Giorgio, A Pesole, PG Crosignani. A levonorgestrel-releasing intrauterine system for the treatment of dysmenorrhoea associated with endometritis: a pilot study. *Fertil Steril* 1999; **72**(3): 505–8. **36**

T Walsh, D Grimes, R Frezieres, A Nelson, L Bernstein, A Coulson, G Bernstein. Randomised controlled trial of prophylactic antibiotics before insertion of intrauterine devices. *Lancet* 1998; **351**: 1005–8. **5**

WHO Collaborative Study of Cardiovascular Disease and Steroid Hormone Contraception. Cardiovascular risk factors and use of oral and injectable progestogen-only contraceptives and combined injectable contraceptives. *Contraception* 1998; **57**(5): 315–24. **45**

WHO Collaborative Study of Cardiovascular Disease and Steroid Hormone Contraception. Cardiovascular disease and use of oral and injectable progestogen-only contraceptives and combined injectable contraceptives. Results of an international, multicentre, case–control study. *Contraception* 1998; **57**: 315–24. **69**

WHO Task Force on Postovulatory Methods of Fertility Regulation. Comparison of three single doses of mifepristone as emergency contraception: a randomised trial. *Lancet* 1999; **353**: 697–702. **100**

WHO Task Force on Postovulatory Methods of Fertility Regulation. Randomised controlled trial of levonorgestrel versus the Yuzpe regimen of combined oral contraceptives for emergency contraception. *Lancet* 1998; **352**: 428–33. **98**

L Zhou, B Xiao. Preliminary analysis of a multicenter clinical trial using Multiload® Cu 375SL for emergency contraception. *Adv Contracept* 1998; **14**: 161–70. **101**

S Ziebland, A Graham, A McPherson. Concerns and cautions about prescribing and deregulating emergency contraception: a qualitative study of GPs using telephone interviews. *Fam Pract* 1998; **15**(5): 449–56. **107**

Part II The menopause

DH Barlow, G Samsoioe, JM van Geelen. A study of European women's experience of the problems of urogenital ageing and its management. *Maturitas* 1997; **27**: 239–47. **240**

NH Bjarnason, K Bjarnason, J Haarbo, C Rosenquist, C Christiansen. Tibolone: prevention of bone loss in late postmenopausal women. *J Clin Endocrinol Metab* 1996; **81**(7): 2419–22. **136**

JS Carpenter, MA Andykowski, M Cordova, *et al.* Hot flushes in postmenopausal women treated for breast carcinoma. *Cancer* 1998; **82**: 1682–91. **181**

MA Cobleigh, FE Norlock, DM Oleske, A Starr. Hormone replacement therapy and high S phase in breast cancer. *J Am Med Assoc* 1999; **281**: 1528–30. **166**

GA Colditz, B Rosner for the Nurses' Health Study Research Group. Use of estrogen plus progestin is associated with greater increase in breast cancer risk than estrogen alone. *Am J Epidemiol* 1998; **147**(Suppl.): 64S. **169**

V Donnelly, PR O'Connell, C O'Herlihy. The influence of oestrogen replacement on faecal incontinence in postmenopausal women. *Br J Obstet Gynaecol* 1997; **104**: 311–5. **242**

WD Dupont, DL Page, FF Parl, *et al.* Estrogen replacement therapy in women with a history of proliferative breast disease. *Cancer* 1999; **85**: 1277–83. **179**

Early Breast Cancer Trialists' Collaborative Group. Tamoxifen for early breast cancer: an overview of randomised trials. *Lancet* 1998; **351**: 1451–67. **162**

B Ettinger, A Pressmens, P Silver. Effect of age on reasons for initiation and discontinuation of hormone replacement therapy. *Menopause* 1999; **6**: 282–9. **217**

SF Evans, MWJ Davie. Low and conventional dose transdermal oestradiol are equally effective at preventing bone loss in spine and femur at all post-menopausal ages. *Clin Endocrinol* 1996; **44**: 79–84. **140**

LJ Fallowfield, SK Leaity, A Howell, S Benson, D Cella. Assessment of quality of life in women undergoing hormonal therapy for breast cancer; validation of an endocrine symptom subscale for the FACT-B. *Breast Cancer Res Treat* 1999; **55**: 89–199. **183**

F Fioretti, A Tavani, S Gallus, S Franceschi, C La Vecchia. Menopause and risk of non-fatal acute myocardial infarction: an Italian case–control study and a review of the literature. *Hum Reprod* 2000; **15**: 599–603. **155**

B Fisher, JP Constatino, DI Wickerham, *et al.* and other National Surgical Adjuvant Breast and Bowel Project Investigators. The NSABP P-1 trial. Tamoxifen for prevention of breast cancer: report of the National Surgical Adjuvant Breast and Bowel Project P-1 Study. *J Natl Cancer Inst* 1998; **90**: 1371–88. **162**

B Fowble, A Hanlon, G Freedman, A Patchefshy, H Kessler, N Nicolaou, J Hoffman, E Sigurdson, M Boraas, L Goldstein. Postmenopausal hormone replacement therapy: effect on diagnosis and outcome in early-stage invasive breast cancer treated with conservative surgery and radiation.. *J Clin Oncol* 1999; **17**: 1680–8. **174**

SM Gapstur, M Morrow, TA Sellers. Hormone replacement therapy and risk of breast cancer with a favourable histology. *J Am Med Assoc* 1999; **281**: 2091–7. **175**

PJ Goodwin, M Ennis, KI Pritchard, M Trudeau, N Hood. Risk of menopause during the first year after breast cancer diagnosis. *J Clin Oncol* 1999; **17**: 2365–70. **182**

GA Greendale, BA Reboussin, A Sie, *et al.* for the Postmenopausal Estrogen/Progestin Interventions (PEPI) Investigators. Effects of estrogen and estrogen–progestin on mammographic parenchymal density. *Ann Intern Med* 1999; **130**: 262–9. **176**

ML Hammar, R Lindgren, GE Berg, CG Mπller, MK Niklasson. Effects of hormone replacement therapy on the postural balance among postmenopausal women. *Obstet Gynecol* 1996; **88**: 955–60. **236**

SE Hankinson, WC Willett, JE Manson, GA Colditz, DJ Hunter, D Spiegelman, RL Barbarieri, FE Spiezer. Plasma sex steroid hormone levels and risk of breast cancer in postmenopausal women. *J Natl Cancer Inst* 1998; **90**: 1292–9. **165**

ST Harris, NB Watts, HK Genant, CD McKeever, *et al.* Effects of risedronate treatment on vertebral and non-vertebral fractures in women with postmenopausal osteoporosis. *J Am Med Assoc* 1999; **282**: 1344–52. **138**

E Hemminki, K McPherson. Value of drug-licensing documents in studying the effect of postmenopausal hormone therapy on cardiovascular disease. *Lancet* 2000; **355**: 566–9. **157**

VW Henderson, A Paganini-Hill, BL Miller, RJ Elble, PF Reyes, D Shoupe, CA McCleary, RA Klein, AM Hake, MR Farlow. Estrogen for Alzheimer's disease in women: randomised, double-blind, placebo-controlled trial. *Neurology* 2000; **54**: 295. **230**

DM Herrington, DM Reboussin, KB Brosnihan, PC Sharp, SA Shumaker, TE Snyder, *et al.* Effects of estrogen replacement on the progression of coronary-artery atherosclerosis. *New Engl J Med* 2000; **343**: 522–9. **152**

S Hizmetli, H Elden, E Kaptanoglu, V Nacitarhan, S Kocagil. The effect of different doses of calcitonin on bone mineral density and fracture risk in postmenopausal osteoporosis. *Int J Clin Prac* 1998; **52**(7): 453–5. **141**

AB Hodsman, LJ Fraher, PH Watson, T Ostbye, LW Stitt, JD Adachi, *et al.* Randomized controlled trial to compare the efficacy of cyclical parathyroid hormone versus cyclical parathyroid hormone and sequential calcitonin to improve bone mass in postmenopausal women with osteoporosis. *J Clin Endocrinol Metab* 1997; **82**(2): 620–8. **139**

LJ Hofseth, AM Raafat, JR Osuch, DR Pathak, CA Slomski, SZ Haslam. Hormone replacement therapy with estrogen or estrogen plus medroxyprogesterone acetate is associated with increased epithelial proliferation in the normal postmenopausal breast. *J Clin Endocrinol Metab* 1999; **84**: 4559–65. **169**

E Hogervorst, M Boshuisen, W Riedel, C Willeken, J Jolles. The effect of hormone replacement therapy on cognitive function in elderly women. *Psychoneuroendocrinology* 1999; **24**: 43–68. **221**

K Holli, J Isola, J Cuzick. Low biologic aggressiveness in breast cancer in women using hormone replacement therapy. *J Clin Oncol* 1998; **16**: 3115–20. **166**

S Hulley, D Grady, T Bush, *et al.* Randomized trial of estrogen plus progestin for secondary prevention of coronary heart disease in postmenopausal women. Heart and Estrogen/progestin Replacement Study (HERS) Research Group. *J Am Med Assoc* 1998; **280**: 605–13. **150**

I Ingram, K Sanders, K Marlene, D Lopez, DJ Hunter. Case controlled study of phyto-oestrogens and breast cancer. *Lancet* 1997; **350**: 990–4. **211**

P Kannu, M Palvanen, J Kaprio, J Parkkari, M Koskenvuo. Genetic factors and osteoporotic fractures in elderly people: prospective 25 year follow up of a nationwide cohort of elderly Finnish twins. *Br Med J* 1999; **319**: 1334–7. **235**

AM Kavanagh, H Mitchell, GG Giles. Hormone replacement therapy and accuracy of mammographic screening. *Lancet* 2000; **355**: 270–4. **176**

C Kawas, S Resnick, A Morrison, R Brookmeyer, M Corrada, A Zonderman, C Bacal, D Donnell Lingle, E Metter. A prospective study of estrogen replacement therapy and the risk of developing Alzheimer's disease: the Baltimore Longitudinal Study of Aging. *Neurology* 1997; **48**: 1517–21. **229**

DC Knight, JB Howes, JA Eden. The effect of Promensil™, an isoflavone extract, on menopausal symptoms. *Climateric* 1999; **2**: 79–84. **209**

MH Komulainen, H Kroger, MT Tuppurainen, AM Heikkinen, *et al.* HRT and vitamin D in prevention of non-vertebral fractures in postmenopausal women; a 5 year randomized trial. *Maturitas* 1998; **31**: 45–54. **135**

SG Leveille, AZ LaCroix, KM Newton, NL Keenan. Older women and hormone replacement therapy: factors influencing late life initiation. *J Am Geriatr Soc* 1997; **45**: 1496–1500. **216**

CL Loprinzi, JW Kugler, JA Mailliard, B LaVasseur, D Barton, P Novotny, S Dakhil, CG Kardinal, BJ Christensen, K Rodger, TA Rummans. Venlafaxine alleviates hot flashes: a North Cent Cancer Treatment Group Trial. *Proceedings of the (36th) Annual Meeting of the American Society of Clinical Oncology*, Vol. **19**, 2000, Abstract 4. **186**

E Lundstrom, B Wilczek, Z von Palffy, G Soderqvist, B von Schoultz. Mammographic breast density during hormone replacement therapy: effects of continuous combination, unopposed transdermal and low-potency oestrogen regimens. *Climacteric* 2001; **4**: 42–8. **206**

C Magnusson, LA Baron, N Correia, R Bergstrπm, HO Adami, I Persson. Breast cancer risk following long-term oestrogen and oestrogen–progestin replacement therapy. *Int J Cancer* 1999; **81**: 339–44. **171**

J Marsden, NPM Sacks, M Baum, RP A'Hern, MI Whitehead. Are randomised trials of hormone replacement therapy in symptomatic breast cancer patients feasible? *Fertil Steril* 2000; **73**: 292–9. **189**

ME Mendelsohn, RH Karas. The protective effects of estrogen on the cardiovascular system. *New Engl J Med* 1999; **340**: 1801–11. **154**

PJ Meunier, JL Sebert, JY Reginster, D Briancon, T Appelboom, P Netter, *et al.* Fluoride salts are no better at preventing new vertebral fractures than calcium–vitamin D in postmenopausal osteoporosis: the FAVO Study. *Osteoporosis Int* 1998; **8**(1): 4–11. **139**

H Mizunuma, H Okano, M Soda, I Kagami, S Miyamoto, T Tokizawa, S Honjo, Y Ibuki. Prevention of postmenopausal bone loss with minimal uterine bleeding using a low dose continuous estrogen/progestin therapy: a 2-year prospective study. *Maturitas* 1997; **27**: 69–76. **143**

H Mizunuma, H Okano, M Soda, I Kagami, S Miyamoto, T Tokizawa, S Honjo, Y Ibuki. Prevention of postmenopausal bone loss with minimal uterine bleeding using low dose continuous estrogen/progestin therapy: a 2-year prospective study. *Maturitas* 1997; **27**: 69–76. **203**

MORE Investigators. Reduction of vertebral fracture risk in post-menopausal women with osteoporosis treated with raloxifene: results from a three-year randomized clinical trial. *J Am Med Assoc* 1999; **282**(7): 637–45. **136**

L Mosca, SM Grundy, D Judelson, K King, M Limacher, S Oparil, R Pasternak, TA Pearson, RF Redberg, SC Smith Jr, M Winston, S Zinberg. Guide to Preventive Cardiology for Women. AHA/ACC Scientific Statement: Consensus Panel Statement. *J Am Coll Cardiol* 1999; **33**: 1751–5. **158**

RA Mulnard, CW Cotman, C Kawas, CH Van Dyck, M Sano, R Doody, E Koss, E Pfeiffer, S Jin, A Gamst, M Grundman, R Thomas, LJ Thal. Estrogen replacement therapy for treatment of mild to moderate Alzheimer disease. A randomised controlled trial. *J Am Med Assoc* 2000; **283**: 1007–15. **232**

PJ Nestel, S Pomeroy, S Kay, P Komesaroff, J Behrsing, JD Cameron, L West. Isoflavones from red clover improve systemic arterial compliance but not plasma lipids in menopausal women. *J Clin Endocrinol Metab* 1999; **84**: 895–8. **210**

N Panay, E Versi, M Savvas. A comparison of 25 mg and 50 mg oestradiol implants in the control of climacteric symptoms following hysterectomy and bilateral salpingo-oophorectomy. *Br J Obstet Gynaecol* 2000; **107**: 1012–6. **197**

KJ Pandya, RF Raubertas, PS Flynn, HE Hynes, RJ Rosenbluth, JJ Kirshner, HI Pierce, V Drugalin, GR Morrow. Oral clonidine in postmenopausal patients with breast cancer experiencing tamoxifen-induced hot flushes: a University of Rochester Cancer Centre Community Clinical Oncology Program Study. *Ann Intern Med* 2000; **132**: 788–93. **185**

I Persson, E Weiderpass, L Bergqvist, R Bergstrπm, C Schairer. Risks of breast and endometrial cancer after estrogen and estrogen–progestin replacement. *Cancer Causes & Control* 1999; **10**: 253–250. **170**

KM Prestwood, M Gunness, DB Muchmore, Y Lu, M Wong, LG Raisz. A comparison of the effects of raloxifene and estrogen on bone in postmenopausal women. *J Clin Endocrinol Metab* 2000; **85**: 2197–2202. **142**

KM Prestwood, AM Kenny, C Unson, M Kulldorff. The effect of low dose micronised 17β-estradiol on bone turnover, sex hormone levels and side effects in older women: a randomised, double blind, placebo-controlled study. *J Clin Endocrinol Metab* 2000; **85**: 4462–9. **202**

SK Quella, CL Loprinzi, DL Barton, JA Knost, JA Sloan, BI Lavasseur, D Swan, KR Krupp, KD Miller, PJ Novotny. Evaluation of soy phytoestrogens for the treatment of hot flushes in breast cancer survivors: a North Central Cancer Treatment Group trial. *J Clin Oncol* 2000; **18**: 1068–74. **185**

SK Quella, CL Loprinzi, JA Sloan, NL Varyht, WL DeKrey, T Fischer, G Finik, N Pierson, T Pisansky. Long term use of megestrol acetate by cancer survivors for the treatment of hot flashes. *Cancer* 1998; **82**: 1784–8. **187**

TR Rebbeck, AM Levin, A Eisen, C Snyder, P Watson, L Cannon-Albright, C Isaacs, O Olopade, JE Garber, AK Goodwin, MB Daly, SA Narod, SL Neuhausen, HT Lynch, BL Weber. Breast cancer risk after bilateral prophylactic oophorectomy in BRCA1 carriers. *J Natl Cancer Inst* 1999; **91**: 1475–9. **178**

PM Ridker, CH Hennekens, N Rifai, JE Buring, JE Manson. Hormone replacement therapy and increased plasma concentration of C-reactive protein. *Circulation* 1999; **100**: 713–6. **157**

K Rodstrom, C Bengtsson, L Lissner, C Bjorkelund. Pre-existing risk factor profiles in users and non-users of hormone replacement therapy: prospective cohort study in Gothenburg, Sweden. *Br Med J* 1999; **319**: 890–3. **156**

RK Ross, A Paganini-Hill, PC Wan, MC Pike. Effect of hormone replacement therapy on breast cancer risk: estrogen versus estrogen plus progestin. *J Natl Cancer Inst* 2000; **92**: 328–32. **172**

S Rozenberg, A Lefever, M Kroll, J Vandromme, M Paesmans, H Ham. Prescription attitudes among gynaecologists towards two particular risk factors of osteoporosis: the patient's age and her bone mineral density. *Maturitas* 1999; **32**: 19–24. **233**

C Schairer, J Lubin, R Troisi, S Sturgeon, L Brinton, R Hoover. Menopausal estrogen and estrogen–progestin replacement therapy and breast cancer risk. *J Am Med Assoc* 2000; **283**: 485–91. **171**

DA Skelton, SK Phillips, SA Bruce, CH Naylor, RC Woledge. Hormone replacement therapy increases isometric muscle strength of adductor pollicis in post menopausal women. *Clin Sci* 1999; **96**: 357–64. **238**

S Stallard, JC Litherland, CM Cordiner, HM Dobson, WD George, EA Mallon, D Hale. Effect of hormone replacement therapy on the pathological stage of breast cancer: population based, cross-sectional study. *Br Med J* 2000; **320**: 348–9. **177**

C Varas-Lorenzo, LA Garcia-Rodriguez, S Perez-Gutthann, A Duque-Oliart. Hormone replacement therapy and incidence of acute myocardial infarction. A population-based nested case-control study. *Circulation* 2000; **101**: 2572–8. **154**

R Vassilopoulou-Sellin, L Asmar, GN Hortobagyi, MJ Klein, M McNeese, SE Singletary, RL Theirault. Oestrogen replacement therapy after localised breast cancer: clinical outcome of 319 women followed up prospectively. *J Clin Oncol* 1999; **17**: 1428–87. **188**

SC Waring, WA Rocca, RC Petersen, PC O'Brien, EG Tangalos, E Kokmen. Postmenopausal oestrogen replacement therapy and risk of AD. A population based study. *Neurology* 1999; **52**: 965. **228**

K Yaffe, LY Lui, D Grady, J Cauley, J Kramer, SR Cummings. Cognitive decline in women in relation to non-protein-bound

General Index

in older women 215–44

in osteoporosis management 129–131, 135,
140–5, 201–4, 233–6

regimens 199–200

routes of delivery 140–1, 194–7, 200–1

sequential 199

side effects 193, 205–7

in urogenital atrophy 198, 241–2, 200–1

venous thromboembolic disease risk 207

human menopausal gonadotrophin (HMG) use
with IUI 278, 279

hydroxyurea, use in cervical cancer 262–3, 266

hysterectomy, use of LNG-IUS as alternative
32–4

hysterosalpingography 270–1

hysteroscopy 270–1

hysterosonography 270–1

I

IGF (insulin-like growth factor) system 29

imaging techniques

pelvic floor 315–17

see also magnetic resonance imaging;
mammography; ultrasonography

imipramine, use in detrusor instability 305

Implanon® 79–80

adverse events 93–5

dysmenorrhoea 92

effect on bone density 82–5

efficacy and pharmacodynamics 88–90

insertion and removal 85–6

pharmacokinetics 87–8

safety and efficacy 80–2

vaginal bleeding patterns 91–2, 93

implant contraception *see* contraceptive implants;
Implanon®; Norplant®

in vitro fertilization *see* IVF

incontinence

cost implications 289

faecal 317–20

effect of HRT 242–3

urinary 289–314

see also vaginal prolapse

infertility 269–85

see also fertility; IUI; IVF

insulin-like growth factor (IGF) system 29

Intac procedure 311

interval debulking surgery in ovarian cancer
252–4, 267

intracytoplasmic sperm injection (ICSI) 282,
285

intranasal oestradiol 198

intraurethral continence devices 299

intraurethral ultrasound 293

intrauterine devices 3–40

use in emergency contraception 98, 101–2,
103, 109, 119–20

use of antibiotic prophylaxis 102

intrauterine insemination *see* IUI

intravaginal continence devices 298–300

intravaginal oestradiol 198, 200–1

Introl intravaginal continence device 299

isoflavones 208, 209–11

see also phyto-oestrogens

IUDs *see* intrauterine devices

IUI (intrauterine insemination) 269, 278

cost-effectiveness 280–2

double 279

IVF (in vitro fertilization) 269

chances of success 274–6

cost effectiveness 280–2

future possibilities 285

multiple pregnancy 273–7

J

Jadelle® 73–4

comparison with Norplant® 77–9

L

lactating women, use of POP 65, 66

laparoscopic surgery

in treatment of endometriosis 272–3

in urinary incontinence 311–12

laparoscopy

role in infertility management 269

transhydrolaparoscopy 271–2

leak point pressure 294–5

'lemon' sign 342

Levonelle-2® 98

levonorgestrel

comparison with desogestrel as POP 60–6

comparison with Yuzpe regimen 98–100

effect on endometrium 29

use in emergency contraception 98–100,
102–3

use in post coital contraception 104

levonorgestrel implants 73–7

comparison of capsule with rod 77–9

see also contraceptive implants; Implanon®;
Norplant®

levonorgestrel intrauterine system *see* LNG-IUS

Livial® *see* tibolone

LNG-IUS (levonorgestrel intrauterine system)
18–20